Operative Manual of Minimally Invasive and LASER Ano-proctology

Sanjay Kumar Singla • Kushal Mital

Operative Manual of Minimally Invasive and LASER Ano-proctology

Tips and Tricks to Improve Outcomes

Springer

Sanjay Kumar Singla
Department of Surgery and Anorectal Surgery
Singla Hospital
Bhiwani, Haryana, India

Kushal Mital
Department of Surgery and Anorectal Surgery
Medicare Hospital
Thane, Maharashtra, India

This work contains media enhancements, which are displayed with a "play" icon. Material in the print book can be viewed on a mobile device by downloading the Springer Nature "More Media" app available in the major app stores. The media enhancements in the online version of the work can be accessed directly by authorized users.

ISBN 978-981-96-6189-3 ISBN 978-981-96-6190-9 (eBook)
https://doi.org/10.1007/978-981-96-6190-9

This Springer imprint is published by the registered company Springer Nature Singapore Pte Ltd.
The registered company address is: 152 Beach Road, #21-01/04 Gateway East, Singapore 189721, Singapore

Foreword

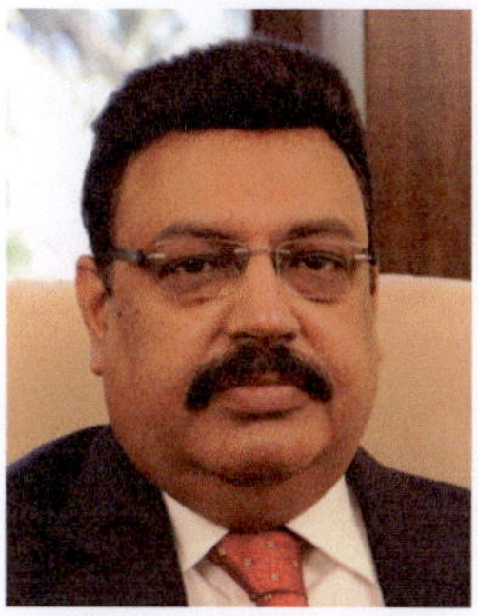

In recent years, advancements in minimally invasive and laser technologies have transformed the field of ano-proctology, providing practitioners with safer, more efficient and patient-friendly solutions for complex ano-rectal conditions. This manual serves as an essential resource, meticulously compiling the latest procedural techniques, guidelines and best practices for minimally invasive and laser treatments in ano-proctology.

Although the development of laser applications in proctology has its limitations, it represents an alternative minimally invasive method in the management of conditions like haemorrhoids, fistulas, fissures and pilonidal disease. Moreover, advancements in high-resolution imaging and endoscopic technology allow for enhanced visualization, ensuring better outcomes with minimal risk.

This practical manual brings together insights from leading experts in the field. Detailed illustrations, procedural steps and troubleshooting tips make it an invaluable guide, offering the knowledge required for effective patient care and improved postoperative outcomes.

Past President: Asia Pacific Federation of Coloproctology
Tokyo, Japan
Past President: Association of Colon and Rectal
Surgeons of India (ACRSI)
Jalandhar, India
Chairman: Fellowship Board of ACRSI
Mumbai, India
Head – Department of Colorectal Surgery
Saifee Hospital
Mumbai, India

Parvez Sheikh

November, 2024

Foreword

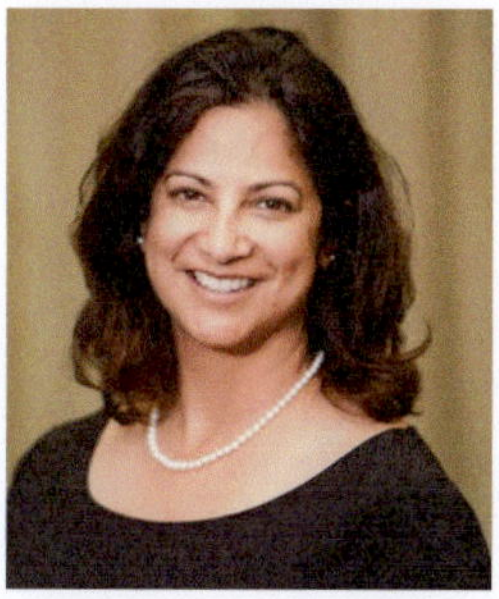

It is an honor to present the foreword to *Minimally Invasive Proctology*, an innovative text edited by Drs. Sanjay Singla and Kushal Mital, pioneers in minimally invasive anorectal surgery. Colorectal surgeons in India have long championed the integration of advanced surgical techniques and educational initiatives, significantly influencing global practices. This work exemplifies their dedication to the field.

The origins of colorectal surgery lie in proctology, with references to anorectal diseases as early as 1250 BC, suggesting practitioners specialized in this area. Despite millennia of attention, curative treatments remain elusive, and anorectal disorders are often underdiagnosed, leading to suboptimal management. Patients frequently endure chronic pain, bowel dysfunction, and reduced quality of life, underscoring the need for greater focus on this area.

Colorectal surgery globally tends to prioritize abdominal pathology, often overlooking the persistent and debilitating nature of anorectal diseases. Senior surgeons are frequently consulted by junior colleagues grappling with complex cases, lamenting missed opportunities to deepen their expertise in anorectal disorders during training.

This text, a testament to the pioneering efforts of the Association of Colon and Rectal Surgeons of India (ACRSI), established in 1977, reflects its commitment to advancing surgical innovation and education. Drs. Singla and Mital have synthesized years of research, clinical trials, and practice into a resource that underscores the value of minimally invasive approaches. Their work not only enhances surgical outcomes but also emphasizes patient-centered care, making it indispensable for both seasoned practitioners and trainees.

As we look to the future of colorectal surgery, the contributions of ACRSI and the editors will undoubtedly continue to shape global surgical practice. This text serves as both an educational cornerstone and an inspiration for ongoing advancements in the treatment of anorectal diseases.

Professor of Surgery, University of California San Diego, San Diego, CA, USA

President, American Society of Colon and Rectal Surgeons, Bannockburn, IL, USA

Sonia L. Ramamoorthy

December, 2024

Foreword

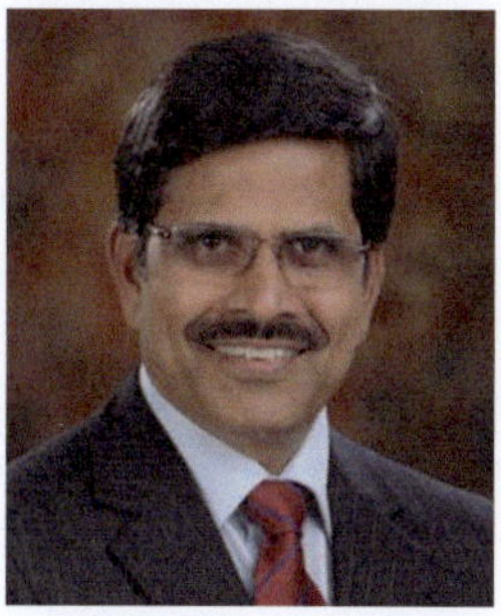

The treatment of anorectal diseases has undergone significant changes recently, driven by advancements in our understanding of pathophysiology and the integration of new technologies. Minimally invasive surgery has emerged as the standard approach for numerous anorectal conditions. However, there remains a shortage of surgeons adequately trained to address issues related to the anorectal area.

The Chapter of the Association of Colon and Rectal Surgeons of India (ACRSI) was established within the Association of Surgeons of India (ASI) in 1977. Since its inception, considerable progress has been made in training young surgeons in the specialized field of colon and rectal surgery. Thanks to the efforts of ACRSI, colorectal surgery has been recognized as a distinct specialty by the National Board of Medical Education in India, and a post-doctoral fellowship programme in colo-proctology is now available for qualified surgeons.

Given the rapid advancements in technology and the evolving understanding of anorectal diseases, there is an urgent need to revise teaching programmes and methodologies. Structured training programmes for laparoscopic colorectal surgery are currently in place, with robotic surgery and artificial intelligence surgery on the horizon. While minimally invasive surgery for abdominal organs and thoracic procedures has made remarkable progress, minimally invasive anorectal surgery is still in its early stages. The authors, drawing from their extensive experience in training for minimally invasive anorectal surgery, have compiled this book, which encompasses a broad range of topics related to the anorectum, including detailed discussions on anatomy, pathophysiology and the latest diagnostic and therapeutic technologies. Relevant classifications for selecting appropriate treatments are also addressed, along with the significance of operating room setup and patient positioning. It is essential for physicians to approach the management of anorectal conditions with empathy. By embracing minimally invasive therapies, whether surgical or non-surgical, practitioners can achieve better outcomes in the treatment of anorectal diseases.

The authors advocate for the training of surgeons in minimally invasive techniques to effectively address prevalent issues such as haemorrhoids, anal fissures, fistula in ano and pilonidal sinus disease. They clarify the specific applications of advanced technologies, including LASER, in the field of ano-proctology, as well as the optimal utilization of diagnostic tools like MRI and endoscopy. The text thoroughly discusses relevant pathological anatomy and physiology, providing a clear outline of the operative steps involved in minimally invasive procedures tailored to various anorectal conditions.

Both authors are actively engaged in the comprehensive training of emerging surgeons in minimally invasive surgical techniques and the use of LASER technology in ano-proctology, both in India and internationally. I have observed that Drs. SKS and KM possess a deep understanding and enthusiasm for educating others in minimally invasive anorectal surgery. I am confident that this book will serve as a valuable resource for practicing anorectal surgeons.

Founder Association of Minimal Access Surgeons of India (AMASI), GEM Hospital
Coimbatore, India
December, 2024

C. Palanivelu

Preface

It often baffles and disappoints us as medical professionals to watch that people still go to quacks for their anorectal problems.

Reasons of people going to such quacks can be multifold:

I. Poverty and lack of health education.
II. People relate to these so-called health providers more as compared to qualified surgeons.
III. On the professional level, surgeons find it a menial job and don't provide services with compassion.
IV. Not many surgeons are properly trained in managing complaints related to anorectal region.

Moreover when we as doctors got trained in general surgery residency, cases related to anorectal region especially benign conditions like haemorrhoids, fissure, perianal abscess and fistula were left in the end of OT list, to be managed or mismanaged by the most junior person in the team, and this practice continues.

To change the scenario, many initiatives are already afoot. Keeping this in mind Chapter of Association of Colon and Rectal surgeons of India (ACRSI) was created within Association of Surgeons of India (ASI) in 1977. A lot has been done since then for training young surgeons in the art and craft of colon and rectal surgery. First training course in colon and rectal surgery was started in 1997 at Ajmer. Fellowship programme of ACRSI (FACRSI) was started in year 1999 at Madurai and 18 Honorary fellows were selected for prestigious fellowship award of Association of Colon and Rectal surgeons of India (FACRSI). This continues to be the best programme under ASI. Annual conferences and workshops are conducted under the aegis of ACRSI to train surgeons.

Recently (with efforts of ACRSI) colorectal surgery has been recognized as a separate speciality by the National Board of Medical education In India and a fellowship programme-.

Fellowship of National Board is being offered to qualified surgeons.

We can create awareness and provide Health Education to public, which we do by rallies, marathons, health-talks, celebrating piles-day and issuing press release from time to time. The authors of this book find that there is a strong need to create special force of skilful surgeons who are compassionate to handle anorectal problems.

With the advancement of technology and the rapidly changing understanding of diseases of anorectal region, there is a need to restructure the teaching programmes and methodology. It is also important to fulfil the desire of better medical services by an ever-increasing section of high middle class in our society. There are structured programmes available for laparoscopic colorectal surgery in different countries. Books and manuals have been prepared for the training of doctors. Specialized colorectal units are recognized as super speciality in some regions of the world. However, other countries still do not recognize it as a sub-speciality.

The authors find that as in the beginning of laparoscopic surgery, training in Laparoscopic surgery was more of industry induced. Slowly, teaching institutes and hospitals picked it up and now its included in surgical curriculum world-wide. Later, minimally invasive surgery (including robotic surgery) of abdominal organs and thorax progressed leaps and bounds.

Doctors should also understand the need to handle anorectum with compassion it requires. If we provide services in this field with minimum morbidity (less- pain, almost no bleeding, minimal incontinence in case of fistula in ano, less days off the work), then only we will win the confidence of masses.

The authors find that the best way to achieve this is to train surgeons in minimally invasive methods to treat common problems faced by people like piles, fissure, fistula in ano and pilonidal sinus disease. We should be able to define the exact role of new technology like LASER in ano-proctology. One should be able to make the best use of already available knowledge and technology (MRI and endoscopy) in this area. It is our endeavour to provide knowhow regarding relevant pathological anatomy and physiology of anorectum before explanation of the operative steps to handle the specific disease.

Both the authors are involved in extensive training of young surgeons in minimally invasive and LASERS in ano-proctology in India and overseas.

One of the authors SKS has prepared a novel animal model from Goat anal canal and pumpkin to train surgeons in ano-proctology and LASER use, especially in management of fistula in ano [1].

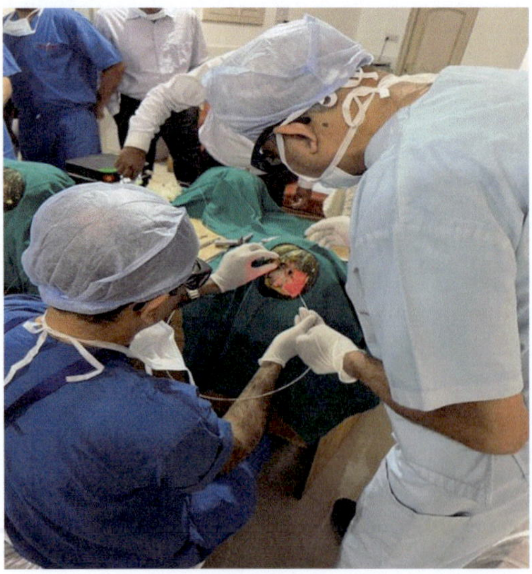

Surgeons honing their skills under supervision, on animal model developed by the author

Another author KM is the force behind IMMAST formerly known as CEMAST, a state of the art training Centre for Minimally access surgeries at Mumbai.

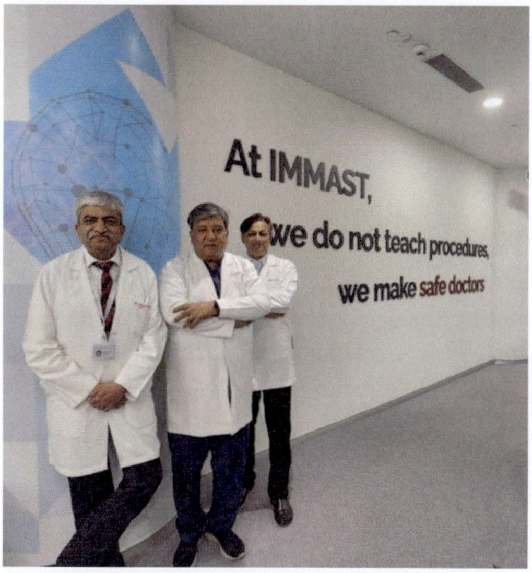
At IMMAST,
we do not teach procedures,
we make safe doctors

The authors at work and the present venture

Hand-drawn sketches and drawings from classroom teaching by authors are part of this book. How to use and keep equipment safe is another concern of the authors. Operative steps have been explained with sketches, clinical photographs and videos from real scenario of operation theatre. Possible complications and their prevention and management have been presented in tabulated form. Pearls of wisdom by previous and present authors have been shelled in "Tips and Tricks" section of different chapters. New concepts for future progress of treatment in tricky situations like fistula in ano have been put forward as food for thought for researchers and aware readers. Novel classification for treatment of pilonidal sinus disease (PSD) (including use of endoscopy and LASER) has been proposed to help reduce morbidity and standardize the management of this chronic illness affecting youth of the society.

A chapter on relatively less-travelled path of minimally invasive Trans anal management of anorectal diseases especially in early malignancy of rectum (TAMIS) has been purposely included to train anorectal surgeons in this field. List of references, suggested reading and viewing material has been provided to expand the knowledge of our worthy readers. Last but not the least every chapter has an algorithm of steps of the procedure for ready reference, on way to OT.

We wish that this book would serve as a guide to young and not that young practitioners of medicine, in the art and craft of MIS in anorectum.

Bhiwani, Haryana, India
drsanjaysingla@gmail.com

Sanjay Kumar Singla

Thane, Maharashtra, India
kushalmital@gmail.com

Kushal Mital

Reference

1. Singla S. Novel animal model from goat ano rectum and pumpkin for training of surgeons in management of fistula in ano. Indian J Colo-Rectal Surg. 2021;4(1):31–2. https://doi.org/10.4103/2666-0784.329673.

Acknowledgements

The completion of this work owes a profound debt to the support, expertise, and encouragement of many remarkable individuals. It is with heartfelt gratitude that I extend my regards to each of them.

To my parents, whose values and guidance have shaped my path. I am immensely grateful to my esteemed mentors, Prof. Amarjit Singh, Dr. Parvez Sheikh, Prof. MC Mishra and Dr. Sharad Karandikar; their wisdom and insight have been a guiding light throughout my career. I am also deeply indebted to my wife, Meenakshi, and children, Sakshi, Kushagra, Sahil and Vivaan; their patience and sacrifice granted me the precious time necessary to pursue this endeavour. Their steadfast support has been both a comfort and an inspiration.

Contribution of my colleague Dr. Kushal Mital is palpable throughout the text.

I am especially grateful to Dr. Taha Mustafa for his invaluable contribution to Chap. 26, which has enriched this work significantly. I am thankful to Dr. Arshad Ahmed for his contribution towards a procedure video (Video 15.4). My special thanks extend to Dr. Rashmi Bajaj and Dr. Aparna Batra, whose meticulous language and aesthetic enhancements brought a refined clarity and cohesion to the manuscript.

This project would not have been possible without the collaborative efforts of numerous colleagues and professionals. I extend my appreciation to Mr. Naren Aggarwal for his foundational role in initiating this work at Springer, and to Ms. Jagjeet Kaur Saini, Ms. Stephanie Sibin and Ms. Sneha Natarajan for their dedication to its final stages.

It is a privilege to recognize the distinguished senior medical professionals who graciously contributed forewords to this work. I am immensely grateful to Dr. C. Palanivelu, a pioneer and leader in minimal access surgery, and Dr. Parvez Sheikh, who is an authority on fistula in ano in this part of the world as well as Dr. Sonia Ramamoorthy, President of the American Association of Colon and Rectal Surgeons for their eloquent endorsements, which lend authority and insight to this book. I am indebted to Dr. Ashok Ladha, Dr. Niranjan Aggarwal, Prof. Hemanga K Bhattacharjee, Dr. Shyam Aggarwal and Dr. Ajit Kukreja for their untiring support of the project.

I will fail in my duty if I don't acknowledge the contribution of two fine ayurvedic surgeons, Padma Shri Prof. M. Sahu from Varanasi and Dr. Mahesh Sanghavi from Mumbai, especially for their contribution in the chapter on Kshar-sootra.

Dr. Surendra Kumar Bansal, an accomplished anaesthesiologist, made all surgeries possible with his dedicated skills.

Swarndeep Kaur and Robin made the operative steps look so vivid with their descriptive drawings.

Finally, I wish to acknowledge Dr. Vinod Jangra for his innovative proposal of including algorithms at the end of each procedural chapter, a feature that enhances the book's utility and accessibility for readers.

Special acknowledgement goes to Atul Sharma, whose diligence in document preparation, collation and video assembly was indispensable in bringing this project to fruition. This book would not have been possible without the hard work of our OT staff Ajit and Rohit, and nurses, Priyanka and Sanju who provide such noble services to our patients.

To everyone who contributed—through time, expertise and support—Thank You. This book stands as a tribute to your commitment to excellence and dedication to advancing this field.

Sanjay Kumar Singla

Disclaimer

Readers are advised to get training under an expert and mentoring with experienced surgeon before they start doing new procedures on their own.

Contents

About the Authors

Dr. Sanjay Singla (MS, FACRSI, FIAGES, FALS) is currently working as a consultant and colorectal surgeon, at Singla Hospital, Bhiwani, and Holy Heart Hospital, Rohtak, India. He is a regular faculty for FACRSI and runs training programs in minimal access and LASERS in anorectal surgeries. He graduated from Government Medical College, Patiala, India. He successfully passed the fellowship examination of the Association of Colon and Rectal Surgeons of India and received a fellowship from the Indian Association of Gastrointestinal Endo-Surgeons for advanced laparoscopic colorectal surgery. He developed an animal model to teach doctors minimal access and LASER surgeries in the anorectum and won the best paper at Fistulacon-2021. He was awarded International Travel Fellowship at Heartlands Hospital NHS Trust Birmingham, England. He was invited as faculty to 19th Annual meeting of the Cairo Colorectal and Pelvic Floor Congress of the Egyptian Society of Colon and Rectum (ESCR), the Mediterranean Society of Pelvic Floor Disorders (MSPFD), and ISUCRS Interim Conference 2025, to deliberate upon his new classification of pilonidal sinus disease. He has authored chapters for medical books and published papers in national and international medical journals. He has also presented at various national and international meetings.

Dr. Kushal Mital (MS, FACRSI) graduated from Medical College Allahabad, India. He is the course director of minimal invasive proctology, IMMAST, Mumbai, and AMASI, GEM, Chennai, India, and he is also practicing colorectal surgery in Mumbai. He has successfully cleared the fellowship examination conducted by the Association of Colon and Rectal Surgeons of India. He has been invited as a faculty for several conferences including the ASUCRS conference in Istanbul, Turkey, in 2022, the ASCRS conference, in Seattle, USA, in 2023, and SMCRCA conference in Merida, Mexico, in 2023. He has authored chapters for medical books and published numerous papers in national and international medical journals. He has authored the book *Common Anorectal Disorders: Surgical Perspective*. He has presented multiple oral and poster presentations at several national and international conferences. He will be president-elect of the Association of Colon and Rectal Surgeons of India from 2025 to 2027.

The original version of the book was revised: Minor corrections in text, figure and table, and 'about the author' section has been updated. The correction to the book is available at https://doi.org/10.1007/978-981-96-6190-9_27

1 How to Set Up Minimally Invasive Ano-proctology Unit and Operative Positioning

Abstract

- What is the need to set up minimally invasive ano-proctology unit?
- Why minimally invasive surgery in ano-proctology is going to stay and will replace broadly the traditional surgery?
- How to do it?
- By creating infrastructure and getting proper training is well explained by pictures and videos.
- Proper operative position is of paramount importance.
- For anorectal surgery, two positions—lithotomy and prone—are important.
- Why, where and how to make these positions have been well explained.
- Prevention of complications due to improper positioning of patient on operation table, has been suggested.
- Use of yellow fin stirrups for lithotomy, how to handle the boot stirrups has been shown with videos.
- A link for web video by manufacturer has been included in suggested video section to make reader familiar with the device before use on the patient.
- Video to show case changing position of anaesthetised patient from supine to prone has been included with captions and voice over.

1.1 Need to Set Up Minimally Invasive Ano-proctology Unit

As we see in last 30 years progress in surgery is mainly in the area of minimal invasion and access, coupled with fibre optics. This development is going to stay because of its obvious advantages of better illumination, magnification, very small wounds and associated scars. It translates in to fine dissection under vision and leads to very less pain, less bleeding, over all decreased morbidity and speedy recovery of the patient. Similarly in ano-proctology, gone are the days of excision of haemorrhoids, large wounds for perianal abscess, fistulae in ano, morbid flap for every case of Pilonidal sinus disease. Not only in benign conditions, even for early cases of anorectal malignant conditions trans anal minimal and endoscopic surgery is coming in a big way.

Supplementary Information The online version contains supplementary material available at https://doi.org/10.1007/978-981-96-6190-9_1. The videos can be accessed individually by clicking the DOI link in the accompanying figure caption or by scanning this link with the SN More Media App.

S. K. Singla, K. Mital, *Operative Manual of Minimally Invasive and LASER Ano-proctology*,
https://doi.org/10.1007/978-981-96-6190-9_1

1.1.1 How to Do It

- Change of mind set of doctors.
- Training of doctors.
- Creating infrastructure of a specialised ano-rectal outpatient and indoor clinic.
- Procurement of equipment and instruments.
  - Examination table (Fig. 1.1) with head low tilt, supports for lithotomy position and cushions for knee chest position.
  - Oxygen supply pipe line.
  - Ceiling examination lights.
  - Sink.
  - Monitor for vitals checking.
  - Ultrasound (US) machines for perineal, transanal and pelvic area.
  - Trolley (Fig. 1.2) for dressings and minor procedures.
  - Electro surgical unit (Fig. 1.3).
  - Suction machine.
  - Fibreoptic light source.
  - Waste bins.
  - Sharps container.
  - Computer.
- Instrumentation for procedures.
- Along with traditional speculums, retractors, probes and blades, we need specialised speculums (Fig. 1.4) like.
  - Park's speculum.
  - Lighted speculums and ano-proctoscopes.
  - Half speculum as provided with Minimal Invasive procedure for Haemorrhoids (MIPH) sets (Fig. 1.5).
  - Chivate's special speculum (Fig. 1.6).
  - Self-retaining proctoscope device by Rojanskul for LIFT (Fig. 1.4).
  - Lighted vaginal speculums (Fig. 1.4).
  - Fibreoptic cables and light source.

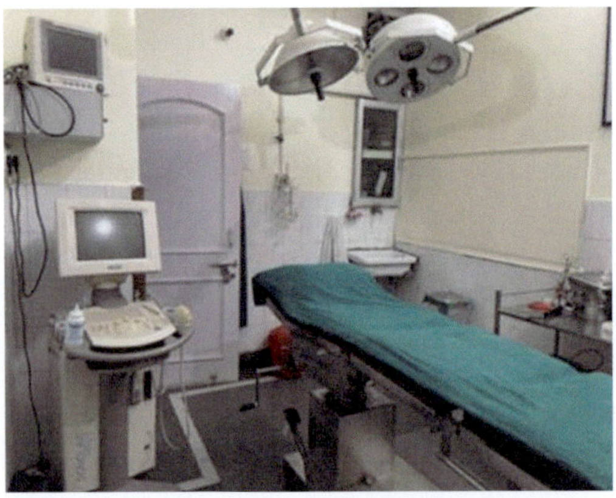

Fig. 1.1 Examination room and minor OT

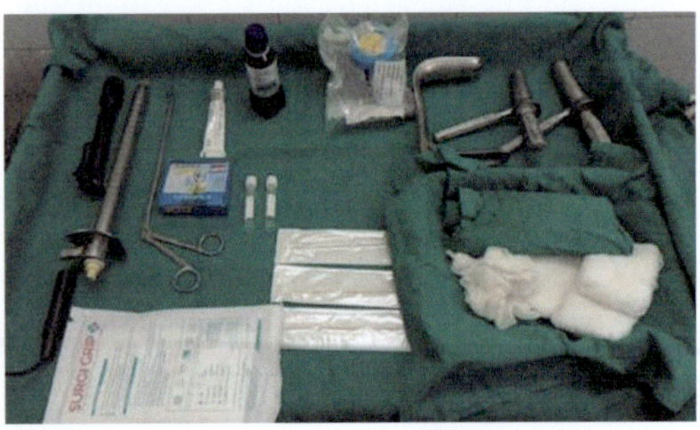

Fig. 1.2 Trolley for examination and dressing

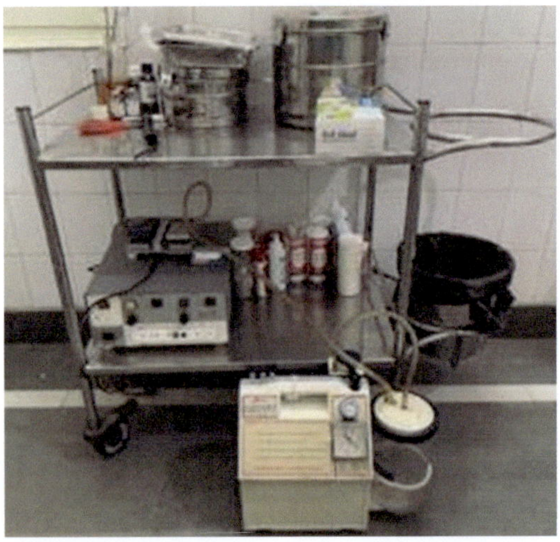

Fig. 1.3 Electrosurgical unit and suction machine

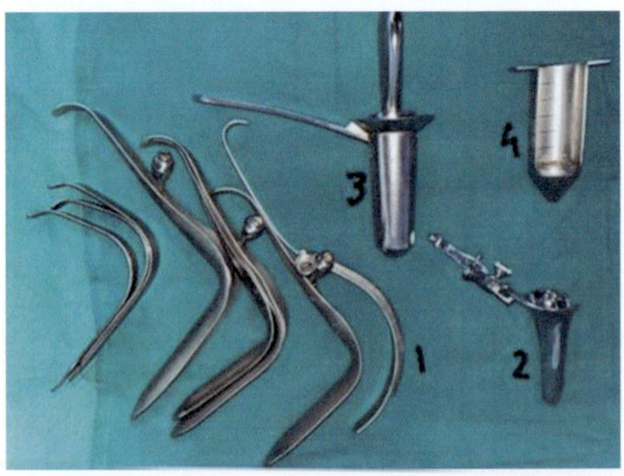

Fig. 1.4 Lighted vaginal speculum 1, Park's speculum 2, proctoscope 3, self-retaining half slit proctoscope designed by Rojanasakul for LIFT

- Retractors like small S shape and self-retaining anal retractors.
- Scopes like.
  - Rigid lighted sigmoidoscope (Fig. 1.7).
  - Flexible sigmoidoscope and colonoscope and associated accessories (Fig. 1.8).
  - Fistuloscope (Meinero's type, Storz) and associated accessories (Fig. 1.9).
- Haemorrhoids sclerotherapy kit (Fig. 1.10).
- Haemorrhoids rubber band ligation kit (Figs. 1.11 and 1.12).
- Skin biopsy punches (Fig. 1.13).
- Energy source.
  - Electrosurgical unit (Fig. 1.3).
  - LASER 1470 Diode LASER Machine (Fig. 1.14).
  - Harmonic and Ligasure optional (Fig. 1.15).
- Micro curettes.
- FiXcision device for coring (Fig. 1.16).
- Long needle holders.

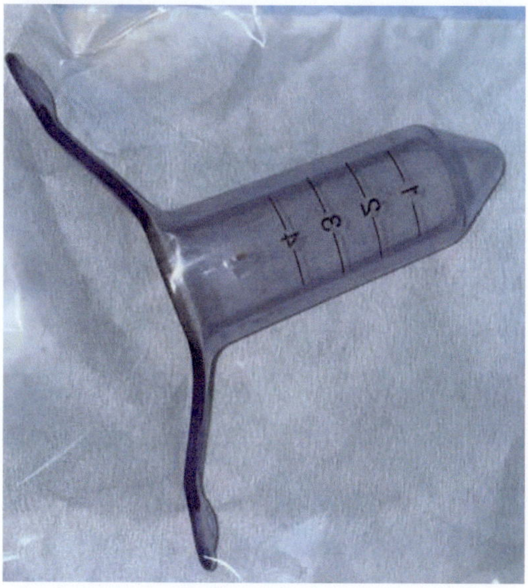

Fig. 1.5 Half speculum for MIPH

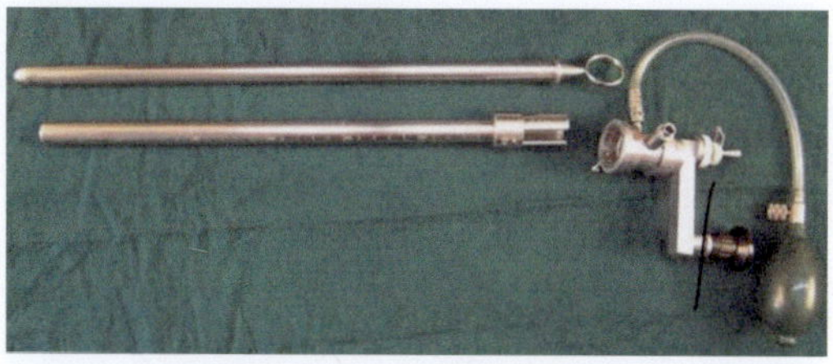

Fig. 1.7 Rigid lighted sigmoidoscope 1.9 cm diameter

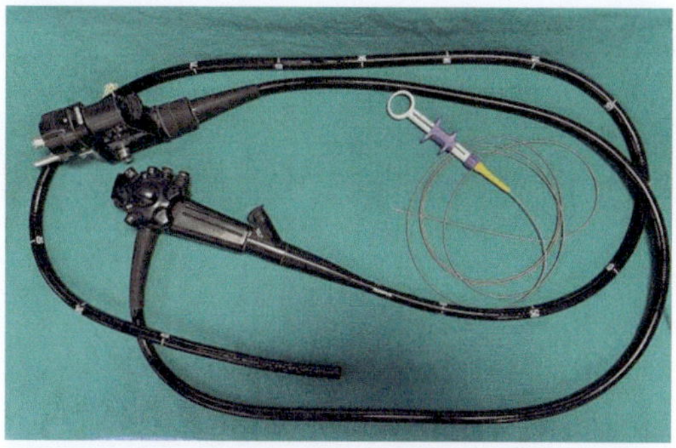

Fig. 1.8 Flexible colonoscope with biopsy forceps

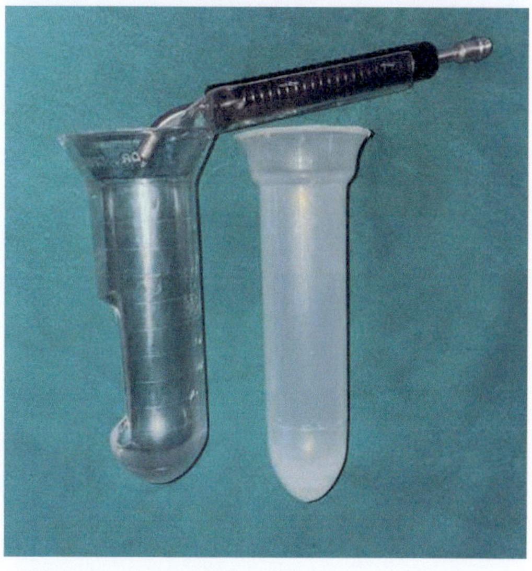

Fig. 1.6 Chivate's speculum with window and obturator

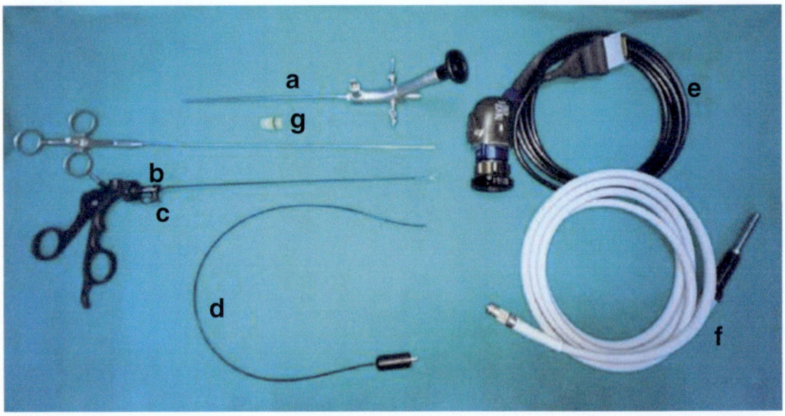

Fig. 1.9 Fistuloscope (A) (Meinero's type Storz) and associated accessories, brush (B), forceps (C), bug bee monopolar electrode (D), camera (E), fibroptic cable (F), water tight washer (G)

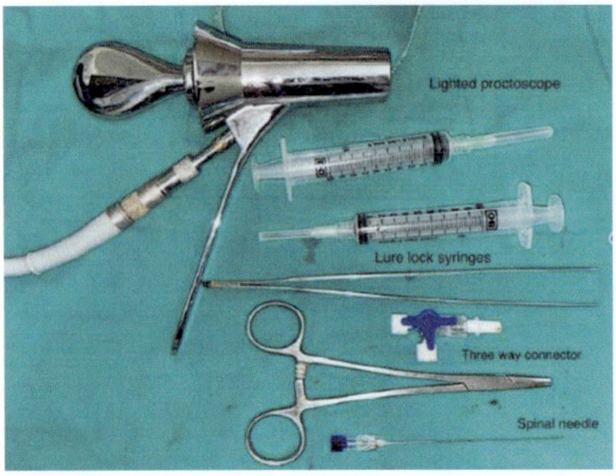

Fig. 1.10 Haemorrhoid foam sclerotherapy kit

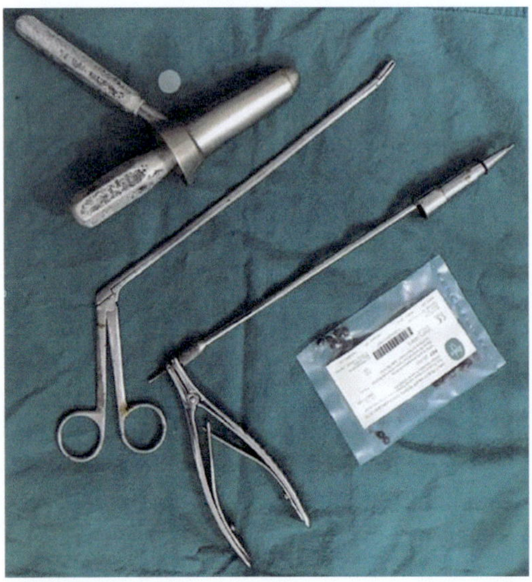

Fig. 1.11 Rubber band ligator set

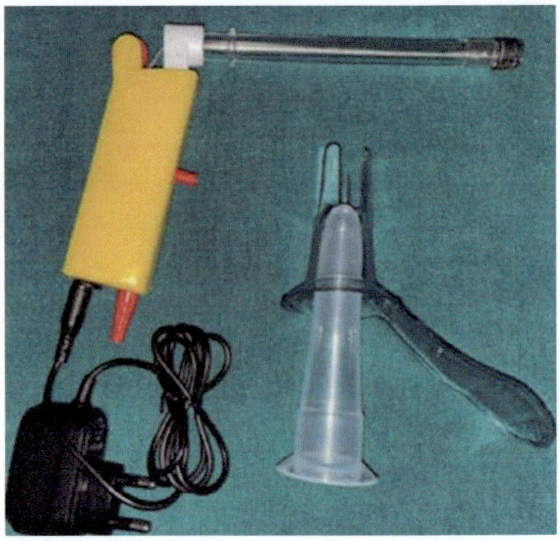

Fig. 1.12 Rubber band ligator set, self-lighted with suction

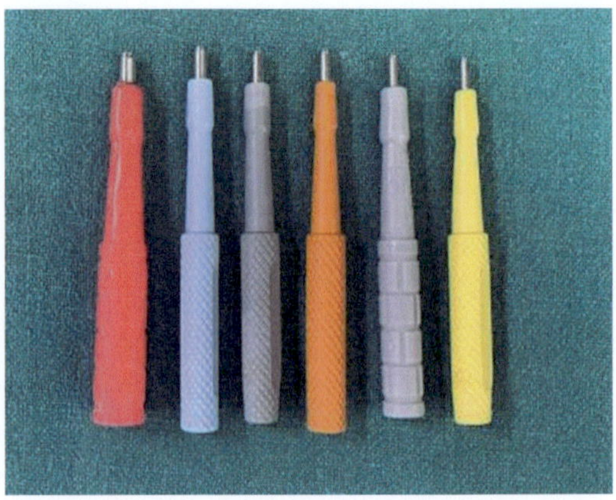

Fig. 1.13 Skin biopsy punches

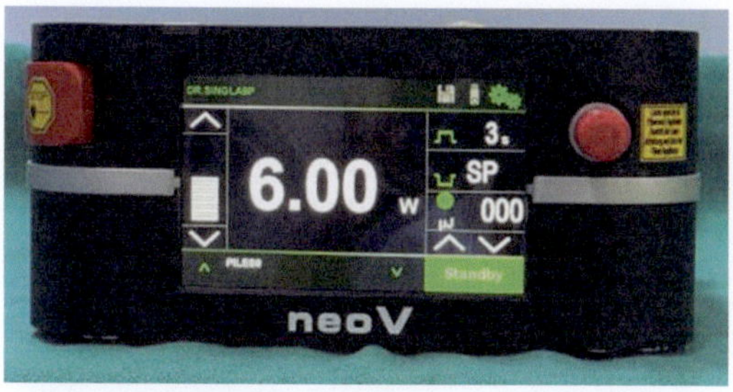

Fig. 1.14 LASER machine 1470 nm diode LASER

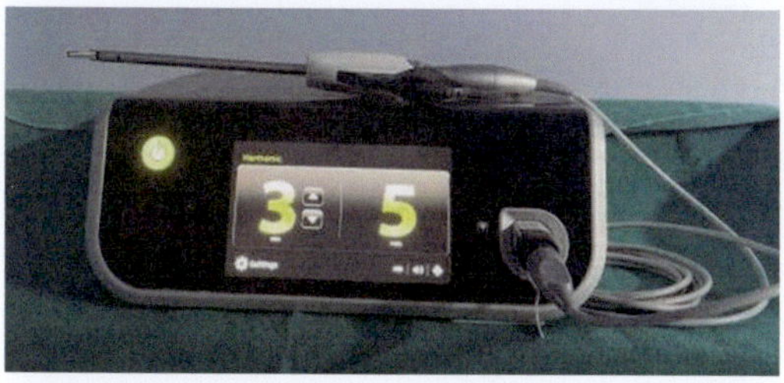

Fig. 1.15 Harmonic and vessel sealer

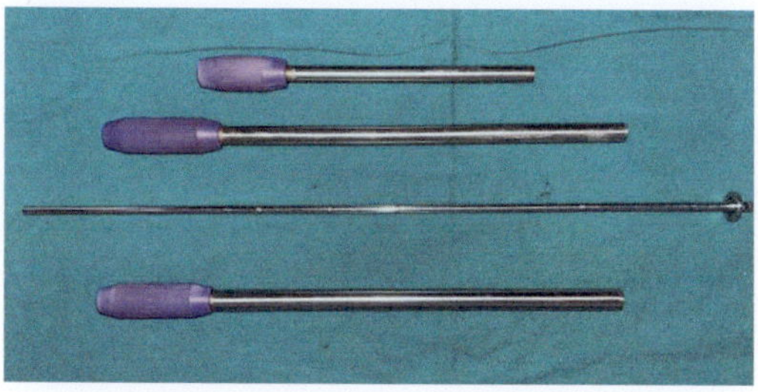

Fig. 1.16 FiXcision devise to core out fistula tract

- Special needles with threads like.
  - 5/8 circle 27 mm round body 2.0 polyglactin suture.
  - 1/2 circle, 30 mm round body needle with 2.0 polyglactin suture.
- Fistula probes and irrigation needle (Fig. 1.17).
- Aneurysmal needle and Lahey's forceps to pass suture, like in case of LIFT (Fig. 1.18).
- Staplers.
  - MIPH stapler (Fig. 1.19).
- Trans anal minimal invasive surgery (TAMIS) instrument sets and platform (Fig. 1.20).

There are currently two approved devices for trans anal access with the TAMIS procedure—the SILS port (Covidien, Mansfield, MA) and the

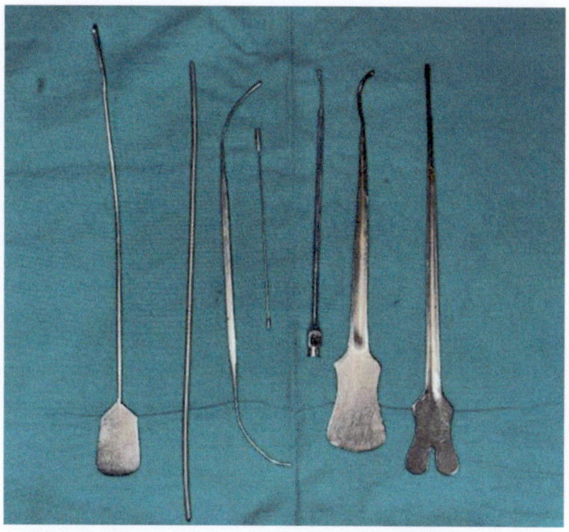

Fig. 1.17 Fistula probes and irrigation needle

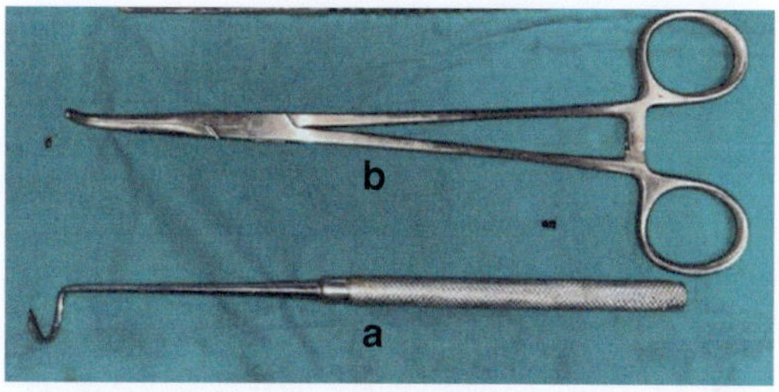

Fig. 1.18 Aneurysmal needle (A) and Lahey's forceps (B)

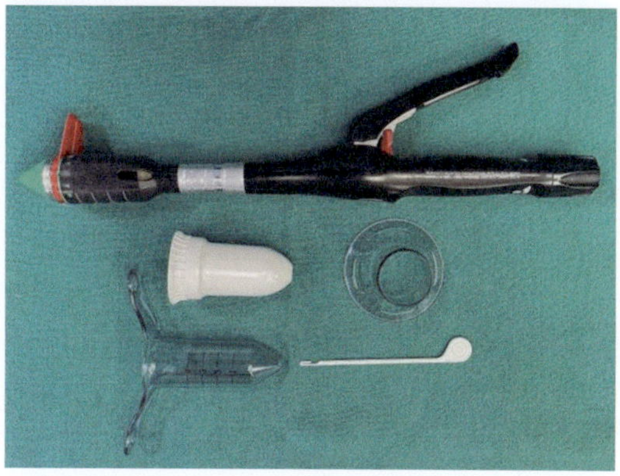

Fig. 1.19 MIPH stapler with accessories

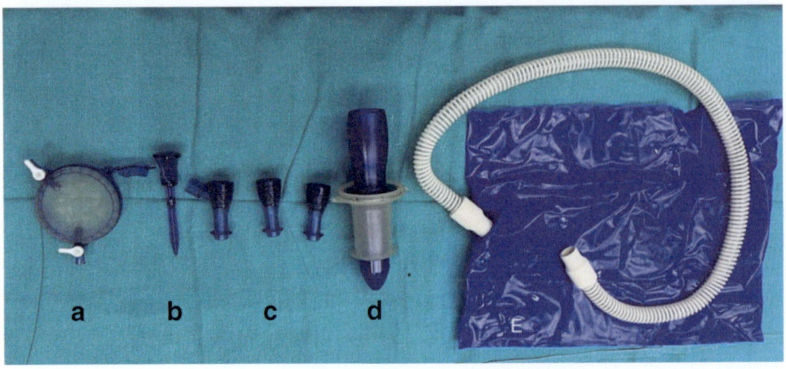

Fig. 1.20 Equipment for TAMIS (GelPOINT Path), (A) gel point cap, (B) obturator, (C) trocars, (D) silicon channel with obturator, (E) reservoir bag

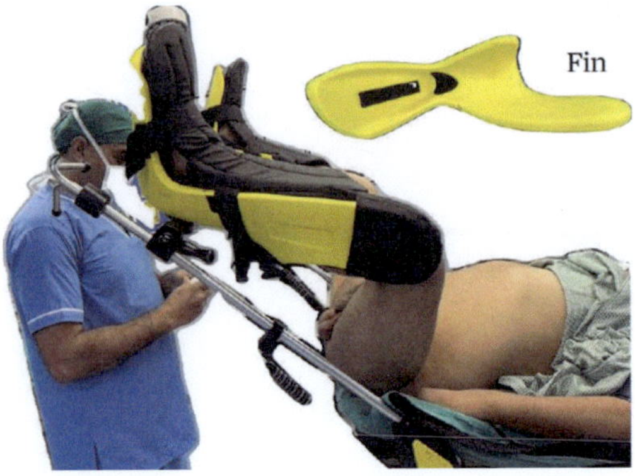

Fig. 1.21 Allen stirrups (yellow fins) Knee flexed supported and well supported calf and foot in boot and self-lifting mechanism to change lithotomy angle

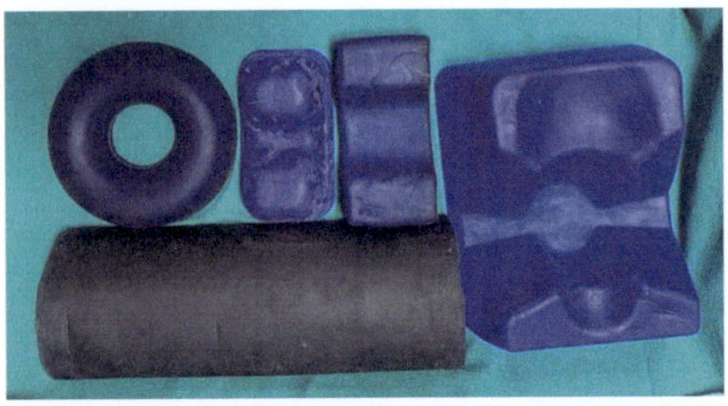

Fig. 1.22 Pads and foam devices for bony protection

GelPOINT Path (Applied Medical, Rancho Santa Margarita, CA).

- Stirrups for lithotomy:
  - Simple candy can type.
  - Boot type Allen (yellow fins) (Fig. 1.21).
- Pads and foams for prone position and bony protection (Fig. 1.22).

1.2 Operative Positioning of the Patient for Anorectal Operations

1.2.1 Lithotomy Position

1.2.1.1 What One Should Know Before Making Position

- Lithotomy (separation of legs with hips flexed) (Fig. 1.23) is the most commonly used position for surgery on anorectum, be it haemorrhoids, fissure, fistula, perianal abscess or TAMIS.
- Lithotomy position can be combined with associated abdominal procedure where perineal access is required:
  - Like abdomino perineal resection (APR) or lower anterior resection (LAR) with low coloanal stapler anastomosis.
  - Complex fistula in ano with extension on to abdominal wall.
- Common complications associated with this position are neuropraxia of the common peroneal nerve and compartment syndrome of the lower extremity. [1]
- Different devices to hold legs in flexed position at knee and hip need proper positioning and padding to avoid joint and nerve injuries.
- For obese patients and patients at risk for venous thrombosis especially during long surgeries, leg compression stockinette or devices are advisable.

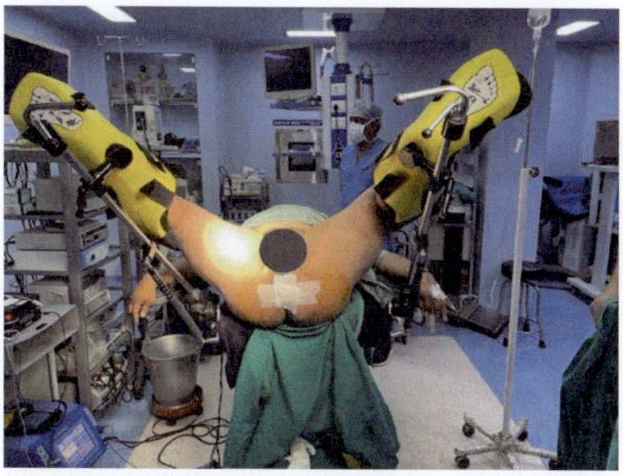

Fig. 1.23 Llithotomy position legs raised and separated

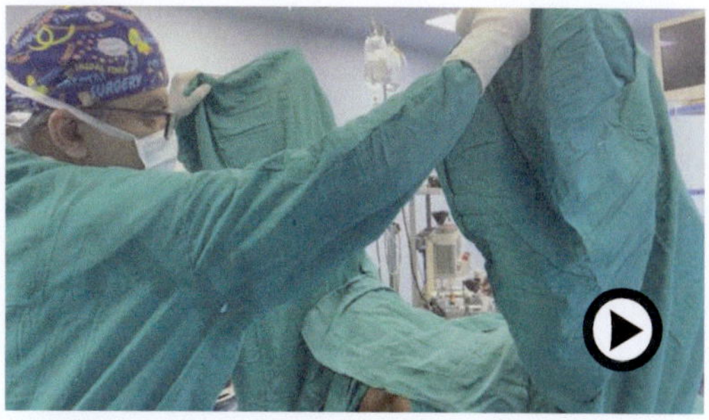

Fig. 1.24 Ease of changing lithotomy without disturbing drapes (▶ https://doi.org/10.1007/000-hpm)

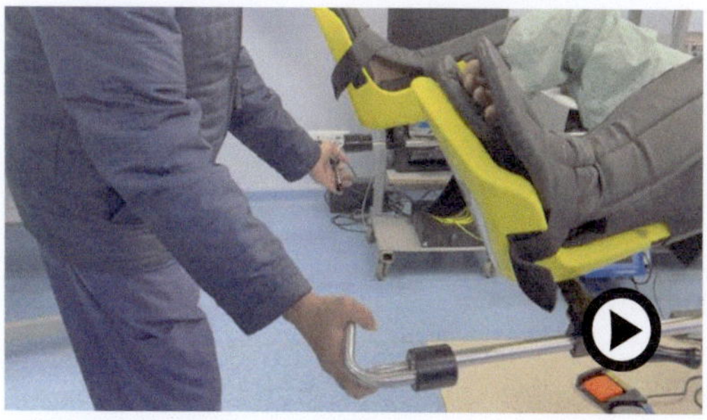

Fig. 1.25 To change the position, unlock the lifting mechanism by bringing knobs close and to fix the position, lock the mechanism by releasing the knobs (▶ https://doi.org/10.1007/000-hpk)

1.2.1.2 Equipment Required for Lithotomy Position

- Leg stirrups.
- Foot boot stirrups (Allen stirrups or yellow fins).
- Operation table with removable attachment for leg portion.
- Padding foam and folded bed sheets to raise the buttocks.

1.2.1.3 Technique

- After anaesthesia (spinal or general), patient lies supine.
- Attach leg supports to table.
- Remove the leg portion attachment.
- Slide the patient down so that perineum hangs over the edge of the table (5–15 cm depending on site of surgery, anus or post to anus as in posterior fistulae) while keeping legs in hand.
- Place both legs in supports simultaneously to avoid torque at junction of spine and pelvis.
- Flexion at knee and hip joint with abduction at hip joint, so that foot, knee and opposite shoulder come in one diagonal line.
- In simple leg stirrups one position is fixed and one has to open locks and fix again after changing position.
- Simple leg stirrups are good for short procedure of 30 min or so as it provides very less support to joints of the leg.
- In simple leg stirrups one strip goes to the ankle and one to mid foot, there is no support to calf and no foot rest.
- Allen stirrups supports leg, foot and knee joint (Fig. 1.21).
- In Allen stirrups with self-lifting hydraulic mechanism one can hold the limbs in any position of flexion and abduction at hip and one can adjust flexion at knee.
- No need to disturb the sterile draping while doing flexion and abduction at hip (Fig. 1.24; Video 1.1).
- To change position, unlock by pressing knobs, releasing knobs leads to locking in a position for safety (Fig. 1.25; Video 1.2).
- One can operate trans-anal and through posterior perineum as well, with ease—like in posterior fistulae going quite posterior towards sacrum.
- In long procedures, one can bring the lithotomy down (bringing legs below the heart level

and decreasing flexion at hip to allow better lower limb perfusion) without disturbing drapes.

- Put both limbs in flexion at knee and keep the feet in boots and adjust rotation at ankle so that foot planter fits nicely in boot which is already padded.
- Slide down leg and boot support so that nothing comes posterior to popliteal fossa.
- Fin is designed so that knee rests comfortably (Fig. 1.21).
- One can adjust the flexion and abduction at hips as necessary.

1.2.1.4 Complications (Table 1.1)

1.2.1.5 Tips and Tricks

- Always procure specific instruments and get proper training for minimally invasive surgery.
- Scopes, LASER machine, harmonic etc., are costly equipment. Always have maintenance contract and ensure after sales service.
- In long procedures one can bring the lithotomy down, to bring legs below the heart level and decreasing flexion at hip to allow better lower limb perfusion (without disturbing drapes).
- Use adequate padding to prevent pressure on bony prominences.

Table 1.1 Complications of lithotomy position

Complication	Prevention	Management
Neuropraxia of common peroneal nerve. Foot drop/ weakness in dorsiflexors of the foot and great toe drop	Proper padding near the fibular head and neck area.	Deflazacort 6 mg twice a day for 5 days.
Compartment syndrome of lower leg/severe and progressive pain leg which increases by passive movement of the ankle.	Lower the leg below heart level and decrease flexion at hip in between the procedure especially if procedure goes beyond 5 h.	Detection Oxygenation Maintain high perfusion Dermato fasciotomy [2]

1.2.2 Prone and Prone Jack Knife (Prone with Flexion at Hip and Legs Spread Apart) Position

1.2.2.1 What One Should Know Before Making Prone Position

Advantages of Prone Position

- Prone position gives good exposure to sacrococcygeal area as in case of pilonidal sinus, posterior perineum between the anal canal and the coccyx. Prone jack knife position is better for simultaneous exposure of the anal canal and sacrococcygeal area as in a case of pilonidal sinus with tract going caudal and one wants to rule out associated fistula in ano.
- While working from within anal canal for anterior fistulae with deep inter sphincteric extension, prone jack knife position gives opportunity to work on floor.
- Position is good for working surgeon and improves exposure for assistants especially.
- Certain surgeons prefer this position for all types of surgery on anal canal especially in the United States of America.

Limitations of Prone Position

- Air way access is obviously limited in prone position, Patient cannot be operated with face mask and oxygen instead needs endotracheal intubation or at least a laryngeal mask.
- Prone position makes a person vulnerable to upper extremity injuries like shoulder dislocation and neuropraxia.
- Arms should be kept above the head while rotating the patient from supine to prone position.
- Padding of pressure points should be adequate.
- Marking around the anus as one is facing a clock like 1'o clock, 2'o clock etc. labelled in supine position get flipped by 180 degree which is self explanatroy in (Fig. 1.26a, b).

1.2.2.2 Equipment Required

- Blankets and sheets as rolls.
- Foam pads and foam head support (Fig. 1.22).
- Pillows.
- Wide straps and tapes.

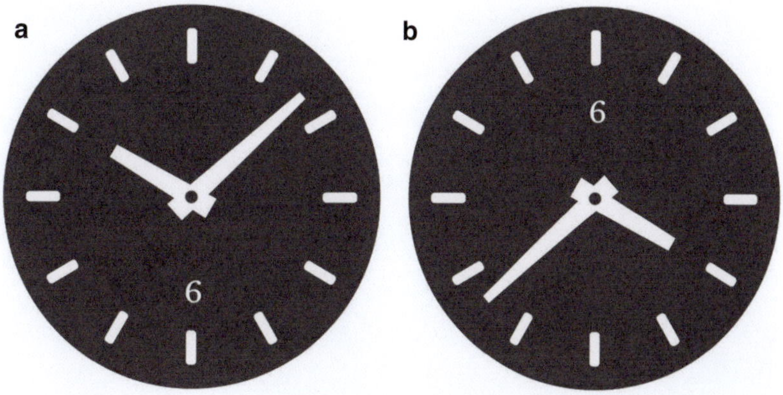

Fig. 1.26 (**a**) Supine and lithotomy position magnetic resonance imaging (MRI) and endo US also reported in this position. (**b**) Prone position all markings change

1.2.2.3 Technique (Video 1.3)

- Arrange head support, sheet rolls for chest and pelvis on OT table (Fig. 1.27).
- Arm rests are also padded well.
- Rail in the patient on trolley.
- Raise the trolley level up to OT table.
- Intubate the patient on trolley.
- Raise upper limbs above head level.
- Rotate the patient gently over to OT table in prone position.
- One person should hold head, another feet. Three persons will lift from shoulder, chest and pelvis and another team of three will receive the patient in prone position on OT table (Fig. 1.28; Video 1.3).
- Check the position of head rest, all pads like chest pads, roll sheet beneath pelvis, support below ankle for feet. Arm rests paddings should be well mounted.
- Buttocks are strapped to wide open the natal cleft as per requirement (Fig. 1.29a, b).
- Break the table below the pelvis to flex the hips to make jack knife position as per requirement (Fig. 1.30).
- Connect the pulse oximeter probe in changed position.
- Let the anaesthesia team settle again.
- Clean and drape the patient with sterile sheets.

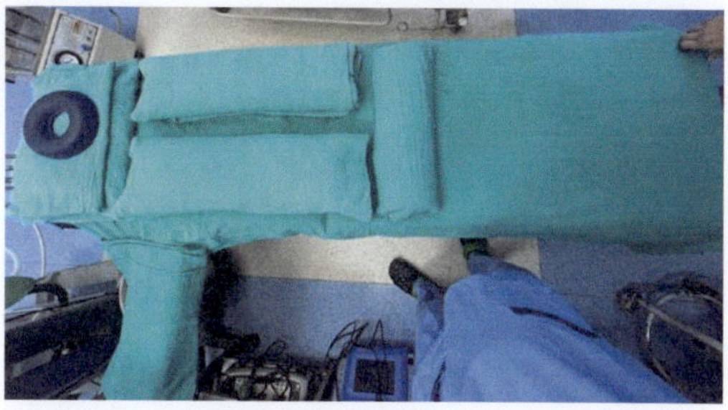

Fig. 1.27 OT table with foam head rest and sheet rolls for chest and pelvis

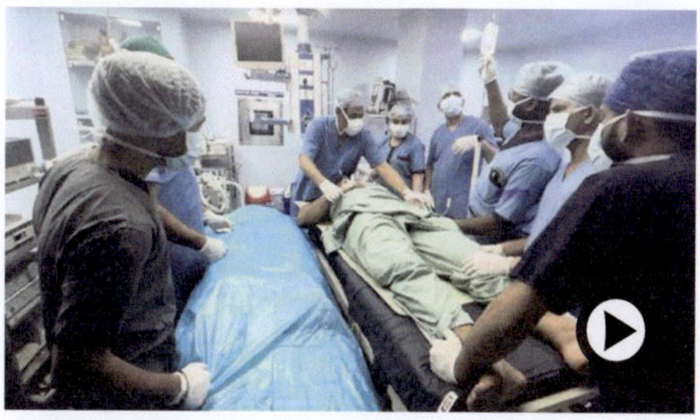

Fig. 1.28 Man power to rotate the intubated patient from supine to prone. Video 1.3 Changing position of anaesthetised patient from supine to prone (▶ https://doi.org/10.1007/000-hpn)

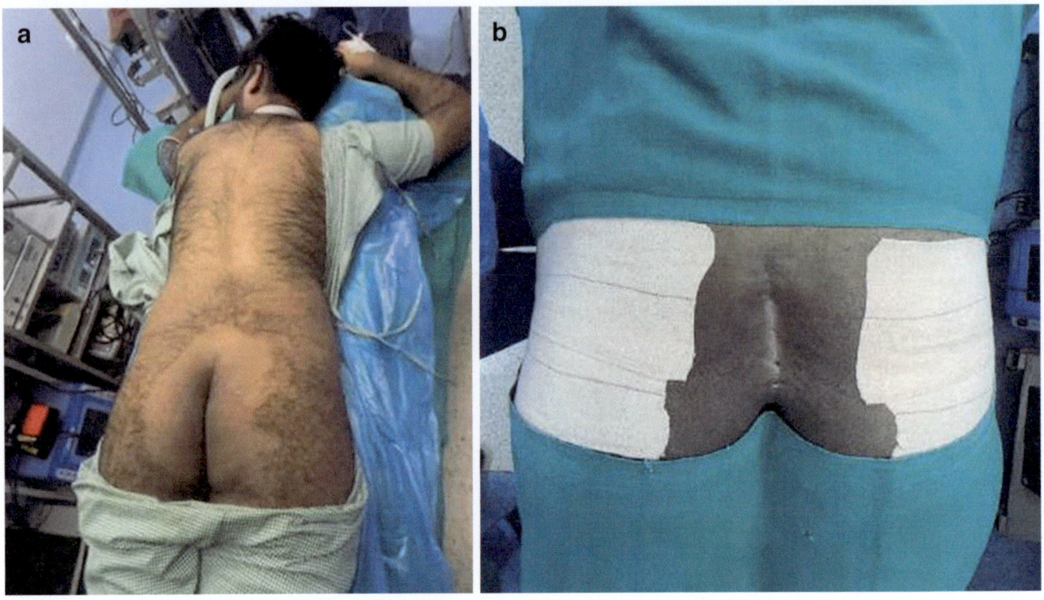

Fig. 1.29 (a) Prone position without straps. (b) Buttocks strapped to open the natal cleft

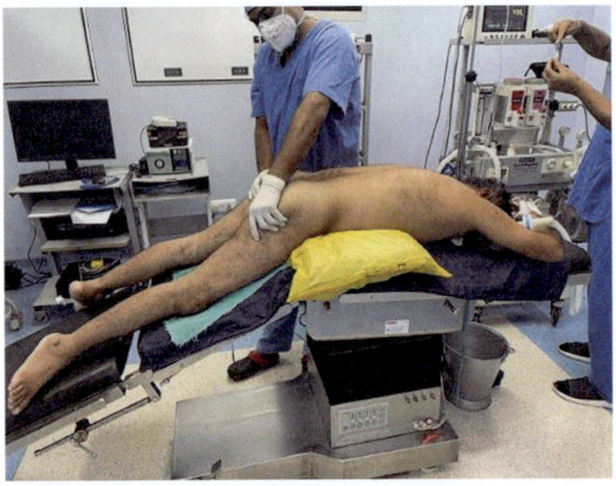

Fig. 1.30 Break the table below the pelvis to make prone to prone jack knife position

1.2.2.4 Tips and Tricks

- Anal and perianal conditions recorded in supine position by o' clock position gets flipped upside down in prone position and all other positions rotate by 180° accordingly.
- Adequate man power should be there in OT before flipping the anaesthetised patient from supine to prone.
- Tell the personal regarding their respective roles while flipping the position.
- Always check placement of endotracheal tube after an anaesthetised patient is flipped from lithotomy to prone position.
- Role of proper padding cannot be overemphasised.

Algorithm for Making Lithotomy

Anorectal procedure requirement for usual lithotomy/hyperextended lithotomy (with increased flexion at hip)
Spinal or GA
Supine position
Bring the patient down
Buttocks come over leg portion of table
Fix the holding blocks of stirrups on side railings
Hold the legs
Remove the lower portion of operating table
Fix yellow fin stirrups

(continued)

Remove under garments of the patient
Flex both hips and knee symmetrically and raise the limbs to put both feet in boots simultaneously
Adjust ankle lever and abduction at hip, so that ankle, knee and opposite shoulder come in one diagonal line and foot rests in the boot comfortably
Adjust calf support so that nothing comes in popliteal fossa

Algorithm for Making Prone Position

Intubate the patient in supine position on trolley
Pump the trolley up, equal to the height of operation table
Bring trolley to the side of operation table
Operation table is well padded
Take the arms of the patient above the level of his/her head
Anaesthetist takes care of endotracheal tube
One nurse takes control of the i/v line
Three people hold the patient one from shoulder, another at lower chest and third at pelvis to flip the patient on to operation table in prone position
Three persons in corresponding position receive the patient in flipped position
Apply rolled sheet as pad below the ankle joint
Reassess the placement of endotracheal tube
Reposition the pulse oximeter
Let the anaesthesia team settle
Clean and drape as required

References

1. Angermeier K, Jordan G. Complications of the exaggerated lithotomy position: a review of 177 cases. J Urol. 1994;151(4):866–8. [PubMed] [CrossRef]
2. Halvachizadeh S, Jensen KO, Pape H-C. Chapter 12 Compartment syndrome due to patient positioning. In: Mauffrey C, Hak DJ, Martin III MP, editors. Compartment syndrome: a guide to diagnosis and management [Internet]. Cham: Springer; 2019.

Suggested Readings

Biswas S, Gnanasekaran I, Ivatury RR, Simon R, Patel AN. Exaggerated lithotomy position-related rhabdomyolysis. Am Surg. 1997;63(4):361–4. PMID: 9124760

Fish DR. Chapter 3 Principles of operative positioning. In: Steele SR, editor. Cleveland clinic illustrated tips and tricks in colon and rectal surgery, vol. 1. Wolters Kluwer; 2020.

Mayilvaganan KS, Singla S. Chapter 35 Setting up of colorectal clinic & examination of an anorectal patient. In: Agarwal N, Sharma PP, Sheikh P, editors. ACRSI text book of colorectal surgery. Jaypee Brothers; 2023.

Suggested Viewing

Video 1.1 by manufacturer before using an unfamiliar device at https://www.youtube.com/watch?v=fudU0yo_VG8

2 How to Manage Benign Anorectal Disorders in a Minimally Invasive Manner? Haemorrhoids Office Procedure Foam Sclerotherapy

Abstract

- Injection foam sclerotherapy, using some of the modern sclerosant, like polidocanol and thin bore-needle through a proctoscope is becoming quite popular to treat almost all grades of haemorrhoids.
- Relevant anatomy is described with clinical photographs.
- Indications, contraindications of the procedure and equipment required for sclerotherapy have been enumerated.
- Procedural details of making foam of sclerosant and application of foam sclerosant in haemorrhoids are well explained with figures, clinical photographs and video.
- Importance of appearance of striation sign is well explained and shown with high-quality pictures.
- It is cost-effective, office-based, quite safe and successful procedure if done properly.
- Complications of the procedure, their prevention and management are presented in tabulated form for easy reference, when required.
- Some pearls of wisdom have been shelled in Sect. 2.6.
- Readers, in search of evidence, can further explore "Suggested Reading" section.
- One can view our multimedia presentation on sclerotherapy and possible complications by opening a link in "Suggested Viewing" section.

Supplementary Information The online version contains supplementary material available at https://doi.org/10.1007/978-981-96-6190-9_2. The videos can be accessed individually by clicking the DOI link in the accompanying figure caption or by scanning this link with the SN More Media App.

S. K. Singla, K. Mital, *Operative Manual of Minimally Invasive and LASER Ano-proctology*,
https://doi.org/10.1007/978-981-96-6190-9_2

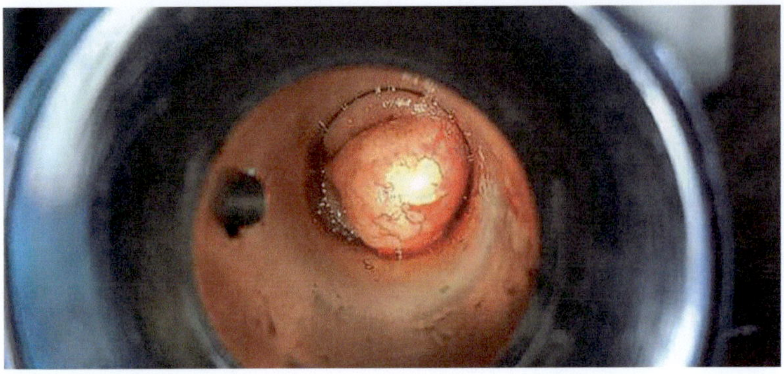

2.1 What One Should Know Before the Procedure

- The mere presence of prominent sub mucosal anal cushions is not an indication for their management (avoid over-treating them after finding a report of prominent anal cushions on colonoscopy).
- Patient should have bleeding or associated protrusion.
- Sclerotherapy means to induce sclerosis (fibrosis) in sub mucosal cushions by means of chemical-induced aseptic inflammation, which, in turn, stops bleeding from diseased sub-mucosal cushions and fixes them to underlying fibres of sphincter.
- Foam increases surface area of the drug-contact, thereby small drug quantity can spread homogeneously in a wider area.
- During COVID-19 pandemic, sclerotherapy of haemorrhoids efficiently helped as a bridge treatment for patients waiting for formal haemorrhoid surgery.
  - *Indications of sclerotherapy.*
    - Best reserved for grade 1 and 2 haemorrhoids, though with modern sclerosing agents it is being used in grade 3 or grade 4 haemorrhoids also [1].
    - Failed medical treatment.
    - Bleeding from haemorrhoids and patient on anticoagulants. Most of the times bleeding stops without stopping intake of anticoagulants. We find this as the best indication of sclerotherapy.
    - Where you do not want to operate like severely anaemic patient with bleeding from haemorrhoids, HIV-positive patients with bleeding from haemorrhoids.
    - According to the guidelines and the manufacturer's information, pregnancy is a contra-indication for sclerotherapy with polidocanol. As per current data, there is no reason for an interruption of pregnancy after sclerotherapy conducted during undetected pregnancy.
  - *Contraindications for sclerotherapy.*
    - External haemorrhoids.
    - Thrombosed or strangulated haemorrhoids.
    - Any acute infection in the area and lower gastrointestinal tract (GI).
    - Hypersensitivity to drug used for sclerotherapy.
- Though quite safe, patient should be counselled for early discomfort and possibility of bleeding and reoccurrence.

2.2 Equipment Required (Fig. 2.1)

- Lighted proctoscope, straight or beveled.
- Fibre optic cable and light source.
- Xylocain jelly.
- Surgical gloves.
- Sclerosing agent (polidocanol ampules).
- Spinal needle 21 gauge.

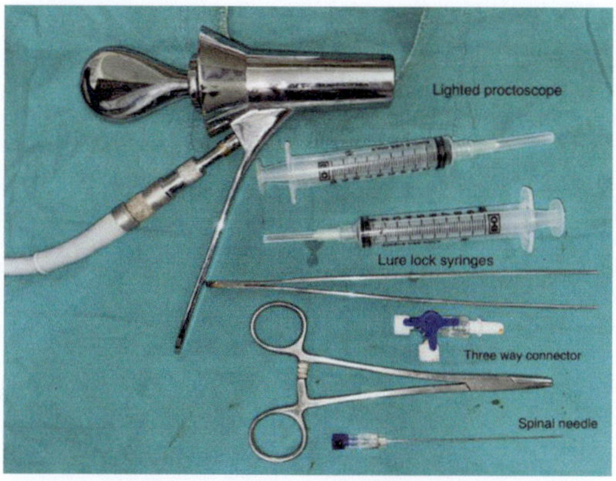

Fig. 2.1 Equipment for foam sclerotherapy

- Syringes 2, 10 cc each with lure lock.
- Three-way lure lock system.
- Long forceps.
- Sterile gauge pieces and cotton balls.
- Resuscitation equipment and oxygen should be available in the room.

2.3 Procedure (Video 2.1)

- We give proctoclysis enema if the rectum is full of stools otherwise no preparation, never inject in case of impacted stools. Ask patient to evacuate after enema.
- Prophylactic antibiotics in patients with prosthetic valves (Bacteraemia 8% cases) [2].
- No anaesthesia except lubricating lignocaine 2% jelly.
- Always do pre-procedure digital rectal examination (DRE), check anatomy and physiology of anal canal and especially any prostatic bulge anteriorly in males.
- Do not depend upon findings of others, do DRE yourself.
- Patient lies in left lateral position with buttocks out of the edge of the table (it opens the space in natal cleft), pants and underwear lowered down to below knee.
- Always cover the patient's anterior parts with bed sheet or large towel especially in a female patient.
- Apply 2% lignocaine jelly in the anal canal and wait for 5 min.

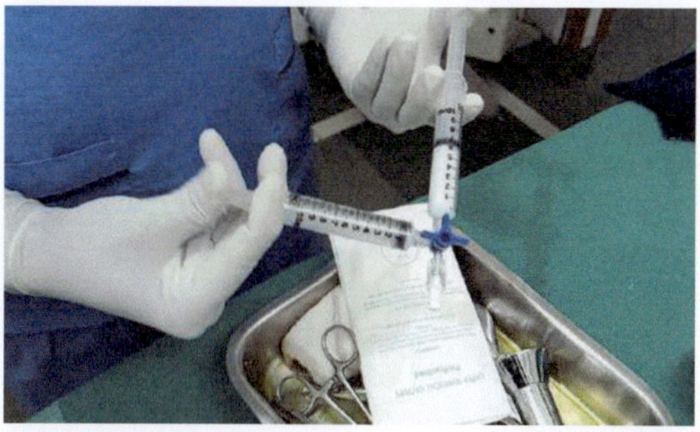

Fig. 2.2 Making foam with Tessari method. Polidocanol:air::1:4

- In the mean time, prepare polidocanol foam by Tessari method (Fig. 2.2) [3].
  - Take two 10 ml lure lock syringes, (to prevent any accidental spillage of drug while creating or injecting foam) fill 2 ml 3% polidocanol in one of them. Take 8 ml air in another syringe and attach them to three-way lure lock system.
  - Mix solution in 1:4 ratio with air with 20 brisk movements and foam is created which remains stable for 2 min.
- One can use 4 ml polidocanol with 16 ml air for large juicy haemorrhoids [1, 3].
- Bend the last 1 cm tip of 21 gauge spinal needle with needle-holder after removing its stylet.
- Put lighted proctoscope in the anal canal gently while asking patient to relax the anal canal.
- Clean the anal canal and inspect the position of haemorrhoids and other landmarks like apex of haemorrhoids and dentate line (Figs. 2.3 and 2.4) while bringing scope out.
- Take the scope back in position and inject almost 3 ml foam at the apex of each major haemorrhoid one by one (this position is well above the dentate line, never ever inject below the dentate line) (Fig. 2.5).
- One may re-emulsify the foam to make it stable before injecting each haemorrhoid.
- We always inject 3.0 clock haemorrhoid first as it is the most dependant in left lateral position and any ooze will not hinder in injecting other areas (Fig. 2.6).
- Drug should be injected in submucosa, striation sign (Fig. 2.7) will appear (mucosa which

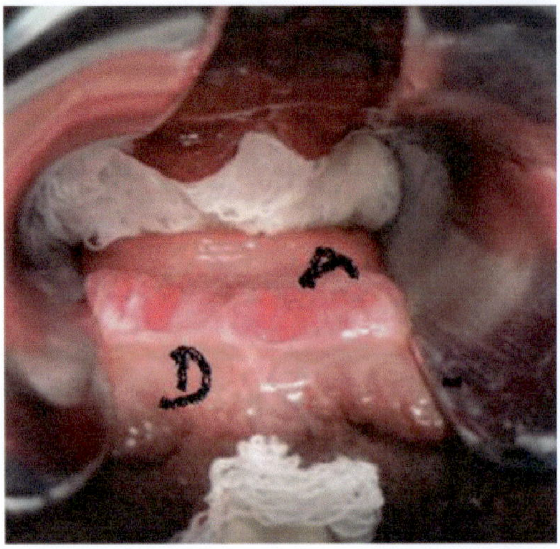

Fig. 2.3 Anal canal with Park's speculum inside showing dentate line (D) and apex of haemorrhoid (A)

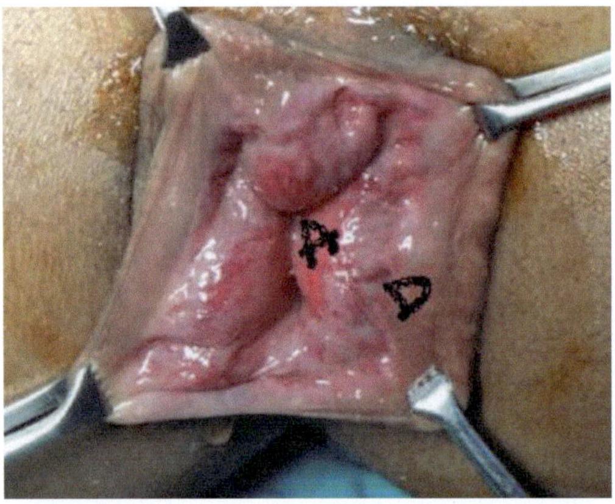

Fig. 2.4 Anal canal showing dentate line (D) and apex of haemorrhoid (A)

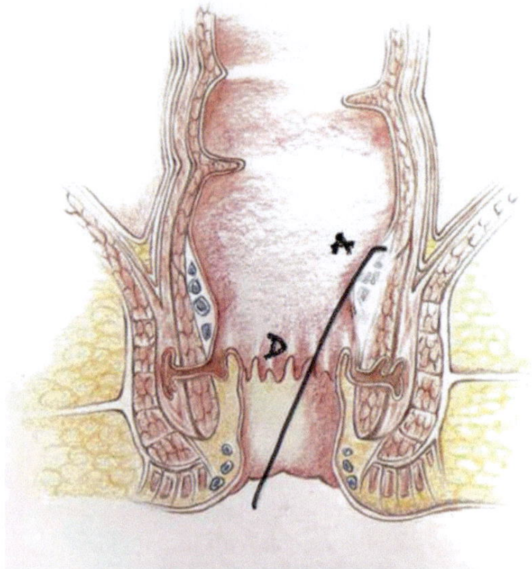

Fig. 2.5 Point of injection—apex of haemorrhoid A well above the dentate line D

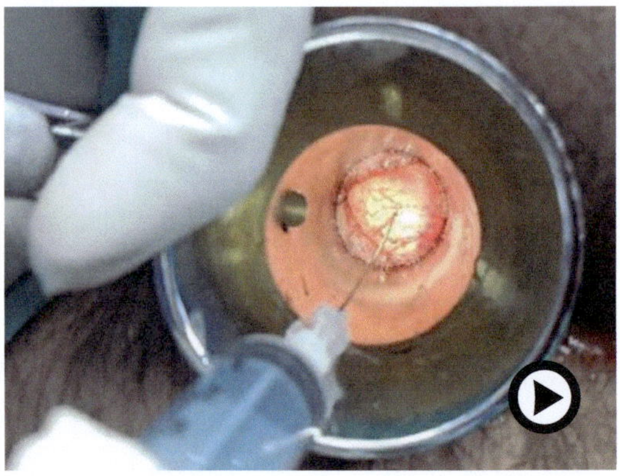

Fig. 2.6 Site of first injection 3.0 clock haemorrhoid in left lateral position
Video 2.1 Foam sclerotherapy of haemorrhoids procedure (▶ https://doi.org/10.1007/000-hpp)

was without any characteristics will swell and random vessels pattern becomes visible over it) that means one is in right place.

- Too superficial injection will blanch the mucosa dead white and may lead to mucosal ulceration and secondary bleeding (Fig. 2.8).
- Too deep injection in muscle will not show up and will lead to some fibrosis of sphincter area.
- Minor ooze from injection site can be controlled by pressure with cotton-ball or gauge.
- Small discomfort while injecting can be further reduced by injecting slowly.
- Any pain-stop and check your injection-site in reference to dentate line.
- Be careful while injecting anterior haemorrhoids, keep bevel of the needle more tangential to avoid any deep injection here, which may lead to urological complications.

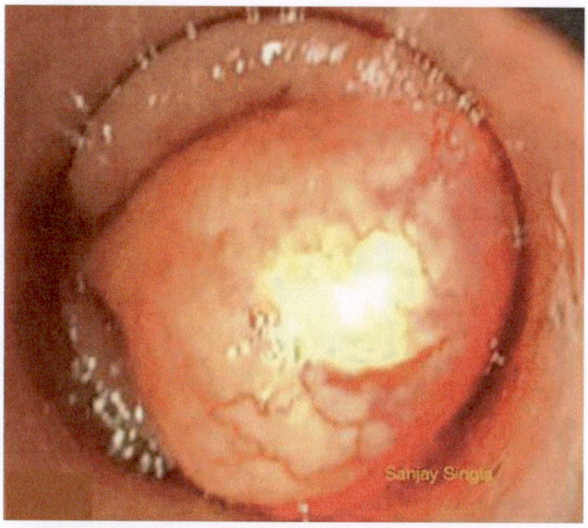

Fig. 2.7 Striation sign, random vessel pattern

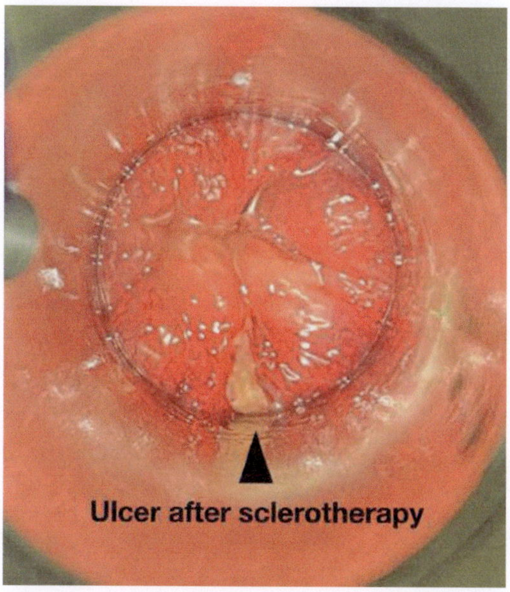

Fig. 2.8 Proctoscopic view of anal mucosal ulceration due to injection of sclerosing agent in the mucosa

- In case of counter-puncture of mucosa, if foam suddenly comes in anal canal, stop there and inject other haemorrhoid first, otherwise foam keeps on leaking from puncture site.
- Always do check proctoscopy and better remove any cotton ball, used to control the ooze.
- Do gentle massage of the area of injection for proper dissemination of the foam.

2.4 Complication of Sclerotherapy (Table 2.1)

Table 2.1 Complications of sclerotherapy

Complication	Prevention	Management
Pain during injection	Always remain above the dentate line and inject slowly	
Bleeding from injection site	Avoid direct puncture of mucosal vessels	Press with cotton-ball or gauge piece
Pain, fever and urinary retention	Call the patient back and check for any infection and treat accordingly	Antibiotics and symptomatic treatment
Beware of this triad		Observe
Urinary symptoms	Keep bevel of needle more tangential while injecting in anterior haemorrhoid to avoid ill-sited injection	Analgesics Non steroidal anti inflammatory drug (NSAIDs)
Lower urinary tract symptoms (LUTS) infection		Antibiotics
Haematuria and haematospermia		
Vasovagal reactions	Reassurance and inject slow	Head low and resuscitate
Rarely necrotising infections	Do not inject in case of infection	Debridement and antibiotics
Very rare, rectovaginal and rectourethral fistula	Be vigilant while injecting anterior Haemorrhoid	Do not be in a hurry to repair. Let inflammation settle

For further details, check suggested readings and videos links given at the end of the chapter.

2.5 Post-procedure Advice to Patients

- Effect may take 1 or 2 days.
- Report back urgently if triad of pain, fever and urinary retention occurs. (Do not advise on telephone, call the patient back.)
- Laxative for a week, avoid straining.
- Diet and defecatory habits modification as for any patient of haemorrhoids.
- Follow-up visit after 3 weeks to check the effect.
- Repeat injection after 6 weeks.
- Advocate Kegel's exercise to prevent protrusion.

2.6 Tips and Tricks

- Never inject in case of impacted stools.
- Do not depend upon findings of others, do Digital rectal examination (DRE) yourself.
- Resuscitation equipment and oxygen should be available in the room.
- Always use lure lock syringes to prevent any accidental spillage of drug while creating or injecting foam.
- One may re-emulsify the foam to make it stable before injecting each haemorrhoid.
- Never bend the tip of spinal-needle with finger, instead use needle holder, remove stylet before one bends the needle.
- Never ever inject below the dentate line.
- Inject 3.0 clock haemorrhoid first as it is most dependant in left lateral position and any ooze will not hinder in injecting other areas.
- In case of counter-puncture of mucosa, if suddenly foam comes in anal canal, stop there and inject other haemorrhoid first otherwise foam keeps on leaking from puncture site.
- Appearance of striation sign ensures right site of injection.
- Beware of triad of pain, fever and urinary retention.

Algorithm for Sclerotherapy

History of bleeding, protrusion
Clinical examination
Investigations colonoscopy in appropriate cases
Indications /contraindications
Counselling
Consent
Pre op. Considerations
Left lateral position
DRE and anoscopy
Making foam of sclerosing agent
Polidocanol: air :: 1:4 2 ml : 8ml
Tessari method
Use lure lock syringes
Inject 3cc foam in apex of each haemorrhoid
Observe for striation sign
Light massage to the submucosal cushions

References

1. Fernandes V, Fonseca J. Polidocanol foam injected at high doses with intravenous needle: the (almost) perfect treatment of symptomatic internal hemorrhoids. GE Port J Gastroenterol. 2019;26(3):169–75.
2. Adami B, Eckardt VF, Suermann RB, et al. Bacteremia after proctoscopy and hemorrhoidal injection sclerotherapy. Dis Colon Rectum. 1981;24:373–4. https://doi.org/10.1007/BF02603422.
3. Xu J, Wang YF, Chen AW, Wang T, Liu SH. A modifed Tessari method for producing more foam. Springerplus. 2016;5:129. https://doi.org/10.1186/s40064-016-1769-5. PMID: 26933628; PMCID: PMC4760956.

Suggested Readings

He A, Chen M. Sclerotherapy in hemorrhoids. Indian J Surg. 2023;85(2):228.

Lohsiriwat V. Hemorrhoids: from basic pathophysiology to clinical management. World J Gastroenterol. 2012;18(17):2009–17. https://doi.org/10.3748/wjg.v18.i17.2009. ArticleCASPubMedPubMed CentralGoogle Scholar.

Mishra S, Sahoo AK, Elamurugan TP, Jagdish S. Polidocanol versus phenol in oil injection sclerotherapy in treatment of internal hemorrhoids: a randomized controlled trial. Turk J Gastroenterol. 2020;31(5):378–83. https://doi.org/10.5152/tjg.2020.19276. [PMC free article] [PubMed] [CrossRef] [Google Scholar].

Miyamoto H, Hada T, Ishiyama G, Ono Y, Watanabe H. Aluminum potassium sulfate and tannic acid sclerotherapy for Goligher grades II and III hemorrhoids: results from a multicenter study. World J Hepatol. 2016;8:844–9. [PMC free article] [PubMed] [Google Scholar]

Salgueiro P, Garrido MMD, Santos RG, Pedroto I, Castro-Poças FM. Polidocanol foam sclerotherapy versus rubber band ligation in hemorrhoidal disease grades I/II/III: randomized trial. Dis Colon Rectum. 2022;65(7):e718–27. https://doi.org/10.1097/DCR.0000000000002117.

Salgueiro P, Rei A, Garrido M, Rosa B, Oliveira AM, Pereira-Guedes T, Morais S, Castro-Poças F. Polidocanol foam sclerotherapy in the treatment of hemorrhoidal disease in patients with bleeding disorders: a multicenter, prospective, cohort study. Tech Coloproctol. 2022;26(8):615–25. https://doi.org/10.1007/s10151-022-02600-5. Epub 2022 Feb 25. PMID: 35217937; PMCID: PMC8879173.

Suggested Viewing

Video 2.1 Abstract of polidocanol foam sclero therapy PFS vs RBL at https://links.lww.com/DCR/B816.

Video 2.2 Polidocanol foam sclerotherapy of haemorrhoids procedure, complications of sclerotherapy—prevention and management at https://www.youtube.com/watch?v=c8B7XpuRdAw.

3 Haemorrhoids: Office Procedure Rubber-Band Ligation

Abstract

- Rubber-band ligation is one of the most successful office-based procedure to tackle early haemorrhoids, which do not require surgery.
- Mechanism of action of bands in controlling bleeding and protrusion has been explained.
- Indications and contraindications of the procedure have been enumerated.
- Various types of banding devices have been mentioned and two common types—manual and suction device—explained with sketches and clinical photographs.
- Ways to prevent pain after banding are explained in depth.
- "Why not to choose banding in patients on anticoagulants" is elucidated well.
- Complications of banding and their prevention and management are presented in tabulated form, for easy access and reference.
- Pearls of wisdom from present and previous authors are grouped in Sect. 3.9.
- Video of the procedure with suction-type banding device has been provided.
- Those interested in evidence can check "References" and "Suggested Reading" sections.

Supplementary Information The online version contains supplementary material available at https://doi.org/10.1007/978-981-96-6190-9_3. The videos can be accessed individually by clicking the DOI link in the accompanying figure caption or by scanning this link with the SN More Media App.

3.1 What One Should Know Before the Procedure

- In banding one ligates mucosa and submucosal tissue well above the dentate line to do a controlled injury. It leads to tissue destruction which heals by fibrosis and eventually fixes the tissue.
- Conventionally, banding is supposed to control protrusion better than sclerotherapy.
- All patients should be cautioned against bleeding from site when banded mucosa sloughs out after 7–8 days.
- Though safe to band all three major haemorrhoids in one sitting, but it may increase the discomfort.

3.2 Indications

- Grade 2 and 3 haemorrhoids (banding becomes difficult if there is no loose mucosa as in grade 1 haemorrhoids).

S. K. Singla, K. Mital, *Operative Manual of Minimally Invasive and LASER Ano-proctology*,
https://doi.org/10.1007/978-981-96-6190-9_3

3.3 Contraindications

- Patients on anticoagulants should be offered sclerotherapy (we do not advocate adjusting the timing of banding as proposed by Nelson) [1].
- Patients of cirrhosis and portal hypertension with bleeding from haemorrhoids are candidates for sclerotherapy [2].
- Concurrent anorectal sepsis.

3.4 Equipment Required for Banding (Figs. 3.1 and 3.2)

- Lighted proctoscope, light source and cable.
- Xylocaine jelly.
- Sterile gloves.
- Long forceps.
- Sterile gauge pieces.
- Band ligator and bands.
  - Conventional ligator (Barron band ligator)
  - Suction ligator (Mc Gown type).
  - Disposable units (O'Regan banding system).
- Syringe with fine needle and saline or xylocaine sol. (Optional).
- Resuscitation equipment and oxygen supply.

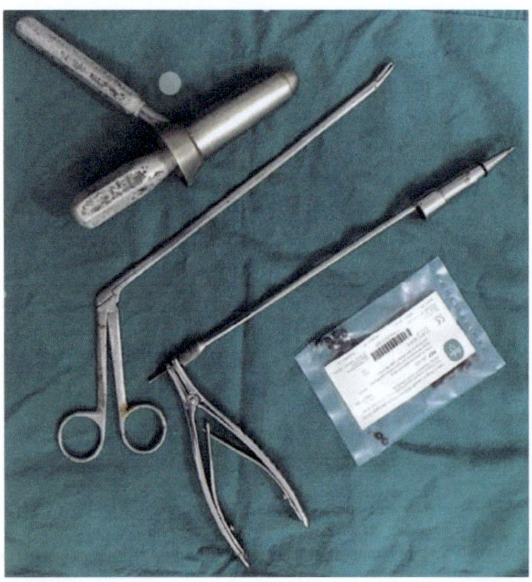

Fig. 3.1 Barron band ligator with bands

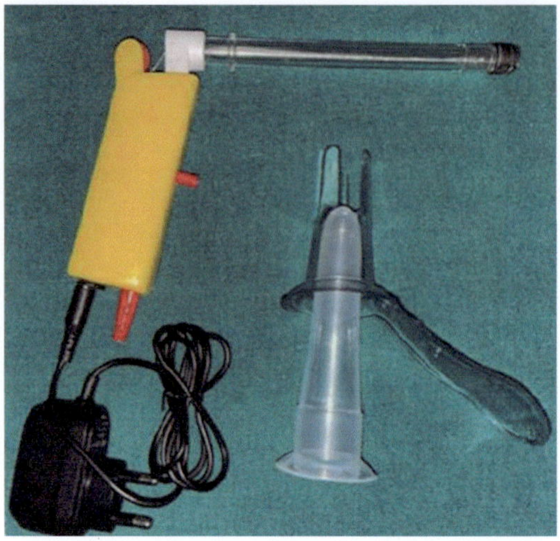

Fig. 3.2 Pre-loaded bands with suction and light source with slit proctoscope

3.5 Procedure

- We give proctoclysis enema if rectum is full of stools, otherwise no preparation, never band in case of impacted stools. Ask patient to evacuate after enema.
- Prophylactic antibiotics in patients with prosthetic valves (Bacteraemia 8% cases) [3, 4].
- No anaesthesia except lubricating lignocaine 2% jelly.
- Always do pre-procedure digital rectal examination (DRE) yourself, check anatomy and physiology of the anal canal. Do not depend upon findings of others.
- Patient lies in left lateral position with buttocks out of the edge of the table (it opens the space in natal cleft) and pants and underwear lowered down to below knee.
- Always cover the patient's anterior parts with bed—sheet or large towel, especially in a female patient.
- Apply 2% lignocaine jelly in the anal canal and wait for 5 min.
- In the meantime, prepare the ligator and put the rubber band over the cone and slide down to mount it on to barrel (Fig. 3.3).
- Put lighted proctoscope in the anal canal gently while asking patient to relax the anal canal.

- Clean the anal canal and inspect the position of haemorrhoids. Look for land marks like apex of haemorrhoids and dentate line while bringing scope out.
- Adjust the level of ano-scope so that one can visualise the haemorrhoids 1.5–2 cm above the level of dentate line (Fig. 3.4).
- Assistant holds the anoscope for the surgeon and maintains the position so that surgeon can see the target at 1.5–2 cm proximal to dentate line (Fig. 3.5).
- Put holding-forceps through the loaded barrel of ligator and catch hold mucosa and submucosa at least 1.5–2 cm above the dentate line, if painful leave it and catch further 0.5 cm proximally (Fig. 3.6).
- Release the band while maintaining the traction on mucosa so that sufficient tissue comes in to the barrel (Figs. 3.7 and 3.8).

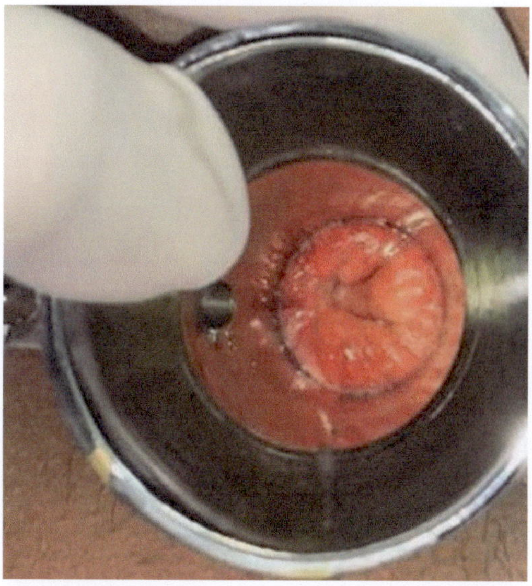

Fig. 3.4 Surgeon visualises the haemorrhoids and adjusts the level of proctoscope to target the tissue 1.5–2 cm proximal to dentate line

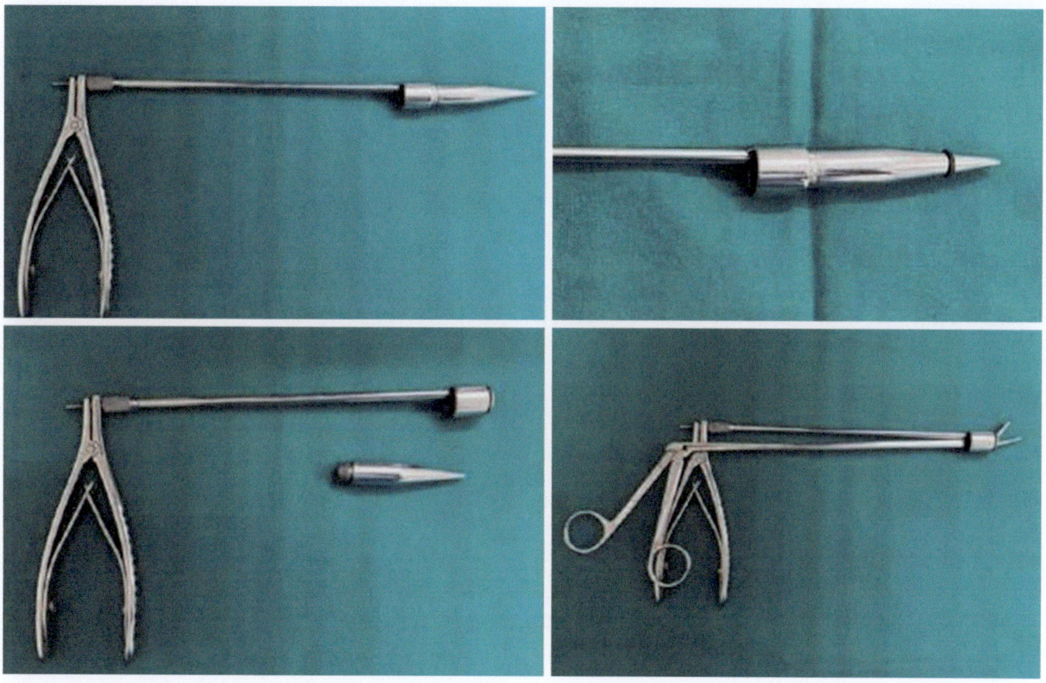

Fig. 3.3 Mount rubber band on the barrel with the help of cone, cone is removed and forceps passes through the loaded barrel

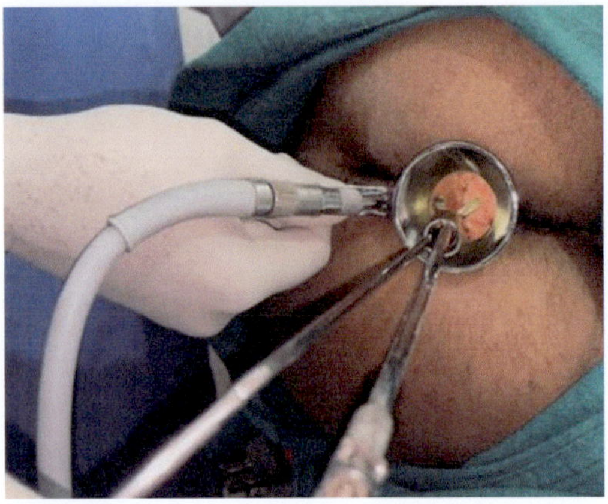

Fig. 3.5 Assistant holds the scope and surgeon is to use both hands to hold the tissue and fire the ligator

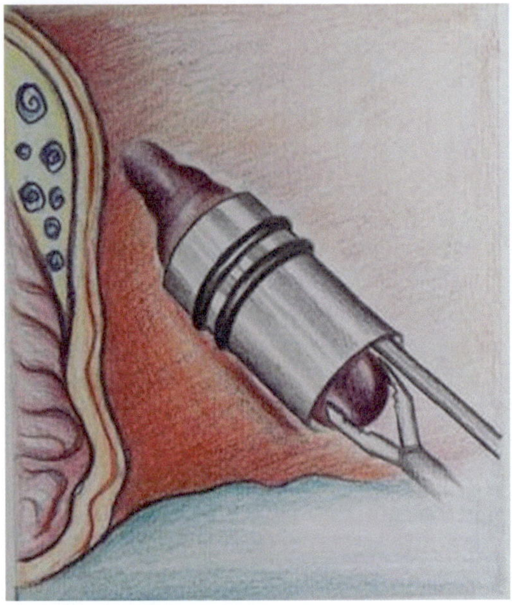

Fig. 3.7 Release the band while maintaining traction on haemorrhoid tissue and pushing barrel towards the wall

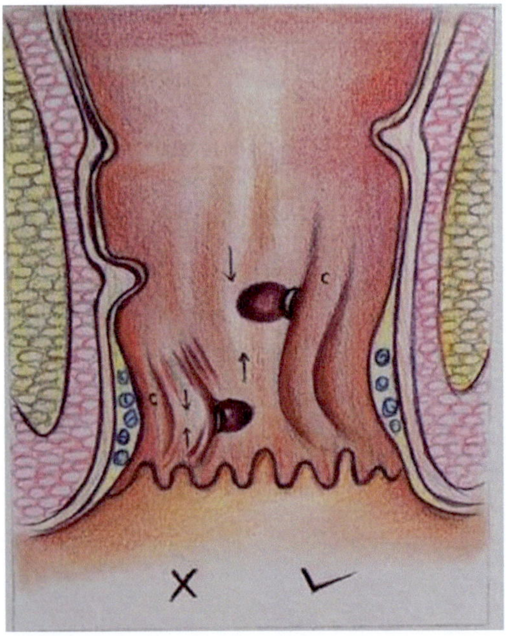

Fig. 3.6 Illustration to show that as one releases the band, some mucosa will be ligated from proximal and some from distal area of catching point (c). Ligated mucosa comes even closer to dentate line

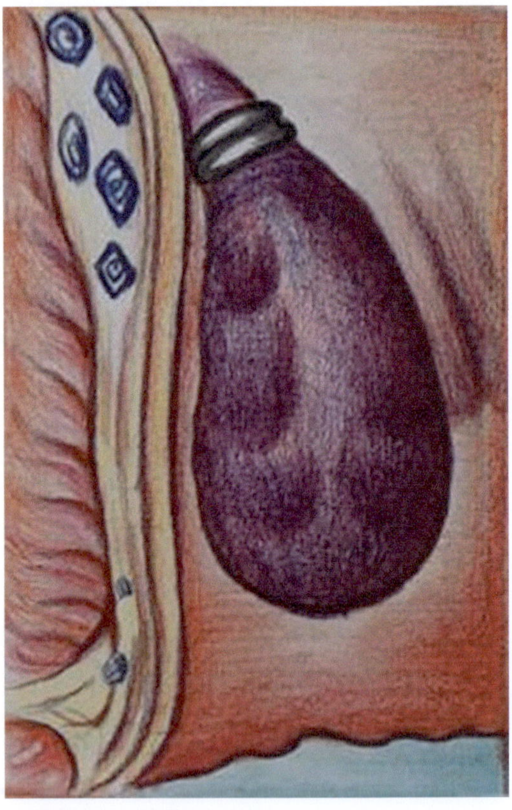

Fig. 3.8 Sufficient tissue ligation

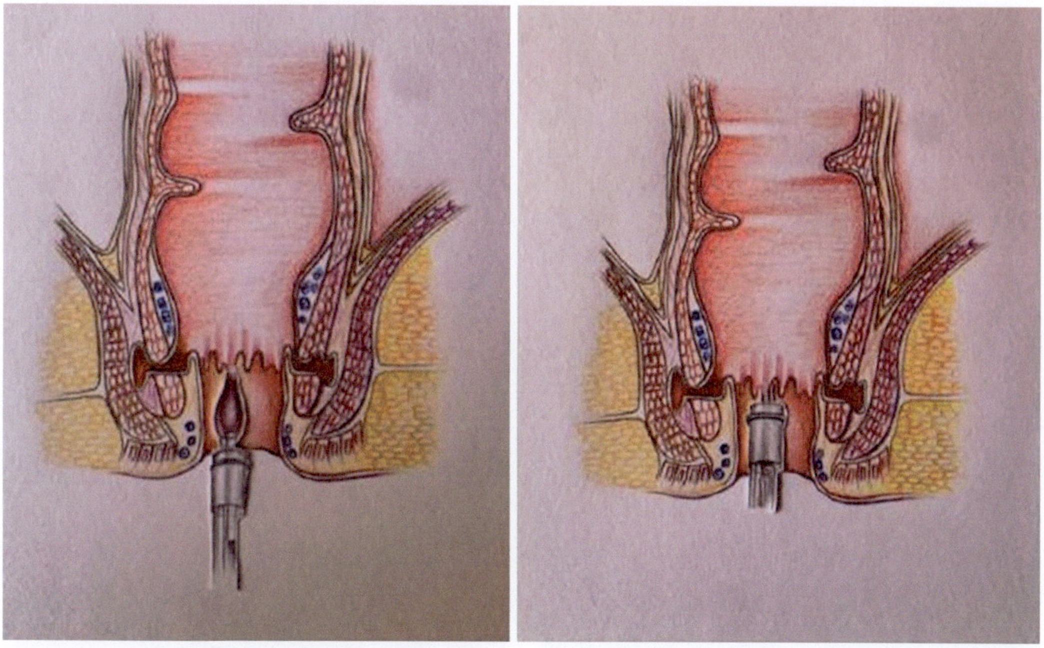

Fig. 3.9 At times, position of haemorrhoids is such that one is to hold the mucosa close to dentate line. Apply traction and push drum towards mucosa if it is painful. Better abandon banding in favour of sclerotherapy, at the apex of such haemorrhoid

- If one is to catch closer to dentate line due to position of haemorrhoids, always test for pain before releasing band, if it is painful, abandon the procedure better use sclerotherapy at the apex of such haemorrhoid (Fig. 3.9).

3.6 Band Ligation with Suction Type Ligator (Video 3.1)

- Another way to use band ligator is with suction (Figs. 3.10 and 3.11).
- Adjust anoscope to see the target area as described earlier.
- With suction-type banding apparatus, operator can band with scope in non-dominant hand, and suction tip with barrel controlled with another hand (Fig. 3.12; Video 3.1).

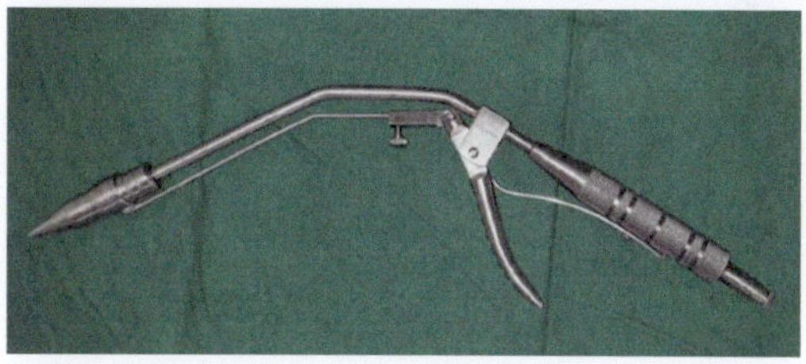

Fig. 3.10 Band ligator with suction

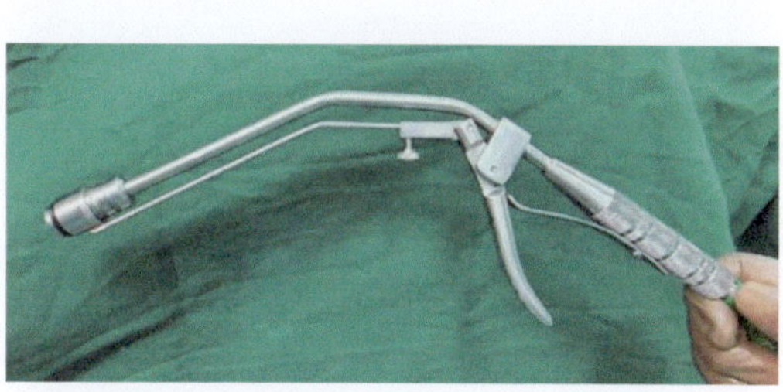

Fig. 3.11 Suction band ligator with rubber band loaded on the barrel

- Suction sucks the target tissue and pressing the clutch on handle releases band over the tissue (Fig. 3.13).
- Only limitation is that the amount of target-tissue which comes in barrel is less than the tissue ligated in manual type band ligator.
- One may inject some normal saline into the banded tissue to increase its volume to prevent slipping of the band (Fig. 3.14).
- We usually band two haemorrhoids in one go (Fig. 3.15). Though it is safe to band more columns, it increases discomfort [5].
- In manual ligator, one is to load bands one by one while preloaded ligator come with multiple bands.
- Local anaesthetic injection if required, is to be given deep to the banded tissue until a bleb large enough to encompass the base of the haemorrhoid is raised, instead giving injection into the devitalised banded tissue [6].
- Bands should be new as old bands may break or loose grip.
- One can make one's own rubber bands by transversally cutting the 12 French Foley's catheter of good quality.
- Do check proctoscopy for any bleeding and slipping of rubber band (Fig. 3.16).

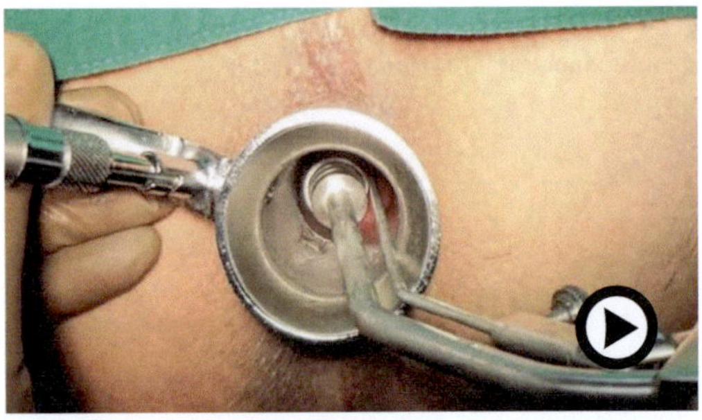

Fig. 3.12 Rubber band ligation by suction band ligator. Anoscope in left hand and ring can be applied with right (single) hand with suction ligator (▶ https://doi.org/10.1007/000-hpq)

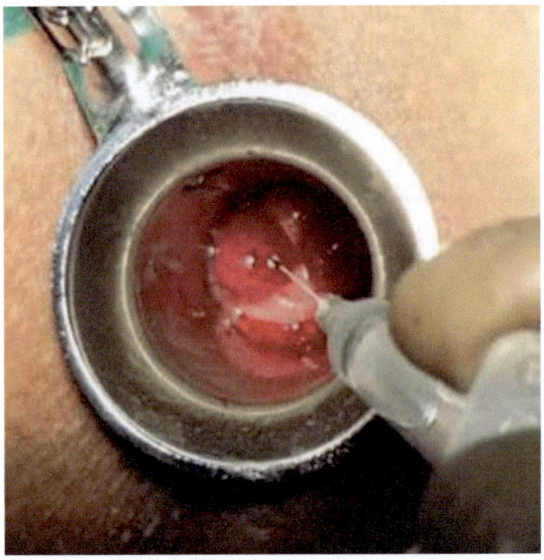

Fig. 3.14 Normal saline being injected into banded tissue to increase its volume to prevent slipping of band

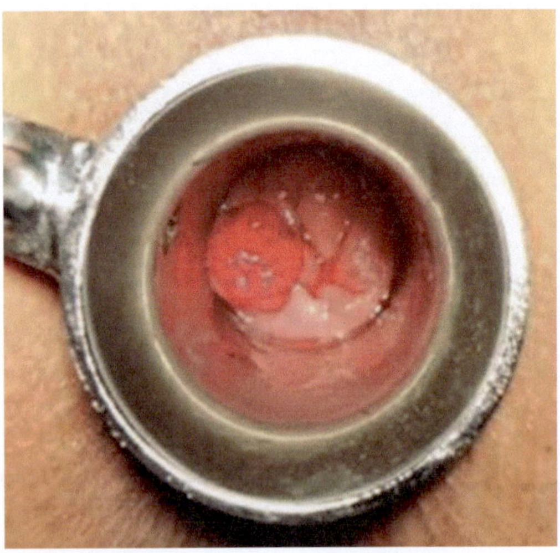

Fig. 3.13 Band ligation of one haemorrhoid well above the dentate line

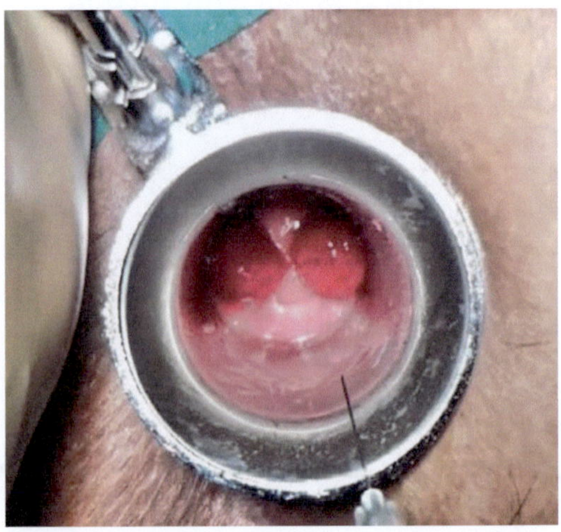

Fig. 3.15 Proctoscopic view of two of the haemorrhoids banded in one go

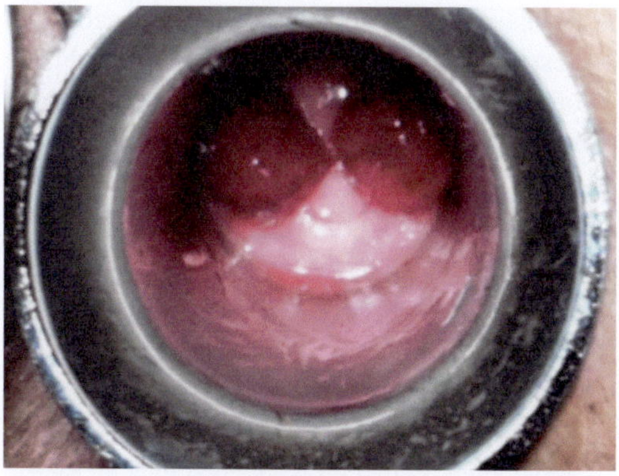

Fig. 3.16 Check proctoscopy after band ligation to detect any bleeding or slipping of bands

3.7 Complication of Banding of Haemorrhoid (Table 3.1)

Table 3.1 Complications of banding of haemorrhoids

Complications	Prevention	Management
Pain	Catch the tissue 1.5–2 cm above the dentate line, if still painful, hold more proximal (Figs. 3.17 and 3.18)	Put bupivacaine sol. in the base of banded tissue to raise a bleb. If still painful cut the band
Bleeding during application	Be gentle with tissue bleeding is less with suction-type ligator	Press with cotton swab or wet gauge
Bleeding after 7–10 days	Cannot prevent but caution the patient. Do not offer band-ligation to patient on anticoagulants	Usually minimal stops itself If excessive-proximal ligature and transfusion as per the need
Perianal sepsis: More common in immunocompromised, severe diabetes or neutropenia	Anorectal washouts before application of bands is suggested, but no support from the literature	Call the patient back if there is triad of pain, fever and urinary retention. Antibiotics and remove the slough/band
Vasovagal reactions	Hold the tissue 1.5–2 cm above the dentate line. If still painful, go more proximal	Ask the patient to lie down when feels giddiness and resuscitate accordingly
Chronic longitudinal anal ulcers	Do not apply band if tissue is not lax enough to come in to the barrel	Give them time to heal
Slippage of bands	Take hold of sufficient tissue and one may inject saline to increase the volume of banded tissue	Reapply the band

3.8 Post-procedure Advice to the Patient

- Laxatives for a week and not to strain while defecation.
- Diet and defecatory advise as for any patient of haemorrhoids.
- In case of pain, fever and urinary retention, call the patient back to hospital urgently and look for any sepsis.
- Caution against bleeding per rectum on seventh or eighth day when mucosa sloughs off. It is usually self-limiting. If more than half a cup of bleed, ask patient to report to the hospital immediately.

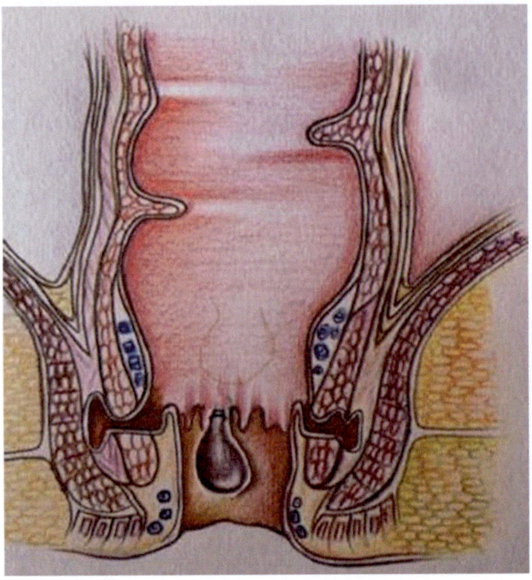

Fig. 3.17 Never apply band so low

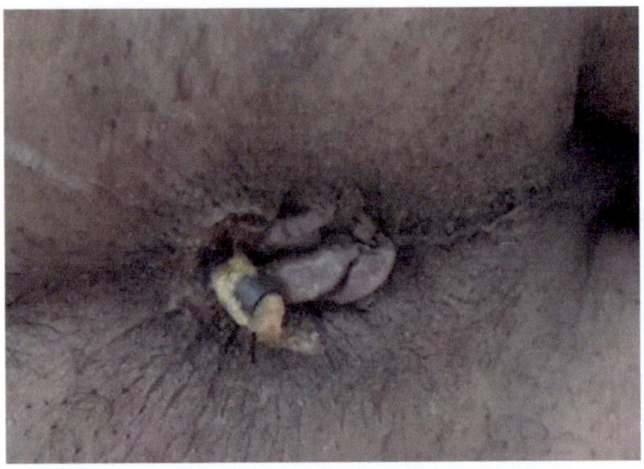

Fig. 3.18 Patient in left lateral position. Very low applied band causing necrosis of pain sensitive area

3.9 Tips and Tricks

- Patients on anticoagulants should not be offered rubber-band ligation, instead sclerotherapy is a better option.
- Never band in case of impacted stools. Ask patient to evacuate after enema.
- Catch hold mucosa and submucosa at least 1.5–2 cm above the dentate line, if painful, leave it and catch further 0.5 cm proximally.
- Assistants may not hold the anoscope in desired position as they cannot see the inside of scope and anoscope slides out. One may learn the technique of holding anoscope in left hand, and performing traction on haemorrhoid and releasing band with (single) right hand as described by Anderson [7].
- Banding with suction device can be done easily by the surgeon without depending on an assistant to hold the anoscope.
- Local anaesthetic injection, if required, to be given deep to the banded tissue, instead giving injection into the devitalised banded tissue.
- Post-procedure, be aware of triad of pain, fever and urinary retention. Call the patient back, no telephonic consultation.

Algorithm for Band Ligation of Haemorrhoids

Clinical history of bleeding and grade 2 or 3 protrusion

DRE and proctoscopy

Prepare the Barron band ligator or suction ligator

Mount rubber band over the barrel of the ligator

Steps for Barren band ligation

Patient in left lateral or lithotomy position

Lubricate anal canal with 2% lignocaine jelly

Put a lighted anoscope in the anal canal and remove the obturator

While withdrawing anoscope, judge the haemorrhoids and target site which should be 1.5–2 cm proximal to dentate line

Assistant holds the anoscope at desired location

Pass the forceps through the barrel and catch hold mucosa and submucosa of the targeted area

Slightly pull the tissue and push the drum of barrel towards mucosa

(continued)

Check that procedure should be pain-free

Close the handle of the ligator as a clutch to download band on to the base of targeted tissue in forceps

Repeat the procedure for another haemorrhoid

Check for any bleeding

Steps for suction type ligator

Anoscope is held in left hand and targeted tissue is selected 1.5 cm to 2 cm proximal to dentate line

With second (right) hand, take suction tip and barrel of the suction ligator on to the mucosa

Apply suction

Check for any pain

Close the clutch handle of suction ligator to put the band at the base of sucked-in tissue

Repeat the procedure for second column of haemorrhoid

One can inject 1 cc normal saline in banded tissue to increase its volume to avoid slipping of band

Check for any bleeding

References

1. Nelson RS, Thomson AG. Risk of bleeding following hemorrhoids banding in patients on antithrombotic therapy. Gastroenterol Clin Biol. 2009;33:463–5.
2. Lohsiriwat V. Treatment of hemorrhoids: a coloproctologist's view. World J Gastroenterol. 2015;21(31):9245–52. https://doi.org/10.3748/wjg.v21.i31.9245, https://www.wjgnet.com/1007-9327/full/v21/i31/9245.htm.
3. Adami B, Eckardt VF, Suermann RB, et al. Bacteremia after proctoscopy and hemorrhoidal injection sclerotherapy. Dis Colon Rectum. 1981;24:373–4. https://doi.org/10.1007/BF0260342238.
4. Tejirian T, Abbas MA. Bacterial endocarditis following rubber band ligation in a patient with a ventricular septal defect: report of a case and guideline analysis. Dis Colon Rectum. 2006;49:1931–3. [PubMed] [Google Scholar].
5. Kubchandani IT. A randomized comparison of single and multiple rubber band ligations. Dis Colon Rectum. 1983;26:705–8. [PubMed].
6. Sajid MS, Bhatti MI, Caswell J, Sains P, Baig MK. Local anaesthetic infiltration for the rubber band ligation of early symptomatic haemorrhoids: a systematic review and meta-analysis. Updat Surg. 2015;67:3–9. [PubMed] [Google Scholar].
7. Anderson AF. A technique for rubber band ligation of internal haemorrhoids. Ann R Coll Surg Engl. 1984;66(5):336. PMID: 6486669; PMCID: PMC2493667.

Suggested Reading

Albuquerque A. Rubber band ligation of hemorrhoids: a guide for complications. World J Gastrointest Surg. 2016;8(9):614–20. Published online 2016 Sept 27. https://doi.org/10.4240/wjgs.v8.i9.614.

4 Haemorrhoids: Non-excisional Procedures Doppler-Guided Haemorrhoidal Artery Ligation/Trans-Anal Haemorrhoidal Dearterilisation (DGHAL/THD) Recto-anal Repair/Mucopexy (RAR/Mucopexy)

Abstract

- Doppler-guided haemorrhoidal artery ligation (DGHAL)/trans-anal haemorrhoidal dearterialisation (THD) is a non-excisional but effective treatment for haemorrhoids.
- As we believe in the vascular theory of haemorrhoids by Aigner, the ligation of haemorrhoidal arteries (called dearterialisation) provide a significant reduction of the arterial overflow to the haemorrhoids.
- Where and how to detect and ligate these vessels, with different types of Doppler-probes, have been well explained with sketches, clinical photographs and videos.
- As arterial ligation suffices for only bleeding haemorrhoids but cases with protrusion of haemorrhoids need either mucopexy or haemorrhoidopexy aka recto anal repair (RAR).
- Mucopexy-plication of the redundant rectal mucosa and submucosa sparing haemorrhoids elevates prolapsing tissue to the anatomical site.
- Surgical technique, peri-operative and post-operative patient management is well explained.
- The details of the surgical procedure are complemented by an operative video and further elucidated by an animated and operative video in "Suggested Viewing" section.
- Complications, though few, have been presented in tabulated form for easy access and reference.
- Words of wisdom by present authors and previous authors have been collected in Sect. 4.6.
- Readers interested in further details are referred to "References" and "Suggested Readings" sections.

Supplementary Information The online version contains supplementary material available at https://doi.org/10.1007/978-981-96-6190-9_4. The videos can be accessed individually by clicking the DOI link in the accompanying figure caption or by scanning this link with the SN More Media App.

4.1 What One Should Know Before the Procedure

Following are the major theories of haemorrhoid development [1].

1. Vascular theory by Aigner [2].
    - Increased diameter of vessels supplying the submucosal cushions.
    - Increased blood supply.
    - Neo vascularisation.
2. Anal cushion-sliding theory by Thomson [3].
3. Rectal-redundancy by Longo [4].
4. Increased pressure on venous outflow from submucosal cushions.

S. K. Singla, K. Mital, *Operative Manual of Minimally Invasive and LASER Ano-proctology*,
https://doi.org/10.1007/978-981-96-6190-9_4

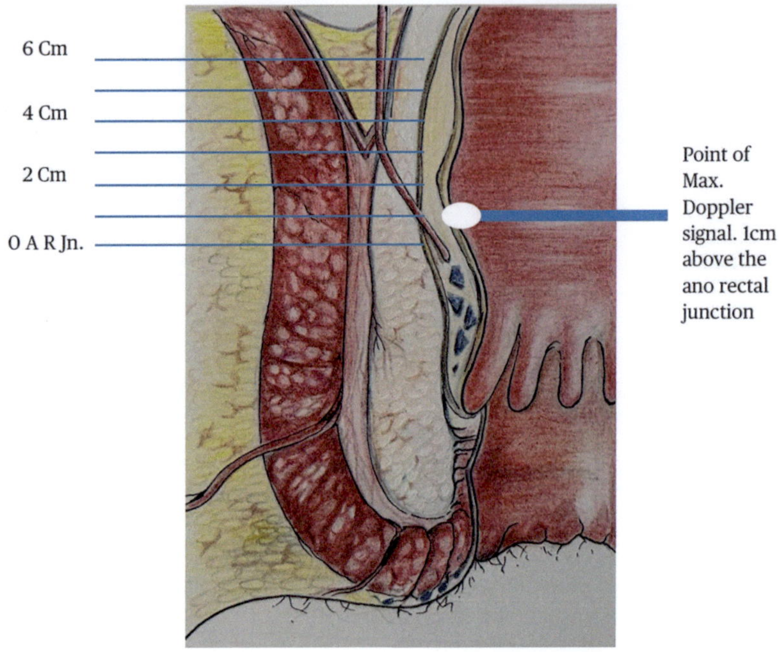

Fig. 4.1 Doppler signal 1 cm above the puborectalis is maximum as blood vessel is only 2 mm deep in submucosa at this place and vessel flow is perpendicular to Doppler signal [6]. This point corresponds to the site of vessel ligation. AR Jn. Anorectal junction on USG top of the puborectalis sling

- A number of inflammatory mediators have also been reported as cause of haemorrhoid disease.
- Haemorrhoids are high flow arterio venous (AV) formation, located just above the dentate line. Principle of Doppler-guided haemorrhoidal artery ligation is
  - To detect flow with Doppler hand held device.
  - To reduce their blood flow by ligating branches of superior rectal artery feeding this AV formation, which is akin to erectile tissue aka corpora cavernosa recti.
- K. Morinaga from Japan ligated haemorrhoidal arteries using a Doppler-device called Moricorn in 1995 [5].
- After this there are evolutions in the instrument.
- Best place to trans-anal ligation of these vessels is 1 cm above the anorectal junction identified by U sling of puborectalis [6].
- If one goes by the laws of physics.
- The Doppler signal's strength is inversely proportional to the cosine of angle between blood flow and the ultrasound waves. Therefore, the greater the angle of the blood-flow in relation to the ultrasound waves (artery towards the peri-rectal tissue or submucosa) (Fig. 4.1), the stronger the Doppler signal will be. Conversely, as the flow alignment with the ultrasound waves increases within the artery passing through the rectal muscle (see Fig. 4.1), the signal strength decreases.
- If patient has only complaint of bleeding then haemorrhoidal artery ligation is sufficient.

4.2 Why and Where One Needs Mucopexy or Recto-anal Repair

- Normally, the submucosal cushions (haemorrhoidal tissue) are loosely attached to circular muscle fibres and internal anal sphincter through the connective tissue stroma of elastic rectal submucosa (Park's ligament) with the help of anchoring fibres from conjoint longitudinal muscle (Treitz's muscle).
- This fixation keeps the sub-mucosal cushions in the anal canal in resting condition.

- During defecation, internal anal sphincter relaxes and sub-mucosal cushions and external vascular plexus pouts as rolling lips.
- It favours venous outflow from the cushions and defecation.
- Once the defecations is over, due to elasticity of rectal mucosa and submucosa, everything goes back inside.
- In individuals with haemorrhoidal disease, submucosal cushions protrude out as a result of altered defecation and weakening of both Park's ligaments and Treitz's muscle.
- Severity of prolapse increases with persistence of straining at defecation leading to engorgement of haemorrhoids and progressive loss of the elasticity of Park's ligament with degeneration of Treitz's muscle.
- Plication of the rectal mucosa and submucosa during mucopexy restores back the prolapsing tissue to its anatomical position.
- Furthermore, inflammation caused by stitches of mucopexy, fixes the plicated mucosa and submucosa to the underlying rectal muscle due to scarring it induces.
- Patient with significant haemorrhoidal prolapse can be subjected to recto-anal repair (RAR) where prolapsing haemorrhoid is hitched up by running suture (Fig. 4.7).
- Vertical mucopexy is done superior to haemorrhoid tissue, thus sparing haemorrhoids altogether [7] (Fig. 4.2).
- When there is circumferential haemorrhoidal prolapse, six column mucopexy at 1, 3, 5, 7, 9 and 11 o' position can be done.
- Patients with bleeding in the earlier phase of the disease, may complain of mucosal and haemorrhoidal prolapse without bleeding in the later phase of haemorrhoidal disease. Such patients should undergo both haemorrhoidal artery ligations (DGHAL)/dearterilisation (THD) and mucopexy.
- Mucopexy can be customised as per length of prolapse - for longer mucosal prolapse making longer running sutures, i.e., up to 5–6 bites at 5 mm apart, otherwise 3–4 bites are sufficient.

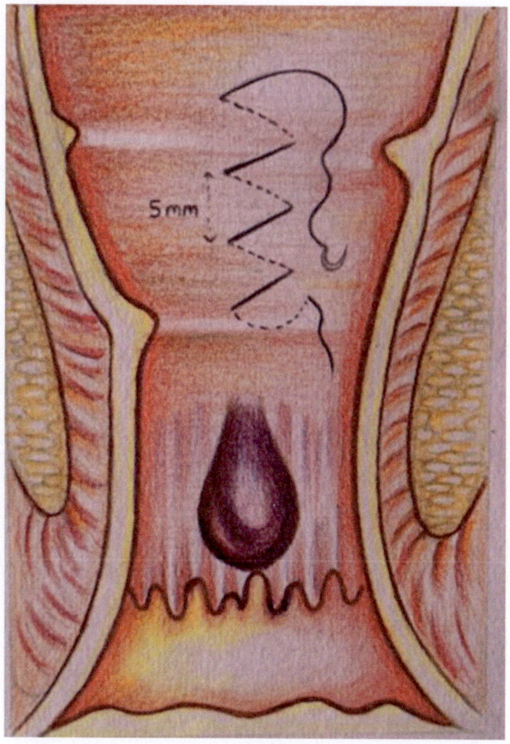

Fig. 4.2 Sketch to show the scheme of proximal bites to do mucopexy. Length of mucopexy can be modified as per prolapse. More prolapse-more bites proximally

4.3 Indications (Fig. 4.3)

- DGHAL or THD may be offered to patients afflicated with active haemorrhoid disease, when diet and defecatory interventions, medicinal therapy and office-procedures such as sclerotherapy and rubber band ligation did not work.
- Grade 3 haemorrhoids—DGHAL with RAR or THD with mucopexy.
- Grade 4 haemorrhoids—DGHAL with RAR or mucopexy and is combined with distal excision of sodden or fibrosed skin.

Recommended treatment of Haemorrhoids Based on severity

Grade 1	Grade 2	Grade 3	Grade 4	Complicated
Dietary,defecatory and lifestyle modification	Dietary,defecatory and lifestyle modification	Dietary,defecatory and lifestyle modification	Dietary,defecatory and lifestyle modification	Dietary,defecatory and lifestyle modification
Medication	Medication			Medication
Office-based procedure (such as sclerotherapy and IRC)	Office-based procedure (such as sclerotherapy, banding and IRC)	Office-based procedure (such as sclerotherapy, banding and IRC)		Multiple thrombectomies and banding
	Failed office procedures Non-excisional operations DGHAL,THD,LASER, MIPH &Chivate's	Non-excisional operation such as DGHAL,mucopexy FGHAL,LASER,MIPH and Chivate's procedures	Non-excisional operation DGHAL,FGHAL,LASER,MIPH and Chivate's With distal excision of fibrosed sodden skin	
		Failed non excisional procedures Excisional operation Hybrid procedures	Excisional operation Hybrid procedures	Excisional operation Hybrid procedures

Fig. 4.3 Various options for treatment of haemorrhoids based on grading of protrusion and severity

4.4 Contra-indications

- Already thrombosed or strangulated haemorrhoids.
- Internal rectal intussusception should not be confused with haemorrhoid prolapse as the former cannot be managed with this technique.
- Active infection in the area or lower gastrointestine (GI).

4.5 Pre-operative Workup

- Preparation as for any case under anaesthesia.
- For high-risk cardiac patients, stop anticoagulants week before or shift on heparin as suggested by cardiologist and then stop heparin a day before.
- Enema 2 h before the procedure and advise patient to pass stools.

4.6 Equipment

- Operation table with stirrups for lithotomy.
- For prone position, rolled-sheets and cushions with tapes for strapping.
- Sterile drapes and gowns.
- Povidine iodine solution.
- Xylocaine jelly, surgical gloves, saline-soaked gauge pieces.
- General equipment trolley, including long needle-holder 10″, long plain forceps, 2.0 polyglactin 910 suture (vicryl) 120 cm length on 27 mm 5/8 circle round body needle (Fig. 4.4).
- Proctoscope equipped with Doppler (Trilogy unit AMI) (Fig. 4.5).
- Product brochure can be viewed at https://www.ami.at/wp-content/uploads/TRILOGY-Product-Brochure-English-2017.pdf.

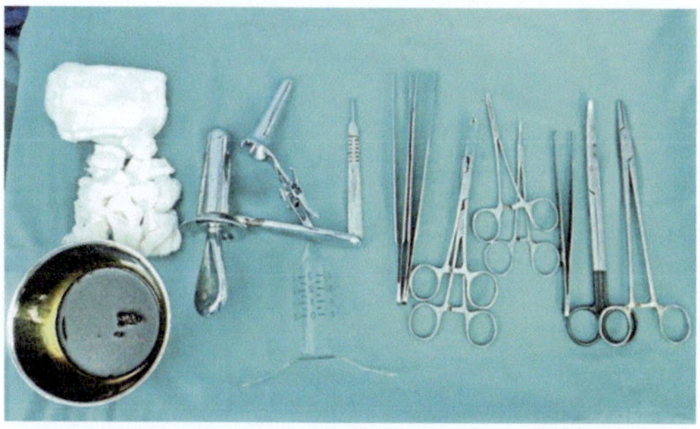

Fig. 4.4 Trolley of general equipment for DGHAL/THD

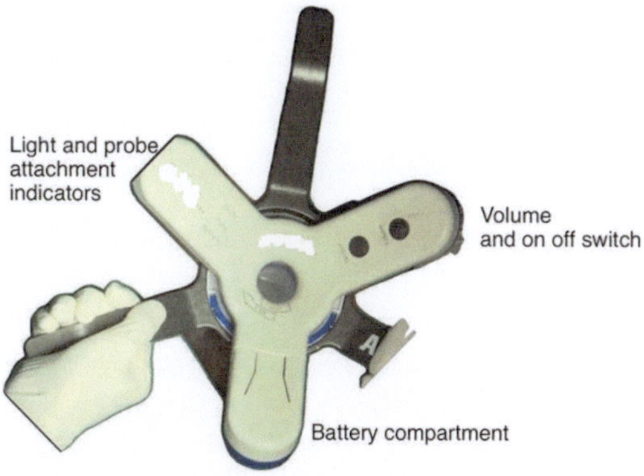

Fig. 4.5 Trilogy unit with bluetooth-enabled speakers. No wires

4.7 Procedure (Doppler-Guided Haemorrhoidal Artery Ligation/DGHAL with Trilogy Unit)

- Patient is put in lithotomy position under low spinal anaesthesia.
- Systolic blood pressure should be above 100–110 mm of Hg for better acoustic signals of Doppler.
- Introduce blue tooth enabled probe (Trilogy unit) into the rectum after adequate lubrication.
- Probe is rotated and moved slowly to search for arteries. One can start from any point.
- Search for the best Doppler signal, which corresponds to the centre of the artery.
- Signals in the distal rectum (just above the haemorrhoid cushions) are relevant for us [7, 8].
- Once the first artery is found, it is ligated through the window given for the purpose in the probe, using 2.0 polyglactin suture on 5/8 circle, 27 mm round body needle (Fig. 4.6).
- The unit is then turned again either clock-wise or anti-clock wise to find more feeding vessels.

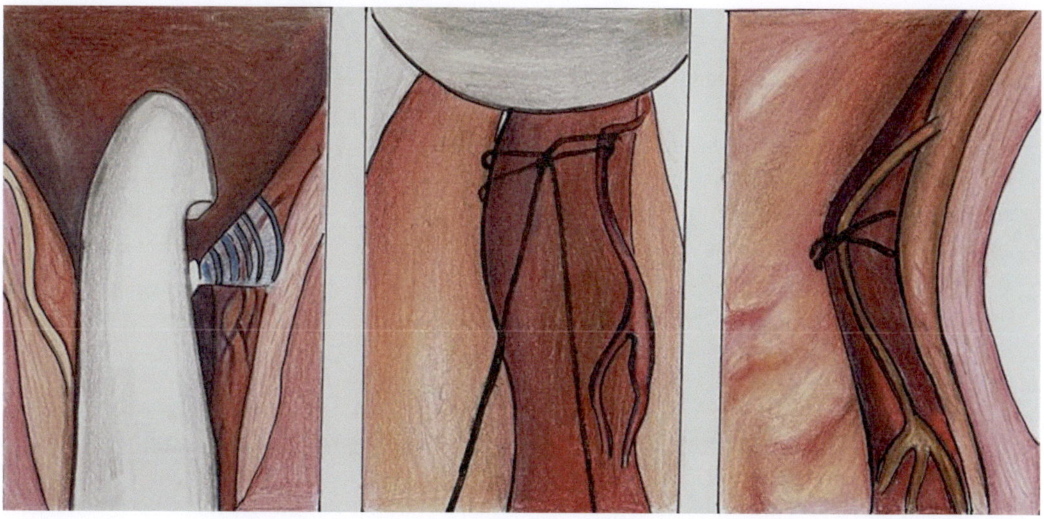

Fig. 4.6 Once the artery is found by Doppler signal it is ligated with suture through the window given for the purpose

- Each artery is ligated as found by the Doppler probe. Five to eight arteries need to be ligated during the whole procedure, usually search for arteries at all odd numbers 1, 3, 5, 7, 9, 11 o'clock positions.
- However, these numbers and position may vary from patient to patient, depending on the respective anatomy. Extent of engorgement of the haemorrhoids also effect the detection of vessels by Doppler.
- DGHAL is sufficient to control bleeding component.

4.8 Recto-Anal Repair (RAR)

- The RAR technique is utilised for managing prolapsing haemorrhoids in the later stages of the disease. RAR includes plication of columns of prolapsed haemorrhoids, performed following the tying off the haemorrhoidal arteries.
- The TRILOGY unit, along with the probe attached, is positioned as it would be for ligation.
- Initially, a stitch is made as close to the top of the prolapsing haemorrhoid as possible (Fig. 4.7).
- The unit and probe are then rotated slightly to expose more mucosa at the end.
- A running suture is initiated and then progressed by slowly turning the device, maintaining a distance of 5–7 mm between each stitch.
- Following the final stitch, the suture material is tied close to the initial stitch, terminating near the dentate line. This action brings the prolapsing tissue up to the original stitch and is then fixed in place with a surgical knot (Fig. 4.8).
- The procedure known as recto-anal repair (RAR) actually consists of performing a haemorrhoidopexy. This method results in increased feeling of tenesmus and a temporary strong urge to have a bowel movement.

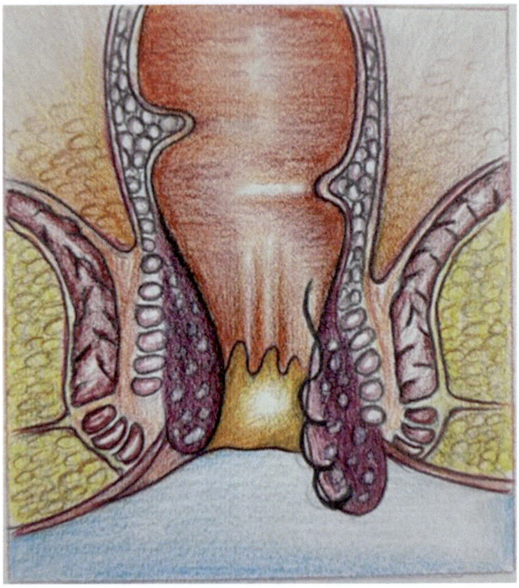

Fig. 4.7 RAR-mucopexy of columns of prolapsing haemorrhoids

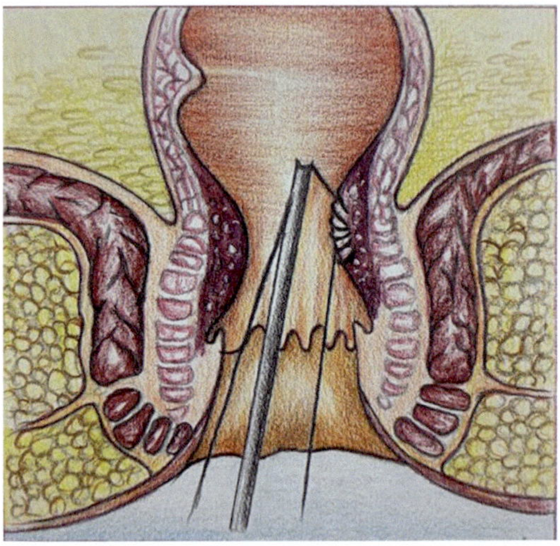

Fig. 4.8 RAR-pulling of prolapsing haemorrhoid in its original position

4.9 Complications (Table 4.1)

Haemorrhoidal de arterialisation THD/DGHAL with other machines by Medtech, THD.

Table 4.1 Complications of DGHAL and RAR

Complications	Prevention	Management
Tenesmus, discomfort or pain in anorectum	Do mucopexy for minimum required columns	Analgesics and NSAIDs
Rectal bleeding post-procedure	Avoid tight suturing during mucopexy, can lead to necrosis of tissue and bleeding	Usually self-limiting
		If excessive, wash the clots and inspect
	Patient is to avoid straining while defecation, both constipation and diarrhoea can break sutures	May need proximal suturing or simple cautery
Re-occurrence	Meticulous operative technique	Bleeding can be managed with sclero or repeated HAL
	Post-operative care to avoid straining	Prolapse by limited excision of mucosa

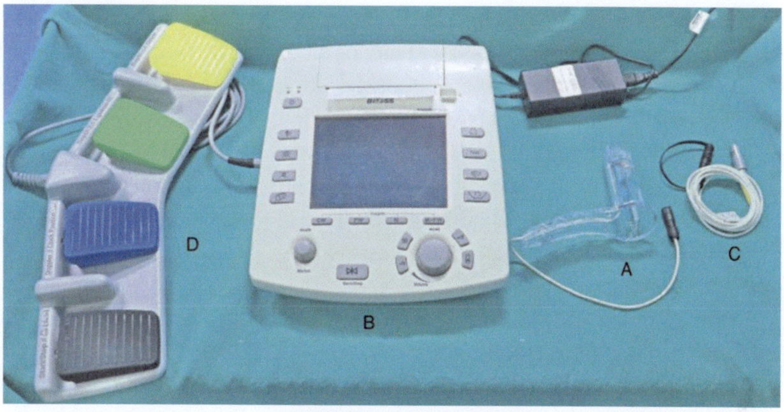

Fig. 4.9 Equipment for DGHAL/THD by Meditech. (A) Self-lighted proctoscope probe with Doppler sensor, reusable and unlimited use. (B) Display board and control panel. (C) Connecting wires for Doppler. (D) Foot control paddles

4.10 Equipment (Fig. 4.9)

- General equipment is same.
- Only Doppler-probe and scope are different and this machine comes with reusable probe with unlimited usage. There is no counter fitted by the company.
- Open slot for suturing is large enough.

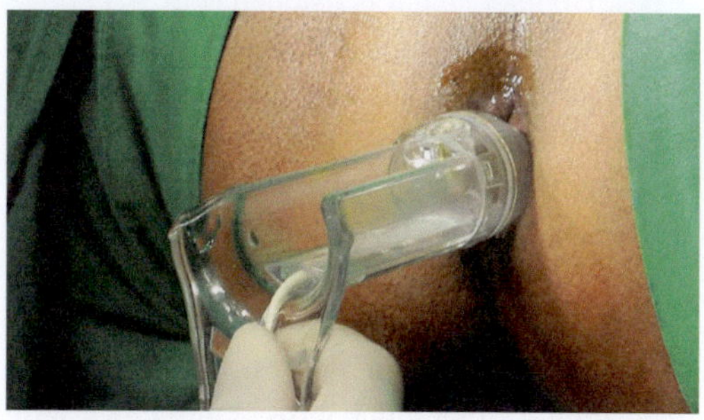

Fig. 4.10 Hand held Doppler probe inside the self-lighted proctoscope

4.11 Procedure (Video 4.1)

Anaesthesia

Low spinal anaesthesia.

Position

Lithotomy.

- Systolic blood pressure should be above 100–110 mm of Hg for better acoustic signals of Doppler.
- Prolapsing piles are assessed and should be reducible.
- Do Digital rectal examination (DRE) and routine anoscopy.
- After adequate lubrication by xylocain jelly, the self-lighted proctoscope fitted with Doppler is negotiated in the anal canal till flange touches the buttocks (Figs. 4.10 and 4.11).

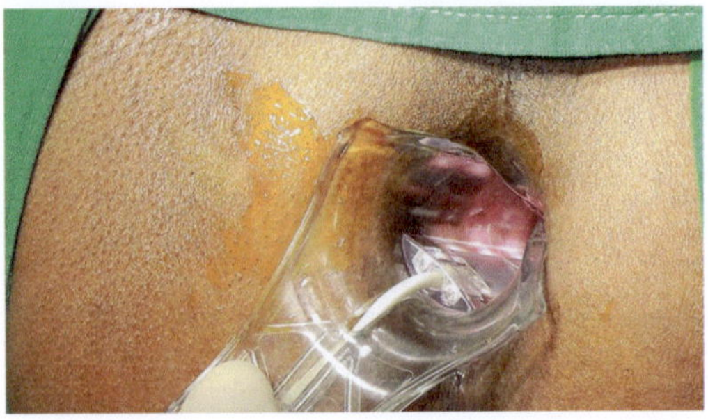

Fig. 4.11 Lubricated probe is inserted and then rotated and withdrawn to find the best acoustic signal of artery supplying the submucosal cushion

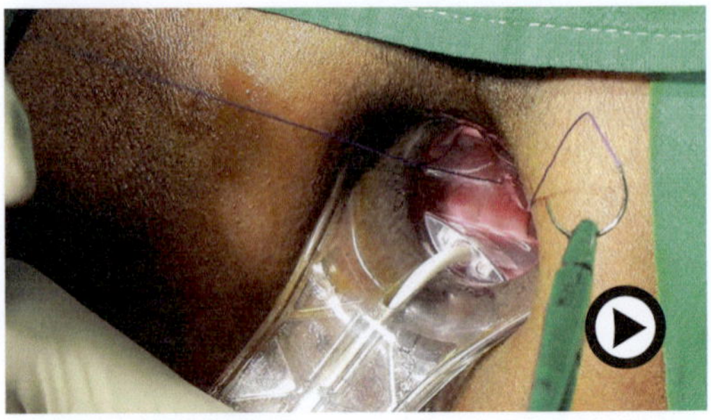

Fig. 4.12 Best audible signal is marked and then vessel at that site is ligated with vicryl 2.0 on 27 mm 5/8 round body needle through a window slot in the proctoscope. Similarly, all detected vessels are ligated, usually 5–8 ligations suffice (▶ https://doi.org/10.1007/000-hpr)

- Turn the Doppler system on.
- Start ligation of audible vessels at any point of the rectal circumference and proceed in a clock-wise or anti-clockwise direction.
- The acoustic signals are checked by slowly rotating and/or tilting the proctoscope around the lower ano-rectum. All odd numbers 1, 3, 5, 7, 9, and 11 o'clock usually have vessels supplying submucosal cushions.
- Doppler probe may detect vessels at places other than odd hour locations.
- The proctoscope is withdrawn distally to the top of haemorrhoid to follow the artery till the best Doppler signal is listened (Fig. 4.11).
- Signals in the distal rectum (just above the haemorrhoid cushions) are relevant for us [7, 8].
- Once the first artery is found, it is ligated through the window given for the purpose in the probe, using 2.0 polyglactin suture on 5/8 circle, 27 mm round body needle (Fig. 4.12; Video 4.1).
- The unit is then taken out, reinserted in next position—either clock wise or anti clock wise to previous position, to further locate other arteries.
- Each artery is ligated at best audible signal site.
- Five to eight arteries need to be ligated during the whole procedure, usually search for arteries at all odd numbers 1, 3, 5, 7, 9, 11 o'clock positions.
- However, these numbers and position may vary from patient to patient, depending on the respective anatomy. Extent of engorgement of the haemorrhoids also effect the detection of vessels by Doppler.
- DGHAL/THD is sufficient to control bleeding component.
- Other instrument by THD S.p.A., Correggio, Italy. company is also used [7].

The most recent proctoscope version (THD Slide®, THD S.p.A., Correggio, Italy) contains a sliding section with the operating window and Doppler-probe, allowing the operator to adjust their position along the device without needing to reposition the proctoscope.

4.12 Proximal Mucopexy of Prolapsing Mucosa Instead of RAR

- In the modified technique, after DGHAL or so-called THD trans-anal haemorrhoidal dearterilisation, mucopexy of redundant rectal mucosa and submucosa is done proximal to haemorrhoid cushion, which lifts the cushion up at its original position (Fig. 4.2).
- The inclusion of mucopexy in THD or DGHAL procedures may decrease the chances of missing arteries that are otherwise undetectable by this method, as the running suture extends up to the top of the haemorrhoids and covers all vessels [8, 9].

- One can run suture from proximal to distal for mucopexy, artery is ligated in most distal suture.
  - After marking the selected site for vessel ligation with stroke of cautery.
  - Take proctoscope window more proximal.
  - Take suture at proximal prolapsing mucosa and submucosa.
  - Start running suture with 5 mm apart bites, picking mucosa and submucosa and proceed proximal to distal.
  - Lower most bites take vessel in the bite by taking one bite proximal and one bite distal to mark made by cautery.
  - Tie both ends and tighten sutures slowly and firmly to hitch up the prolapsing tissue to elevate the haemorrhoid cushion up in the anal canal [7].
- One can ligate the vessel first, then take running suture from distal to proximal for mucopexy (Fig. 4.2).
- It is a total haemorrhoid-sparing technique and is supposed to decrease tenesmus and post-procedure bleeding due to necrosis of tissue involved in mucopexy.

4.13 Post-procedure Advice to the Patient

- Diet and defecatory advice as for any patient of haemorrhoids like diet rich in fibre and fluids.
- Stool softeners in the form of mild laxatives for 3 months.
- Avoid prolonged straining while defecation.
- Patient can feel some tenesmus and discomfort which can be more in case of mucopexy.
- Mild pain and discomfort can be controlled with oral analgesics.
- Patient should be cautioned of small amount of mucous and reddish mucinous discharge from anus due to inflammatory reaction of sutures.
- Patients suffering from chronic diarrhoea or irritable bowel syndrome should be placed on a pre-operative controlled diet along with probiotics [10].
- Patients with chronic inflammatory bowel disease must continue their medicines.
- Usually patient is called for inspection after 7 days of the procedure, DRE examination is done at the end of 1 month and proctoscopy follows after 3 months.

4.14 Tips and Tricks

- Systolic blood pressure of the patient should be above 100–110 mm of Hg for better acoustic signals of Doppler.
- According to a key research done by Ratto et al. [6], the Doppler signal is easily detected at 4–6 cm proximal to the anorectal junction, not present at the middle site, and once again noticeable at the site close to the Ano rectal junction (ARJ) (just 1 cm; proximal to ARJ).
- At this distal site, within last 2 cm of lower rectum vessel is only 2 mm deep to mucosa and is best suited for vessel ligation.
- After ligation at maximal Doppler signal in distal rectum just 1 cm above the anorectal junction, still one can hear the signals due to crumpling of mucosa and submucosa and certain vessels coming close to the probe due to stitching. Ignore these signals and better switch off the Doppler device once we select the best signal site in distal rectum.
- When mucopexy is included in haemorrhoidal artery ligation (THD or DG-HAL), the possibility of missed arteries may be lower as the running suture is usually continued by transfixing the mucosa and submucosa at the level of anorectal junction, thus picking the arterial branches feeding the haemorrhoids [6].
- While doing mucopexy, distance between each stitch should be 5–7 mm. Less distance will increase the chances of mucosal necrosis and increased distance will make large folds prone to suture-break on straining.

Algorithm for Doppler Guided Haemorrhoidal Artery Ligation (DGHAL) or Trans Anal Haemorrhoidal Dearterilisation (THD) for Treatment of Haemorrhoids

Clinical assessment
Indications/contrindications
Preoperative preparation
Proctoclysis enema 2 hrs before
Lithotomy under spinal/GA
DRE and anoscopy
Doppler probe with self-lighted proctoscope inserted in anal canal
Doppler switched on
By rotation, tilt and distal slide of proctoscope, best acoustic signal site is selected and marked vessel in submucosa is ligated with 2.0 polyglactin suture on 27 mm 5/8 round body needle with rotation movement of wrist
All audible vessels on Doppler at best acoustic signal site which is usually within 2 cm of distal rectum are ligated

Algorithm for Recto Anal Repair (RAR)

Indication-prolapsing haemorrhoids
After DGHAL with same proctoscope, take bite proximal to apex of haemorrhoid with 2.0 polyglactin 27 mm 5/8 round body needle
Take a running suture going distally with bites 5 mm apart to include haemorrhoidal cushion
Stop just proximal to dentate line
Tie distal free end of suture with proximal end and tighten the suture slowly and firmly to hitch up the prolapsing tissue

Algorithm for Mucopexy

Indication-prolapse of haemorrhoids with DGHAL/THD
After marking the selected site for vessel ligation with stroke of cautery, take proctoscope window more proximal
Take suture at proximal prolapsing mucosa and submucosa
Take running suture with 5 mm apart bites picking mucosa and submucosa
Lower most bites take vessel in the bite by taking one bite proximal and one bite distal to mark made by cautery
Tie both ends and tighten sutures slowly and firmly to hitch up the prolapsing tissue to elevate the haemorrhoid cushion up in the anal canal
Or
After ligating the vessel, one can take running suture from distal to proximal
Length of running suture (bites taken to plicate the tissue) can be adapted as per length of prolapse
Tie the suture and tighten slowly and firmly to plicate the prolapsing mucosa and elevate the haemorrhoids at anatomical position

References

1. Lohsiriwat V. Hemorrhoids: from basic pathophysiology to clinical management. World J Gastroenterol. 2012;18(17):2009–17. https://doi.org/10.3748/wjg.v18.i17.2009. PMID: 22563187; PMCID: PMC3342598.
2. Aigner F, Bodner G, Gruber H, Conrad F, Fritsch H, Margreiter R, Bonatti H. The vascular nature of hemorrhoids. J Gastrointest Surg. 2006;10(7):1044–50. https://doi.org/10.1016/j.gassur.2005.12.004. PMID: 16843876.

3. Thomson WH. The nature of haemorrhoids. Br J Surg. 1975;62:542–52. [PubMed] [Google Scholar].
4. Longo A. Treatment of hemorrhoids disease by reduction of mucosa and haemorrhoidal prolapse with a circular suturing device: a new procedure. In: Proceedings of the 6th world congress of endoscopic surgery, Rome, Italy. 3–6 June 1998. [Google Scholar].
5. Morinaga K, Hasuda K, Ikeda T. A novel therapy for internal hemorrhoids: ligation of the hemorrhoidal artery with a newly devised instrument (Moricorn) in conjunction with a Doppler flowmeter. Am J Gastroenterol. 1995;90(4):610–3. [PubMed]
6. Ratto C, Parello A, Donisi L, Litta F, Zaccone G, Doglietto GB. Assessment of haemorrhoidal artery network using colour duplex imaging and clinical implications. Br J Surg. 2012;99:112–8.
7. Ratto C. THD Doppler procedure for hemorrhoids: the surgical technique. Tech Coloproctol. 2014;18:291–8. https://doi.org/10.1007/s10151-013-1062-3.
8. Ratto C, Donisi L, Parello A, Litta F, Doglietto GB. Evaluation of transanal hemorrhoidal dearterialization as a minimally invasive therapeutic approach to hemorrhoids. Dis Colon Rectum. 2010;53(5):803–11. https://doi.org/10.1007/DCR.0b013e3181cdafa7.
9. Aigner F, Bodner G, Conrad F, Mbaka G, Kreczy A, Fritsch H. The superior rectal artery and its branching pattern with regard to its clinical influence on ligation techniques for internal hemorrhoids. Am J Surg. 2004;187(1):102–8. https://doi.org/10.1016/j.amjsurg.2002.11.003. PMID: 14706597
10. Ratto C, Parello A, Litta F, De Simone V. Dearterialization of hemorrhoids and mucopexy: techniques and results. In: Ratto C, Parello A, Litta F, editors. Hemorrhoids. Coloproctology, Springer: Cham; 2018; vol 2. https://doi.org/10.1007/978-3-319-53357-5_34.

Suggest Readings

Miyamoto H. Minimally invasive treatment for advanced hemorrhoids. J Anus Rectum Colon. 2023;7(1):8–16. https://doi.org/10.23922/jarc.2022-068. PMID: 36743466; PMCID: PMC9876604.

Oglat AA, Matjafri MZ, Suardi N, Oqlat MA, Abdelrahman MA, Oqlat AA. A review of medical Doppler ultrasonography of blood flow in general and especially in common carotid artery. J Med Ultrasound. 2018;26(1):3–13. https://doi.org/10.4103/JMU.JMU_11_17. Epub 2018 Mar 28. PMID: 30065507; PMCID: PMC6029191

Walega P, Romaniszyn M, Kenig J, Herman R, Nowak W. Doppler-guided hemorrhoid artery ligation with Recto-Anal-Repair modification: functional evaluation and safety assessment of a new minimally invasive method of treatment of advanced hemorrhoidal disease. ScientificWorldJournal. 2012;2012:324040. https://doi.org/10.1100/2012/324040. Epub 2012 Apr 1. PMID: 22547979; PMCID: PMC3324335

Suggested Viewing

Animation Video 4.1 by manufacturer of the device, THD S.p.A., Correggio, Italy. https://youtu.be/ZNPMT8mFyhY.

Another Video 4.2 link of the procedure on the patient. https://onlinelibrary.wiley.com/action/downloadSupplement?doi=10.1111%2Fcodi.16134&file=codi16134-sup-0001-VideoS1.mp4.

5 Haemorrhoids: Non-excisional Procedures Finger-Guided Haemorrhoidal Artery Ligation, Mucopexy and LASER Haemorrhoidoplasty (FGHAL, Mucopexy and LHP)

Abstract

- Surgery to treat haemorrhoids without excising them saves anatomically and physiologically important anal transition zone mucosa and submucosal cushions. No anoderm is damaged there by decreasing possibility of any anal stenosis to zero.
- Almost all excisional procedures lead to excessive pain.
- Indications and contraindications for the procedure are outlined in detail with clinical photographs.
- Different steps of the procedure.
  - Haemorrhoidal artery ligation after palpating the vessel pulse with finger instead of Doppler is fully explained with clinical photographs and videos and substantiated with literature evidence.
  - Mucopexy of redundant mucosa and submucosa distal to proximal, with same suture is well demonstrated.
  - Principal of LASER energy given to shrink and fix this AV malformation (diseased sub-mucosal cushions—aka haemorrhoids) is elaborated.
  - Arteries which escape usual pattern of distribution and ligation, may be taken care by direct LASER into the submucosal cushions.
  - Stress on right LASER, right fibre, right dose and right route of entry into submucosal cushion has been given to make the procedure safe and effective.
- Procedure details are supplemented with two videos by two different operators.
- LASER dosage is presented in a table for ready reference.
- Complications, their prevention and management is summarised in tabulated form for easy access.
- Pre-, peri- and post-operative aspects of the procedure have been explained well.
- Section 5.13 may help to improve efficacy and results.
- Seekers of further knowledge can find some useful reading material in "References" and "Suggested Readings" sections.
- Overall results of hybrid procedure of FGHAL, mucopexy, LHP and excision of sodden, fibrosed skin component are quite comparable to formal ligation and excision with added advantage of almost no pain, no requirement of dressings, fast recovery with early resumption for day-to-day activities.
- Who knows it becomes a GOLD standard one day?

Supplementary Information The online version contains supplementary material available at https://doi.org/10.1007/978-981-96-6190-9_5. The videos can be accessed individually by clicking the DOI link in the accompanying figure caption or by scanning this link with the SN More Media App.

S. K. Singla, K. Mital, *Operative Manual of Minimally Invasive and LASER Ano-proctology*,
https://doi.org/10.1007/978-981-96-6190-9_5

- Algorithm of operative steps, printed at the end of the chapter, is a ready reference on way to operation room (OR).

5.1 Why Non-excisional Procedures for Haemorrhoids

- Submucosal cushions contribute 15% towards continence of stools, so we want to save them.
- Mucosa of anal transition zone covers submucosal cushions, which is physiologically very important as area has specific receptors which sense quality of stools during faecal sampling there by contributes to maintain continence.
- Since the advent of Milligan Morgan procedure (1937), we have not been able to decrease the associated post-operative pain.
- Long healing-time and dressings required after the excisional procedures are cumbersome.
- Results of non-excisional procedures are quite satisfactory in terms of very less pain, almost no bleeding and early return to work though slightly less control over protrusion act excision in long term [1].

5.2 What One Should Know Before the Procedure

- During defecation, internal anal sphincter relaxes and sub-mucosal cushions and external vascular plexus pouts as rolling lips.
- It favours venous outflow from the cushions and defecation.
- Once the defecations is over, due to elasticity of rectal mucosa and submucosa, everything goes back inside.
- In patients with haemorrhoidal disease, due to altered defecation and progressive disruption of both the connective tissue stroma (Park's ligaments) and anchoring system (Treitz's muscle), submucosal cushions prolapse out and are known as haemorrhoids.
- Severity of prolapse increases with persistence of straining at defecation, engorgement of haemorrhoids, progressive loss of the elasticity of the rectal submucosa and degeneration of Treitz's muscle.

5.3 Recent Concept of Pathophysiology of Haemorrhoids

- Vascular theory by Aigner [2, 3].
  - Increased vessel diameter.
  - Increased blood supply.
  - Neo vascularisation.
- Anal-cushion sliding theory by Thomson 1975 [4].
- Rectal redundancy by Longo [5].
- Increased pressure on venous outflow from submucosal cushions.

So the treatment is tailored-

- To detect the vessels feeding haemorrhoids.

One way we have already learnt in the last chapter, i.e., by Doppler guidance. Scientific literature is controversial on utility of Doppler guidance especially when mucopexy is also done with DGHAL [6, 7].

Another way is by palpating vessels with finger in the anal canal. One can easily palpate haemorrhoidal artery pulse after little experience.

- To decrease the blood supply by ligation of haemorrhoidal branches of superior rectal vessel [8].
  - Best place to ligate superior haemorrhoidal vessels is 1 cm above the anorectal junction as 99% of vessels have entered submucosa there and are only 2 mm deep to mucosa [9].
- Mucopexy is done to pull the anal cushions up and then fix them there by giving LASER energy in submucosal cushions which also

further decreases blood supply by shrinkage effect.

- Submucosal cushions are AV formations with high flow in case of haemorrhoids, by doing vessel ligation before doing LASER, we are converting them into low flow AV formation which increases the effects of LASER energy.
- Also Aigner et al. 2004 showed that besides the submucosal branches of the superior rectal artery, additional transmural vessels pierce the muscular layers of the rectum to supply the corpus cavernosum recti [3].
- This observation might explain the persistence of haemorrhoids after ligation of submucosal vessels. Giving LASER energy in submucosal cushions might handle these vessels.
- If there are circumferential haemorrhoids, (rectal redundancy) then we can choose either
  - MIPH as suggested by Longo.
  - Six columns mucopexy or
  - Chivate's procedure/trans-anal suture mucopexy for haemorrhoids [10].

5.4 Indications

- Procedures are better reserved for grade 3 haemorrhoids (Fig. 5.1).
- For grade 4, one has to add excision of non-reducing fibrosed or sodden skin component (Figs. 5.2 and 5.3).
- Failed office procedures for grade 2 haemorrhoids.

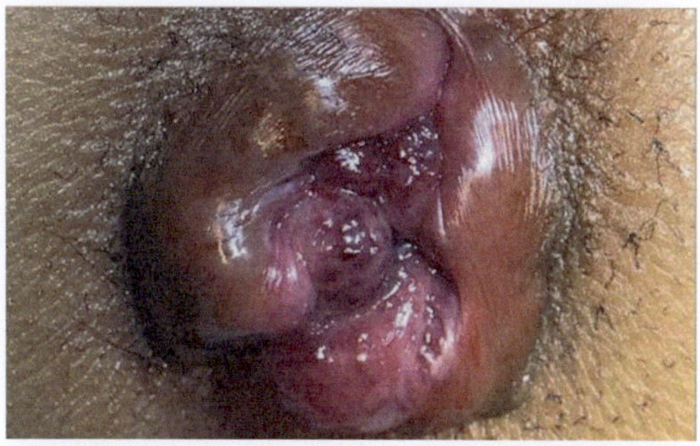

Fig. 5.1 Grade 3 haemorrhoids

Fig. 5.2 (**a**, **b**) Grade 4 haemorrhoids. (**c**) After HAL and LHP excision of skin component is required

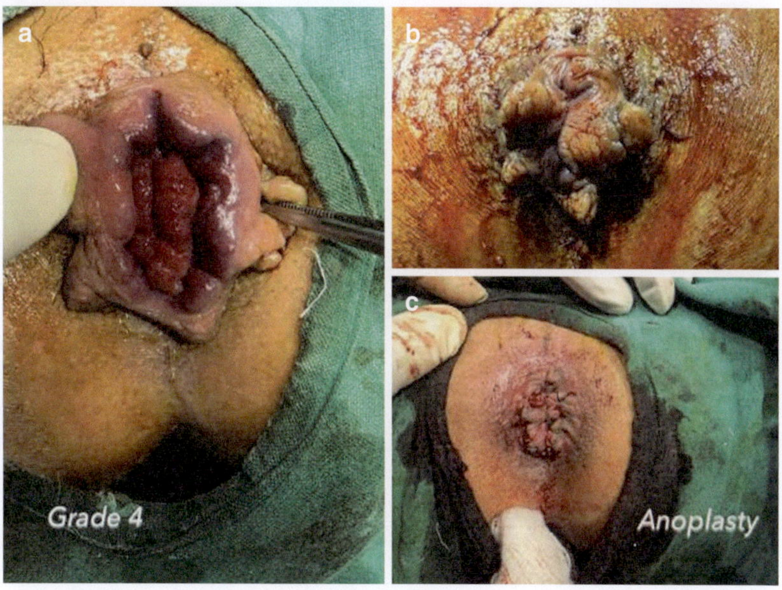

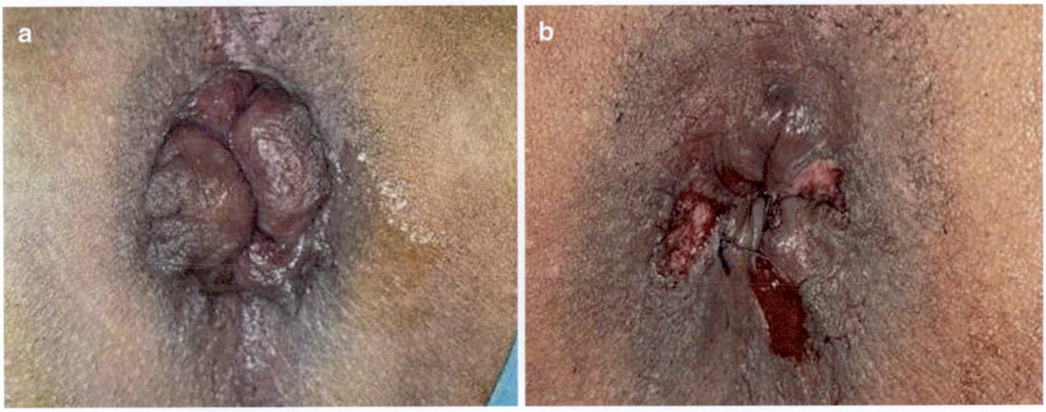

Fig. 5.3 (**a**) Grade 4 haemorrhoids. (**b**) After HAL and LHP only skin component excised sparing anoderm

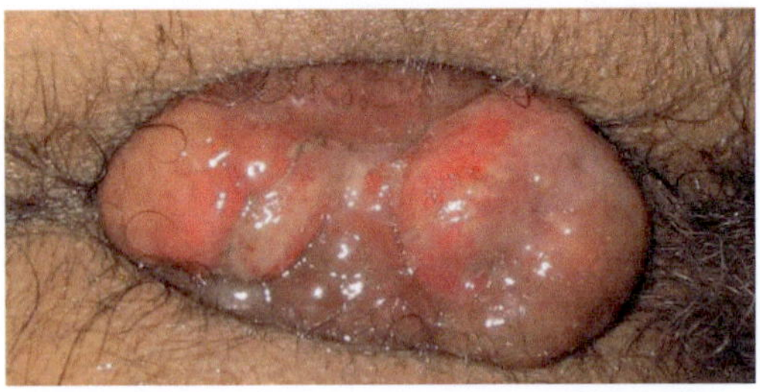

Fig. 5.4 Strangulated haemorrhoids need excision

5.5 Contra-Indications

- Already thrombosed or strangulated haemorrhoids (Fig. 5.4).
- Active infection in the area or lower Gastrointestinal tract (GI).

5.6 Pre-operative Considerations

- Preoperative workup as for any case under anaesthesia.
- For high risk cardiac patients, stop anticoagulants week before or shift on heparin as suggested by cardiologist and then stop heparin a day before.
- Enema 2 h before the procedure and advise patient to pass stools.

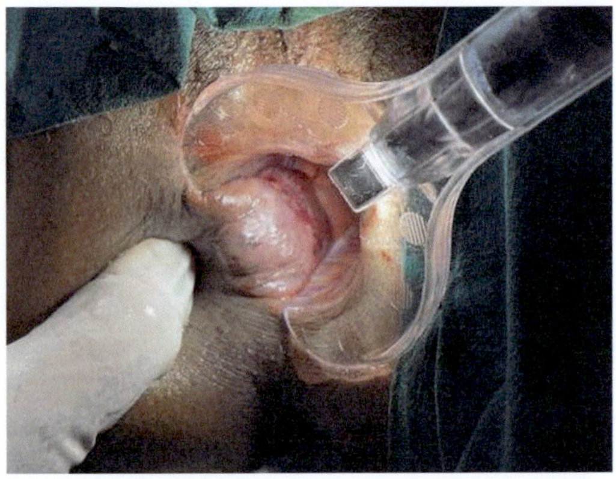

Fig. 5.5 Lighted proctoscope with attachment for fibroptic cable/battery-driven light source makes working quite comfortable

5.7 Equipment Required

- Operation table with stirrups for lithotomy.
- For prone position, rolled sheets and cushions with tapes for strapping.
- Sterile drapes and gowns.
- Povidine iodine solution.
- Xylocaine jelly, surgical gloves, saline-soaked gauge pieces.
- Proctoscope and light source. Lighted operating proctoscopes make life easy (Fig. 5.5).
- Long needle holder 10″, long plain forceps, 2.0 polyglactin 910 suture (vicryl) 120 cm length on 27 mm 5/8 circle round body needle.
- LASER machine 1470 diode LASER with accessories (Fig. 5.6).

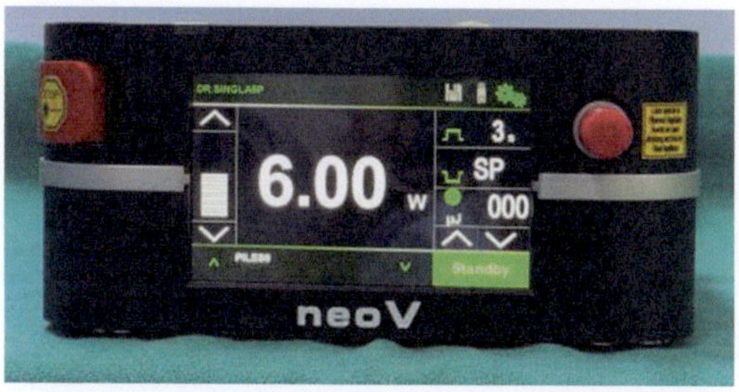

Fig. 5.6 LASER machine 1470 diode LASER

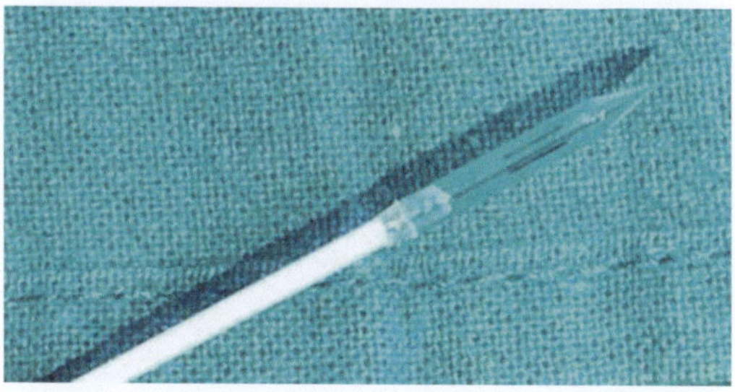

Fig. 5.7 LASER fibre with conical tip

- LASER fibre with conical tip for haemorrhoids (Fig. 5.7).
- Eye protective glasses.
- Ice-filled finger cot.

5.8 Anaesthesia

Spinal, perianal pudendal block/a simplified easily reproducible pudendal nerve-block technique for anorectal surgery (SEPTA) [11].

5.9 Position

Supine, lithotomy or prone with buttocks strapped.

5.10 Procedure [12]

- Inspection of the area, under anaesthesia and in lithotomy, protrusion may increase by one degree.
- DRE with lubricated gloves.
- Proctoscopy and clean the anal canal.
- One can judge the protrusion by putting a long gauge piece in anal canal and the withdrawing it.

5.10.1 First Part of the Procedure Finger-Guided Haemorrhoidal Artery Ligation (FGHAL) or Total Haemorrhoidal Dearterilisation (THD) Without Doppler

- Palpate for pulse of haemorrhoidal arteries. It is good idea to palpate with right-hand index finger on right side of the patient and with left-hand index finger on left of the patient. Make a note of position of palpable vessels in your cortex diary. Mark with electro cautery (Fig. 5.8).
- Put a well-lubricated half speculum/lighted operating proctoscope inside the anal canal, inspect for dentate line and haemorrhoids (Fig. 5.5) and again palpate the haemorrhoidal artery in one sector.
- Mount 27 mm 5/8 circle round body-needle with 120 cm long 2.0 polyglactin 910 suture, on a long needle-holder and hold needle-holder from outside to make a prone position at wrist (Fig. 5.9).
- Start ligating Right Posterior (Rt. Post.) (7'o) palpable vessel 1 cm above anorectal ring by keeping needle-tip perpendicular to rectal mucosa and just rotate your wrist along the curvature of needle, do not push the needle too much. Needle will pass through mucosa and submucosa.

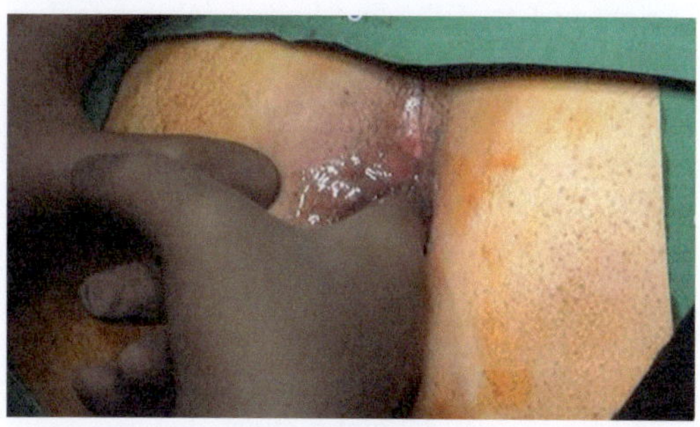

Fig. 5.8 Palpation of haemorrhoidal artery for FGHAL

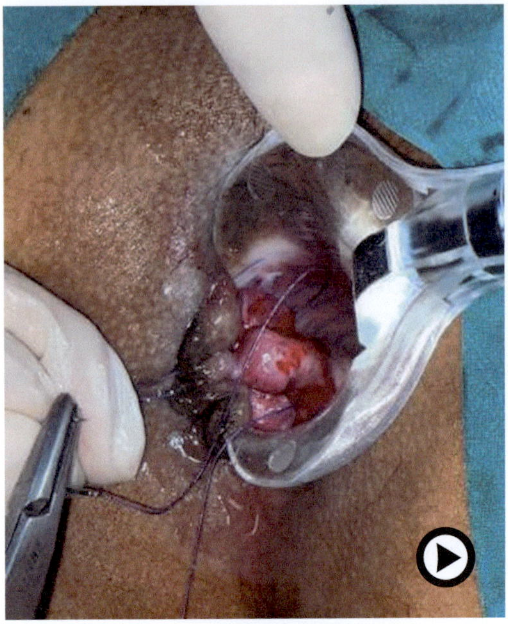

Fig. 5.9 Ligation of palpable vessel with polyglactin 2.0 suture on 5/8 round body 27 mm needle
Video 5.1 Finger-guided haemorrhoidal artery ligation (FGHAL) and lateral internal sphinctrotomy (LIS) in a case of grade III haemorrhoids with fissure in ano (▶ https://doi.org/10.1007/000-hpt)

- Catch both threads and pull slightly to lift the mucosa and now take second bite 5 mm proximal to first one to make figure of 8 and apply surgical knot.
- If prolapse is more, one can do mucopexy by taking two or three more proximal bites at 5 mm distance and tie the ends of threads to pull the prolapsing mucosa and subsequently submucosal cushions (Fig. 5.10).
- Check the absence of pulse—distal to ligation. If still pulse is there, one can ligate few mm right or left of the first ligature as per feel of the pulse.
- Ligate all palpable vessels one by one. Usually four to five ligations suffice.
- For anterior ligation, one may have to press a large haemorrhoid with back of the forceps for visibility.
- One can do additional mucopexy of any prolapsing column of mucosa.
- In case of circumferential piles, one can do up to six-column mucopexy, i.e., at 1, 3, 5, 7, 9 and 11 o'clock positions.

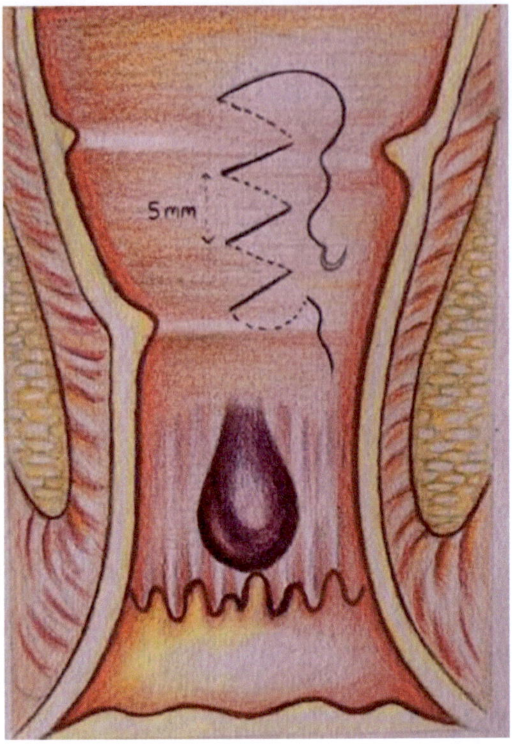

Fig. 5.10 Sketch to show the proximal bites to do mucopexy

Table 5.1 Setting of LASER machine and energy

Type of LASER and fibre	Purpose	Energy in watts (W)	Pulse in seconds (s)
1470 Diode LASER Conical fibre	Puncture anoderm to enter in sub mucosal cushion	6	1
Same	Delivery of energy in the cushions	6	3

5.10.2 Second Part of the Procedure LASER Haemorrhoidoplasty

- Wear LASER-protective glasses.
- Connect the conical fibre to the LASER machine and use the energy settings as shown in Table 5.1.

$$\text{Total of } 6 \times 3 = 18\,\text{J at one point}$$

$$\text{One cushion 9 points in fan shape manner at three stations} = 18 \times 9 = 162\,\text{J}$$

Three cushions or total in anal canal delivered energy does not exceed 500 J

- Put the conical-fibre in its handle, bring tip out and lock it. Activate the LASER fibre.
- Keep tip of conical fibre at anoderm just below the dentate line and deliver 6 W energy for 1 s to puncture and negotiate the tip of LASER fibre in submucosa just proximal to the upper end of the haemorrhoid by slow rotatory movements, never force the fibre (Fig. 5.11).
- If external vascular channels are prominent, then enter at anoderm cutaneous junction (Fig. 5.12).
- Keep LASER fibre parallel to the anal canal walls so that tip remains in the centre of the submucosal cushion, which can be judged by intensity of navigation light glow. Tip too close to mucosa (glow increases) will burn mucosa and tip deep towards internal sphincter (glow goes away) will injure some muscle fibres.

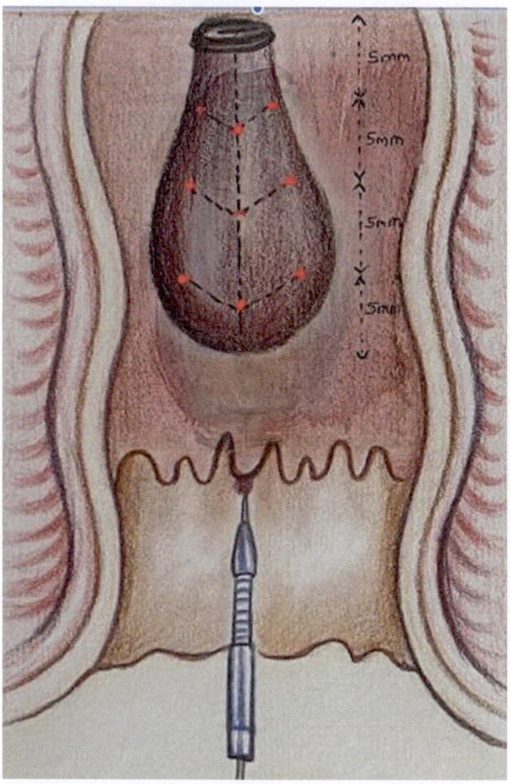

Fig. 5.11 Sketch to show entry point of LASER conical fibre tip below the dentate line and 9 point LASER energy delivery sites within the submucosal cushion for even distribution

- Deliver 6 W for 3 s in the midline and same to the right and left in a fan shape manner, then withdraw fibre for 5 mm and again deliver 6 W for 3 s in the midline and same to the right and left in a fan shape manner, still withdraw LASER fibre for 5 mm again and deliver 6 W for 3 s in midline and on right and left in fan shape manner (Fig. 5.11).
- While delivering energy, go on rotating LASER fibre to avoid sticking.
- Keep cold saline-soaked gauge over the cushion and puncture site and press for 3 min. It serves dual purpose of dissipating heat and controls any blood ooze.
- Repeat the procedure for other two haemorrhoids.
- Do check proctoscopy and clean the anal canal.
- Any ooze, control with pressure with gauge.
- Put finger cot filled with ice in the anal canal.
- Fix a gauge piece with suture on the outer part of finger cot so that it can be pulled out after 10 min in the post-operative area by nurse.

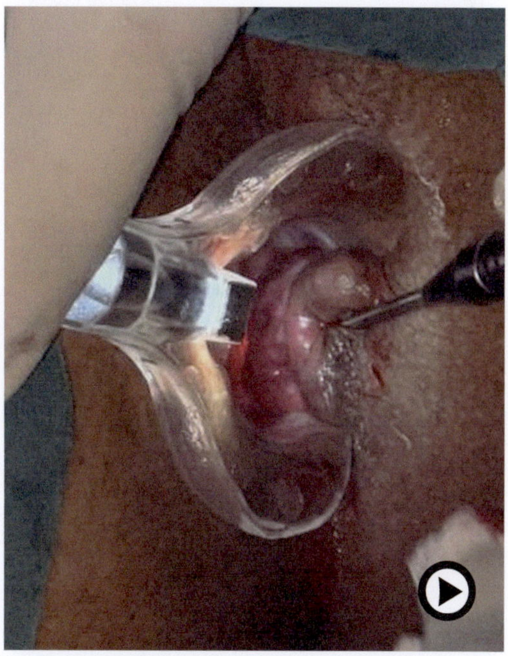

Fig. 5.12 LASER fibre with conical tip inserted at anoderm skin junction as external vascular channel was prominent and anoderm is lifted from internal sphincter-Video 5.2 FGHAL in a case of grade III haemorrhoids (▶ https://doi.org/10.1007/000-hps)

5.11 Complication of FGHAL (Table 5.2)

Table 5.2 Complications of the FGHAL mucopexy and LHP

Complications	Prevention	Management
Surface bleeding from puncture site	Locate the vessel by palpation and avoid it	Press for 3 min
Submucosal bleeding starts while passing suture due to injury to little large vessel and mucosa starts ballooning suddenly	Locate the vessel by palpation and avoid it	Pull both the strings of suture tight and take a large proximal bite and ligate. Press with a large piece of gauge for 3 min then rotate the speculum to work in opposite direction so that the area of bleeding will remain compressed further. If still there is evidence of bleeding take a proximal ligature with 1/2 circle 30 mm needle 2.0 suture
Counter-puncture of mucosa by LASER fibre	Do not apply force while navigating LASER fibre through the submucosa while delivering energy in submucosa. Remain parallel to wall of anal canal	Withdraw fibre by 5 mm and finish the delivery of energy in that cushion and then apply pressure with cold saline-soaked gauge piece for 3 min
Mucosal burns	Remain parallel to anal canal axis and never ever exceed the recommended dose of LASER. Don't think that haemorrhoids will shrink on table	Keep cold saline soaked gauge over the area or ice-filled finger cot
Tip of the LASER fibre slips in to handle	Do not force while advancing fibre tip in submucosa and check for wear and tear of plastic washer in its lock mechanism	Unlock handle of LASER fibre advance the tip and re-lock firmly
Tenesmus, discomfort or pain in anorectum	Do mucopexy for minimum required columns	Analgesics and NSAIDS
Reoccurrence	Meticulous operative technique.	Bleeding can be managed with sclero or repeated HAL
	Post-operative care to avoid straining.	Prolapse by limited excision of mucosa

5.12 Post-procedure Advise to the Patient

- Diet with adequate fibres and fluid using fruits and vegetables.
- Restrain from straining during defecation.
- Use commode and flex-hip by putting foot-elevator stool (Fig. 5.13).
- Laxative for 6 weeks.
- Mild pain and discomfort can be controlled with oral analgesics.
- Patient should be cautioned of small amount of mucous and reddish mucinous discharge from anus due to inflammatory reaction of sutures.
- Patient can feel some tenesmus and discomfort which can be more in case of increased length of mucopexy.
- Kegel's exercise to strengthen anal tone.

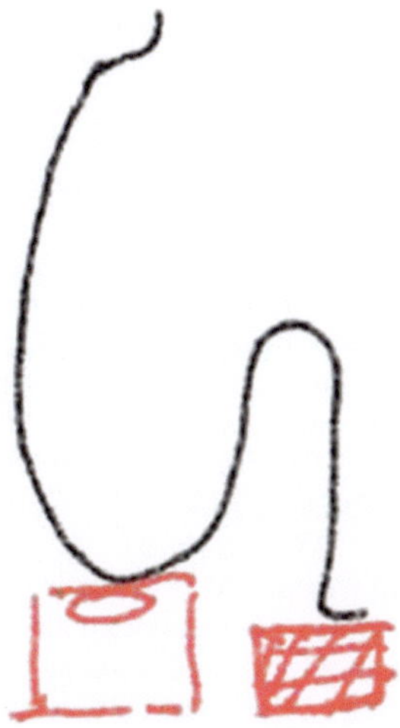

Fig. 5.13 Use of foot elevator stool

5.13 Tips and Tricks

- Under anaesthesia and in lithotomy protrusion of piles may increase by one degree, be careful.
- Systolic blood pressure of the patient should be above 100–110 mm of Hg for better appreciation of the pulse by finger.
- Always palpate right side arteries 7–11 o'clock position with right hand finger and left side arteries from 1 to 5 o'clock position with left hand index-finger and palpate just above the puborectalis sling that is almost 1 cm proximal to anorectal junction (ARJ).
- Vessel-ligation should be just 1 cm above the ARJ or pubo rectalis sling, high ligation leads to failure.
- While ligating vessel, hold needle-holder from outside as we hold a laparoscopic needle holder and just rotate at wrist.
- For anterior ligation, one may have to press a large haemorrhoid with back of the forceps for visibility and ask to increase Trendelenburg position.
- Always wear LASER-protective glasses before using LASER.
- Never push LASER-fibre with force in the submucosal cushion.
- *Ensure.*
- Right LASER fibre (conical tip LASER fibre).
- Right site of entry (always take a direct and shortest route to enter fibre in to submucosa, i.e., from anal lumen side not from intersphincteric space).
- Right dose of energy to be used, never over shoot (Table 5.1).
- Remain parallel to anal canal while delivering LASER energy, one can be guided by intensity of LASER glow.
- Use cold normal saline-filled gauge pieces to press the entry site of LASER fibre and cushion to dissipate the heat.
- Always do check proctoscopy at the end of the procedure.

Video of the procedure (Videos 5.1 and 5.2).

Algorithm for FGHAL Mucopexy and LHP

Clinical assessment
History examination and DRE
Indication/contraindication
Lithotomy/prone
Low spinal anaesthesia
Assess degree of prolapse by putting long gauge in the anal canal and then withdrawing it
Palpate all sectors of anal canal to feel the pulse of haemorrhoidal arteries
Ligate all palpable vessels 1 cm above the anorectal junction
Do proximal mucopexy at every ligated site by running suture and taking bites at an interval of 5 mm proximal to initial bite
Adapt length of mucopexy to the extent of protrusion of haemorrhoid
Prepare for LASER haemorrhoidoplasty (LHP)
Wear LASER protective eye glasses
Fix conical fibre in handle
1470 nm diode LASER 6 watts energy 1 second pulse for entry in to submucosal cushion
Enter just below the dentate line

(continued)

Navigate LASER fibre tip till apex of the haemorrhoid
Deliver 6 watts energy for 3 second pulse = 18 joules in midline
Then same energy on right and left of mid line in fan shape manner
Withdraw the LASER probe by 5 mm
Again deliver same amount of energy in midline and Rt. and Lt. of midline, in fan shape manner
Withdraw fibre for 5 mm again
And repeat the delivery of same energy in mid line and Rt. and Lt.
Withdraw the LASER fibre out of the haemorrhoid
Press the puncture site with cold saline filled gauge piece for 3 minutes
Do final check anoscopy
Excise any skin tag
Inject 5–10 cc methylene blue 1% solution in bupivacaine around skin wound whenever any excision is done below the dentate line
Put finger cot of surgical gloves full of ice, inside the anal canal for 10 minutes

References

1. Denoya P, Tam J, Bergamaschi R. Hemorrhoidal dearterialization with mucopexy versus hemorrhoidectomy: 3-year follow-up assessment of a randomized controlled trial. Tech Coloproctol. 2014;18(11):1081–5. https://doi.org/10.1007/s10151-014-1219-8. Epub 2014 Sept 24. PMID: 25248418; PMCID: PMC4246126.
2. Aigner F, Bodner G, Gruber H, Conrad F, Fritsch H, Margreiter R, Bonatti H. The vascular nature of hemorrhoids. J Gastrointest Surg. 2006;10(7):1044–50. https://doi.org/10.1016/j.gassur.2005.12.004. PMID: 16843876.
3. Aigner F, Bodner G, Conrad F, Mbaka G, Kreczy A, Fritsch H. The superior rectal artery and its branching pattern with regard to its clinical influence on ligation techniques for internal hemorrhoids. Am J Surg. 2004;187(1):102–8. https://doi.org/10.1016/j.amjsurg.2002.11.003. PMID: 14706597.
4. Thomson WH. The nature of haemorrhoids. Br J Surg. 1975;62:542–52. [PubMed] [Google Scholar].
5. Longo A. Treatment of hemorrhoids disease by reduction of mucosa and haemorrhoidal prolapse with a circular suturing device: a new procedure. In: Proceedings of the 6th world congress of endoscopic surgery, Rome, Italy. 3–6 June 1998. [Google Scholar].
6. Bonomo LD, Falletto E, Cuccomarino S, Nicotera A, Jannaci A. Hemorrhoidal artery ligation for the treatment of grade II–III hemorrhoids: is it worth the use of Doppler guide in long-term follow-up?: a single-center cohort study. Ann Surg Open. 2023;4(2):e296. https://doi.org/10.1097/AS9.0000000000000296. PMID: 37601476; PMCID: PMC10431348.
7. Alemrajabi M, Akbari A, Sohrabi S, Rezazadehkermani M, Moradi M, Agah S, Masoodi M. Simple mucopexy and hemorrhoidal arterial ligation with and without Doppler guide: a randomized clinical trial for short-term outcome. Ann Coloproctol. 2023;39(4):351–6. https://doi.org/10.3393/ac.2022.00017.0002. Epub 2022 May 16. PMID: 35570403; PMCID: PMC10475797.
8. Morinaga K, Hasuda K, Ikeda T. A novel therapy for internal hemorrhoids: ligation of the hemorrhoidal artery with a newly devised instrument (Moricorn) in conjunction with a Doppler flowmeter. Am J Gastroenterol. 1995;90:610–3. [PubMed].
9. Ratto C, Parello A, Donisi L, Litta F, Zaccone G, Doglietto GB. Assessment of haemorrhoidal artery network using colour duplex imaging and clinical implications. Br J Surg. 2012;99:112–8.
10. Chivate SD, Killedar MM, Ladukar LD, Vardhani GS, Kavathe SK, Kanekar SR. Transanal suture mucopexy for hemorrhoids. Dis Colon Rectum. 2022;65(5):742–9. https://doi.org/10.1097/DCR.0000000000002191. PMID: 34958048; PMCID: PMC8985695.
11. Ladha A, Garg P, Puranik C. A simplified easily reproducible pudendal nerve block technique for anorectal surgery (SEPTA) – a video vignette. Color Dis. 2018;20(9):829. https://doi.org/10.1111/codi.14261. Epub 2018 Jun 8. PMID: 29770547.
12. Singla S. Hemorrhoidal artery ligation, laser hemorrhoidoplasty, and LIS in a case of grade 3 hemorrhoids and chronic anal fissure. Indian J Colorectal Surg. 2021;4(2):56–7. https://doi.org/10.4103/2666-0784.330171.

Suggested Readings

Gupta K, Agarwal N, Mital K. Clinical outcomes in patients with hemorrhoids treated by finger guided hemorrhoidal artery ligation with laser hemorrhoidoplasty: a retrospective cohort study. J Adv Med Med Res. 2021;33(18):143–52. https://doi.org/10.9734/jammr/2021/v33i1831064.

Lohsiriwat V. Hemorrhoids: from basic pathophysiology to clinical management. World J Gastroenterol.

2012;18(17):2009–17. https://doi.org/10.3748/wjg.v18.i17.2009.

Lohsiriwat V. Anatomy, physiology, and pathophysiology of hemorrhoids. In: Ratto C, Parello A, Litta F, editors. Hemorrhoids, Coloproctology. Cham: Springer; 2017. https://doi.org/10.1007/978-3-319-51989-0_2-1.

Naniksingh Kukreja A. Hemorrhoids. In: Anorectal disorders – from diagnosis to treatment. IntechOpen; 2023. Available from: https://doi.org/10.5772/intechopen.1002689.

Trigui A, Rejab H, Akrout A, et al. Laser utility in the treatment of hemorrhoidal pathology: a review of literature. Lasers Med Sci. 2022;37:693–9. https://doi.org/10.1007/s10103-021-03333-x.

Suggested Viewing

Video 5.1 link from paper reference 11 "codi14261-sup-0001videos1.mp4". https://doi.org/10.1111/codi.14261.

6 Haemorrhoids: Minimally Invasive Procedure for Haemorrhoids (MIPH)/Procedure for Prolapsed Haemorrhoids (PPH)/Stapled Haemorrhoidopexy (SH)

Abstract

- Dr. Longo A, with a concept that haemorrhoids prolapse due to redundancy of rectal mucosa and submucosa as a whole, devised this haemorrhoid-sparing technique to reposition the prolapsed tissue back to its normal anatomical position.
- Instead of haemorrhoids, proximal 2–3 cm loose strip of mucosa and submucosa is excised and spontaneously stitched to pull the tissue up in upper anal canal.
- Components of the circular stapler used for the procedure and steps of the procedure are well explained by sketches and clinical photographs.
- To further make the point clear, animation video by one of the manufacturers and an operative video on our live patient has been included for viewing.
- Pearls of wisdom are shelled in Sect. 6.10.
- Because of decreased pain and early recovery, minimally invasive procedure for haemorrhoids (MIPH) is the most adopted and studied procedure for treating haemorrhoids since late 1990s, after Milligan Morgan and Ferguson procedure. At the same time, some peculiar complications have raised eye-brows also.
- Complications of MIPH, their prevention and management have been grouped in table form for ease and ready reference.
- Readers are instructed to check "References" section and are suggested some reading materials for in-depth knowledge on the subject.
- Algorithm of steps at the end of the chapter fulfills the need to refresh the steps on way to operation room (OR).

6.1 What One Should Know Before the Procedure

- Minimal invasive procedure for haemorrhoids (MIPH) or procedure for prolapse and haemorrhoids (PPH) or stapled haemorrhoidopexy (SH) is a haemorrhoid-sparing procedure, where a circumferential 2–3 cm strip of lower rectal mucosa and submucosa is resected by a circular stapler and resected-ends are staple stitched to reduce the prolapsing haemorrhoid cushions in the upper anal canal.
- Procedure was devised by Dr. Longo.A with a concept that haemorrhoids prolapse due to redundancy of rectal mucosa and submucosa as a whole.
- Initial reports were encouraging as procedure was quite painless as compared to haemor-

Supplementary Information The online version contains supplementary material available at https://doi.org/10.1007/978-981-96-6190-9_6. The videos can be accessed individually by clicking the DOI link in the accompanying figure caption or by scanning this link with the SN More Media App.

S. K. Singla, K. Mital, *Operative Manual of Minimally Invasive and LASER Ano-proctology*,
https://doi.org/10.1007/978-981-96-6190-9_6

rhoid excisional procedures and was adopted world-wide in late 1990s.

- Recurrence of prolapse and bleeding is more as compared to Milligan Morgan and Ferguson procedure.
- Actual problem with the procedure is that once the anvil of stapler goes in, actual staple resection and staple stitching is a total blind procedure.
- Over the years, reports of some peculiar complications like bleeding, sepsis, rectal perforations and peritonitis leading to death, forced many not to choose this procedure as procedure of choice for dealing with internal haemorrhoids. Recent guidelines of the American Association May 2024 state "Stapled hemorrhoidepexy is not routinely recommended as a first-line surgical treatment for internal haemorrhoids, given its marginal efficacy and significant risk-profile. Strength of recommendation: conditional based on moderate-quality evidence" [1].

6.2 Indications

- Circumferential prolapsing haemorrhoids.
- Grade 3 haemorrhoids.

6.3 Contraindications

- Any infection in the area.
- Strangulated internal haemorrhoids.
- Anal stenosis leading to technical difficulty.

6.4 Equipment

- Operation table with stirrups for lithotomy.
- For prone position, rolled sheets and cushions with tapes for strapping (optional).
- Sterile drapes and gowns.
- Povidine iodine solution.
- Xylocaine jelly, surgical gloves, saline soaked gauge pieces.

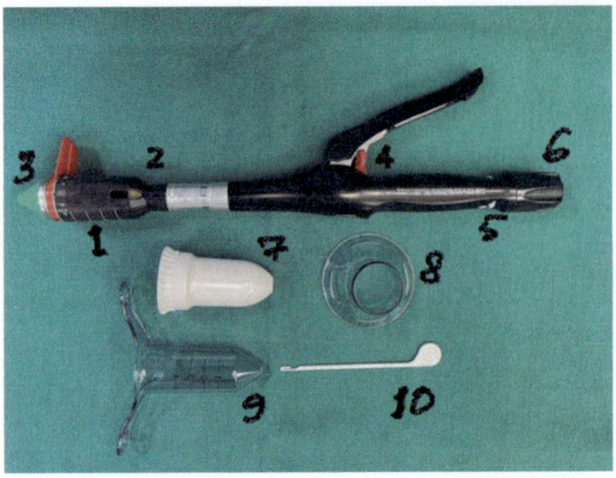

Fig. 6.1 Circular stapler for PPH. (1) The proximal end has markings for the insertion at the adequate depth. (2) Two side openings called suture or thread ports allow the retrieval of ends of purse-string sutures. (3) Anvil which is fixed thus avoiding unnecessary detachment. (4) Side safety knob. (5) Gap setting scale. (6) Closing knob. (7) Obturator. (8) Circular anal dilator (CAD). (9) Purse string suture anoscope or half speculum. (10) Suture retrieval device or suture threader (ST)

- Circular stapler (Fig. 6.1).
  The circular stapler PPH 03 has certain specific features adapted for its use in MIPH or PPH. 2 mm Titanium staples burry in mucosa and height of the closed staples is only 0.75 mm, thus ensuring haemostasis.
- 2.0 Prolene monofilament suture in a 25 mm 5/8 atraumatic needle for purse string suture.

6.5 Peri-operative Preparation

- Proctoclysis enema 2 h before the procedure and ask patient to evacuate.
- Prophylactic antibiotics ofloxacin and metronidazole combination are given with induction of anaesthesia.

6.6 Position of the Patient

- We prefer lithotomy position.
- Some surgeons prefer prone position as it wide opens the peri-anal area.

6.7 Anaesthesia

- Spinal anaesthesia for the lithotomy.
- General anaesthesia for the prone position.

6.8 Procedure

- Slightly dilate the anal canal by inserting a lubricated obturator with gentle right–left rotating movements.
- Then withdraw obturator.
- Manual anal dilatation is not necessary.

6.8.1 Application of Circular Anal Dilator

- Afterwards, the Circular Anal Dilator (CAD33) with the obturator intact is introduced into the rectum. Additional lubricating gel should be applied to avoid any friction which may lead to abrasions and bleeding.
- The CAD is kept in place by passing four anchoring sutures through the skin into the designated slots and securing them. Placing stitches near the anus maximizes the effectiveness of reducing prolapsed haemorrhoids. Figures 6.2 and 6.3 depicts the same information.
- Again, remove the obturator and check for the complete reduction of prolapsing haemorrhoids and position of dentate line through the transparent walls of the CAD.
- Height of CAD is 3 cm and it should cover the dentate line.
- If due to buttocks and android pelvis, CAD is not fitting into the anal canal well, one can cut it from right and left sides keeping only anterior and posterior part as flanges.
- Reduce any skin-fold caught between the CAD and the anorectal wall using a gauge swab.
- If one is to pull perianal skin margin to facilitate introduction of CAD, never pull skin in the area of haemorrhoidal prolapse instead in between the prolapsed areas.
- CAD must be positioned correctly for a successful operation.

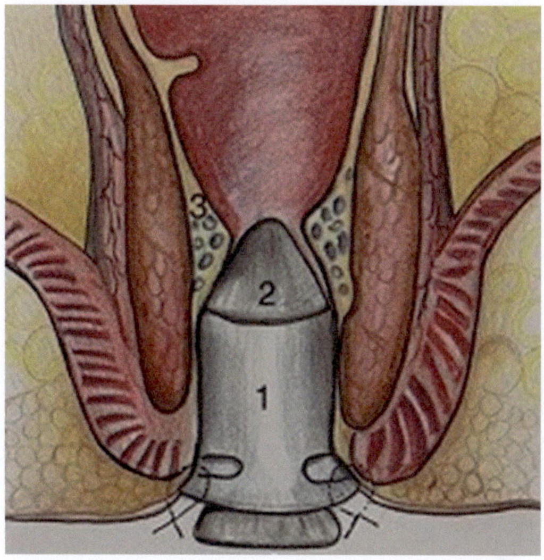

Fig. 6.2 Fixation of circular anal dilator (CAD) to perianal canal skin. (1) CAD. (2) Obturator. (3) Internal haemorrhoids

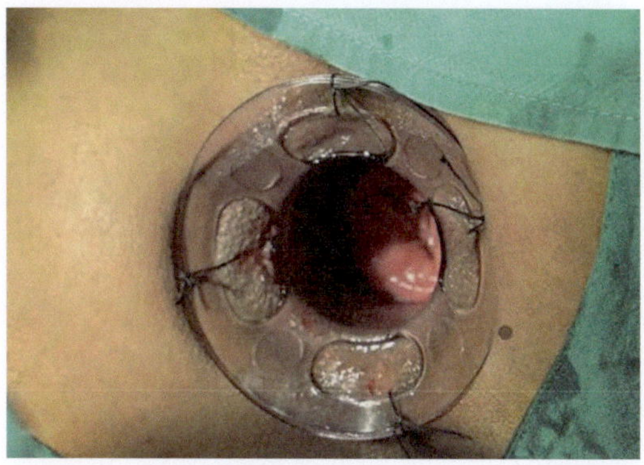

Fig. 6.3 Circular anal dilator fixed with anchoring sutures

6.8.2 Application of Purse-String Suture

- The purse-string suture anoscope (PSA33), commonly called as half speculum, is passed through the CAD.
  - It features a 90° wide opening that is sufficient for a fold of mucosa to stick out, enabling the placement of a purse-string suture above the internal haemorrhoids.
- The suture-bites have to be placed at least 3–4 cm above the dentate line. Upper end of the anoscope where it takes the shape of a

cone is a good guide to start suture (Figs. 6.4 and 6.5).

- Only mucosa and submucosa should be included in the suture bite. Suturing level should be same in whole circumference otherwise traction will be irregular.
- A bite that penetrates through all layers can result in anorectal narrowing or recto-vaginal fistula.
- It also increase the chances of peri-rectal sepsis.
- Before next bite, purse-string ano scope or half speculum has to be removed and reinserted after adequate rotation.

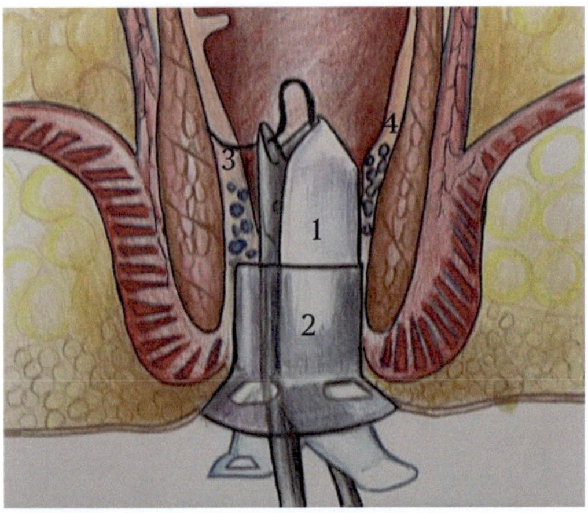

Fig. 6.4 Placement of a purse-string suture through the anoscope (1) pursuing suture anoscope PSA 33Anoscope. (2) Circular anal dilator. (3) Purse-string suture. (4) Internal haemorrhoids

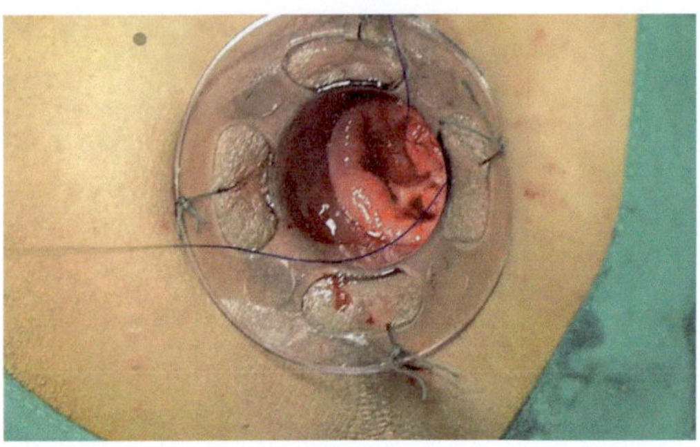

Fig. 6.5 Circular purse string suture passed at least 3–4 cm above the dentate line or 2 cm above the apex of haemorrhoids so that when fired, staple line should not include haemorrhoids

- A rotation of purse string ano scope inside the rectum could cause the mucosa to twist axially leading to application of uneven purse-string suture.
- Check proper placement of purse-string in submucosa by putting finger through and pulling threads of purse string, nowhere bare thread should touch the finger.
- For female patients, it is necessary to conduct a per-vaginal examination at this point to confirm that the purse-string has not attached to the back vaginal wall. If there are doubts about the vaginal participation or effectiveness of the purse-string, it should be removed and reinserted.
- The purse-string suture is kept loose so that the anvil can be placed beyond purse string.

6.8.3 Passing Stapler Beyond Purse String (Figs. 6.6 and 6.7)

- The anvil is inserted past the purse-string when the stapler is fully open. Avoid pulling on the suture ends in order to prevent the loop from tightening. The stapler needs to be taken out and the suture needs to be untied in that

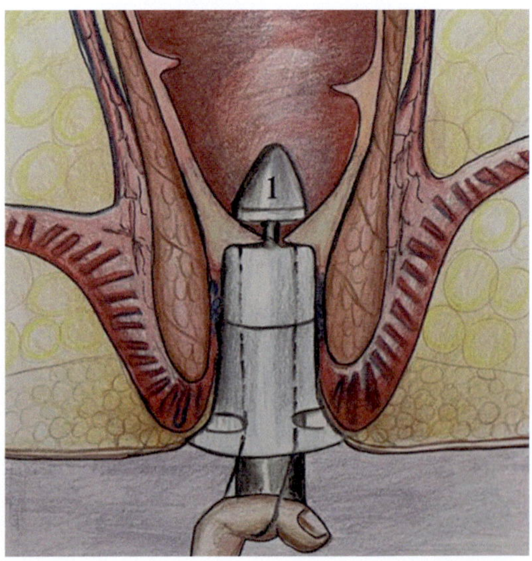

Fig. 6.6 (1) Anvil beyond the purse string, loop of purse-string pulled while distal knob is rotated to close the stapler

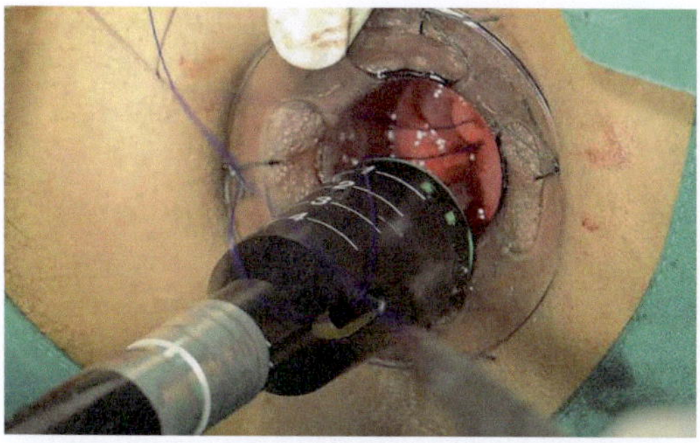

Fig. 6.7 Anvil is passed beyond the purse-string

situation. A forced entry could result in the wall tearing and forming gaps.

- Next, the trocar is encircled by the purse string which is secured with a basic knot. There is a danger of the loose loop being sliced by the circular knife. After the threads are pulled out from lateral ports, the ends are crossed and tied loosely to make a loop for traction.

6.8.4 Closure of the Stapler

- Ensure an adequate counter-traction on threads by hooking the loop with finger as shown in Fig. 6.8. The stapler is partially closed by rotating the distal end knob, continuous traction on the sutures accommodates the mucosal fold between the anvil and the shaft. A correct axial positioning of the device is essential. The correct depth of the instrument is indicated by the 4–5 cm line being at the anal verge. The device is closed until the orange indicator is in the green range. Hold stapler in locked position for a minute to milk out tissue-fluid before firing the stapler.
- It is important to make sure the stapling device is properly aligned with the axis of the anal canal.
- At this stage, it is important to verify that the head of the instrument does not contain the posterior vaginal wall.

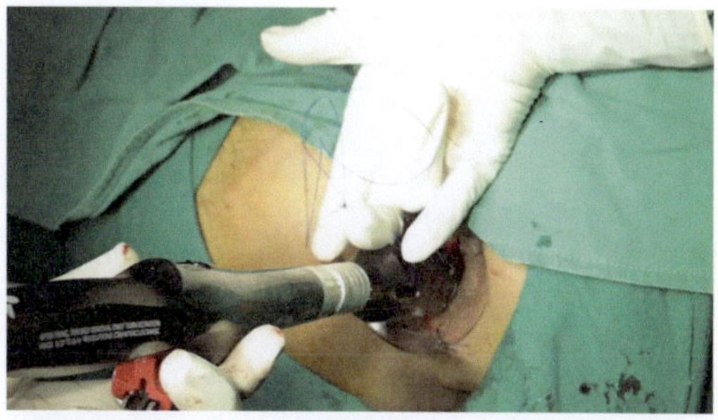

Fig. 6.8 Hooking the thread loop on finger for adequate traction on tissue to bring it in housing of the circular cutter of the stapler. Note the safety knob is in position. Stapler is progressively closed by rotating the distal knob, also note the alignment of the instrument in line with axis of anal canal

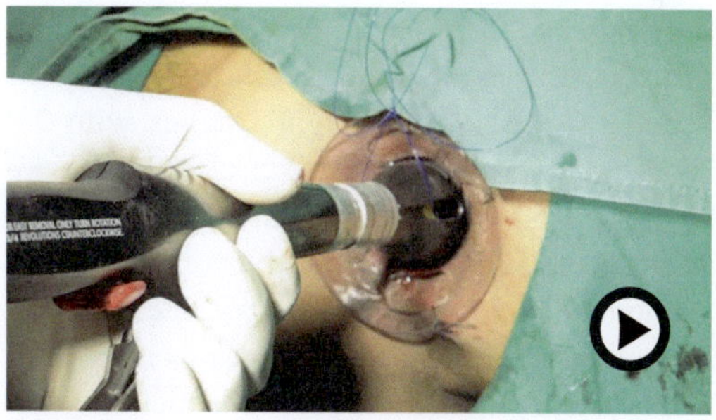

Fig. 6.9 Safety knob released to close the handle in single go (▶ https://doi.org/10.1007/000-hpv)

6.8.5 Firing the Stapler

- The safety knob is unlocked and the handle is shut while applying consistent pressure. Close the handle smoothly and continuously to ensure proper operation, as indicated by a distinct "cracking" noise (Fig. 6.9).
- Release the anvil by turning knob anticlockwise only 180–270°. A larger gap between the anvil and shaft could result in the suture-line getting caught between anvil and the top of the dilator.
- PPH stapler is extracted by slow side-to-side movements.
- The stapler is opened and the resected specimen is checked for the completeness of the

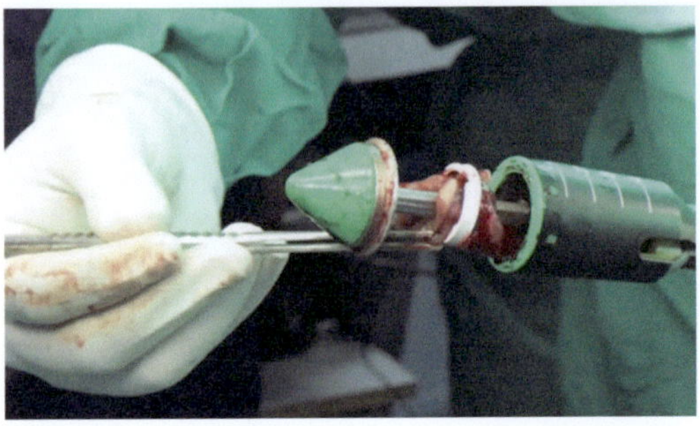

Fig. 6.10 Opened stapler to show the resected specimen

tissue ring so called complete doughnut (Fig. 6.10).

- We keep the CAD still inside the anal canal and ensure complete haemostasis before removing the CAD.
- In case of a staple-line failure, it must be fixed using figure-of-eight stitches with 2.0 absorbable suture on a 1/2 circle 30 mm needle. Using clips could result in ischaemic necrosis and subsequent bleeding. Use of monopolar or bipolar electrocautery is not recommended due to the risk of burns from the energy transmitted by the metallic staples. Gauge packaging done locally is not effective in managing bleeding from the staple line.
- Never leave the patient with any ooze from staple line. Fix it there and then.
- Do check ano-scopy and clean any collected blood.
- A thin gauze ribbon can be inserted into the rectum above the stitching area, with one end outside the anus. In this way, blood will be absorbed through the gauze by capillary action. If there is no bleeding, the ribbon can be gently pulled out after a few hours.
- Certain surgeons leave tube of Mallecots catheter in anal canal with some roll gauge wrapped around it, with same purpose.
- Whatever we use to show up the bleeding, ensure removal of any anal wick or catheter before patient gains senses in the area.
- Monitoring of vitals like pulse rate is a must to check for any ongoing bleeding.
- Other treatments can be done for additional anal conditions along PPH, like Lateral internal sphinctrotomy (LIS) for fissure or excision of skin tags.

6.9 Post-operative Management

- Monitoring of vitals especially pulse-rate for early detection of any post-operative bleeding.
- Check for any retention of urine.
- Intravenous (IV) paracetamol should suffice to control pain.
- Patient can be discharged same evening or next day, especially old age patients after ensuring normal bladder evacuation.
- Oral nonsteroidal anti-inflammatory drugs (NSAIDs) for 5 days.
- Laxatives for 5 days.
- Antibiotics ofloxacin and metronidazole for 5 days.
- Any increase in pain, fever, retention of urine or inability to pass stools should be notified urgently and patient called back to hospital for assessment.

6.10 Tips and Tricks

- The perfect patient would have both prolapsed piles and the presence of internal rectal prolapse, whether it be mucosal or full-thickness.
- At the start of the procedure, the surgeon needs to manually reduce the external prolapse while using a gauge swab to insert CAD. Failure to do so will result in the external prolapse persisting after resection, which will yield an unsatisfactory outcome.
- Most of complications are due to defective passage of purse-string, so be careful about level, depth and completeness of suture line.
- Fire the staple in one quick go to avoid laceration of mucosa.
- Every staple line failure must be fixed using figure-of-eight stitches with a 2.0 absorbable suture on a 30-mm needle with 1/2 circle. The use of clips can result in ischaemic tissue death and subsequent bleeding. Using mono-

polar or bipolar electrocautery is not recommended due to the risk of burns from the metallic staples transmitting energy. Local packing is inefficient in controlling staple line bleeding.

- Never leave the patient with any ooze from staple line. Fix it there and then.
- The surgeon needs to know about a variety of devices and be skilled and trained to choose the right one based on the patients' characteristics and the size of the prolapse.
- Any fibrosed or sodden prolapsed tissue at the end of the procedure needs manual excision, though it will increase pain. Counselling before procedure is must in such cases.

6.11 Complications of the MIPH/Stapler for Haemorrhoidopexy (SH) (Table 6.1)

We find that after the Milligan Morgan and Ferguson technique, Longo's stapler haemorrhoidopexy is the most widely applied and studied technique in the late 1990s worldwide, so obviously more details are available.

Certain peculiar complications associated with the procedure raise the eyebrows.

For details of complications of stapler, suggested reading: At https://link.springer.com/content/pdf/10.1007/s10151-008-0391-0.pdf.

Table 6.1 SH complications, prevention and management

Complications	Prevention	Management
Suture-line bleeding or suture-line failure (tissue gap)	Follow meticulously level and depth of purse-string suture	Post-op anoscopy must. Figure of eight sutures 2.0 absorbable on 1/2 circle 30 mm needle to close the staple-line break
	Fire staple in single flow snap. Slow firing leads to laceration effect. Check the completeness of doughnut	
Post-op. bleeding	Follow meticulously operative details of passing purse-string and firing staple in one go.	Resuscitate the patient. In OT, wash the area and apply figure-of-eight sutures 2.0 absorbable on 1/2 circle 30 mm needle to stop bleeding, do not use cautery or clips.
	Never leave any ooze unattended. Check it there and then on table.	Gauge cannot tamponade significant bleeding
Late on set or chronic pain	Purse string suture should be at least 2–2.5 cm proximal to haemorrhoids apex or 3–4 cm proximal to dentate line.	Various interventions, such as partial lateral internal sphincterotomy, pudendal nerve surgery, staple removal or local anaesthetic application, have been proposed as potential treatments for long-lasting pain without a definitive solution.
	Depth of sutures should not include any smooth muscles of rectal wall.	
	Inflammation due to staples as a possible cause cannot be prevented.	Removal of whole staple-line and mucosal repair by suturing (agraphectomy) [2, 3]
Defective urgency	Purse-string should be 3–4 cm proximal to dentate line. Should not involve haemorrhoid tissue.	Passes with time.
		Counselling
Anal fissure	Avoid mucosal folds in staple line	Remove staples [4]
Anal stenosis Figure 6.11	Prevent full thickness bites in purse-string and too high purse string	Dilatation or as usually stenosis is diaphragmatic type one can cut it open safely in posterior midline
External vascular thrombosis	Reduce any prolapsing tissue properly while putting CAD	Laxatives and oral flavanoids
Rectal perforation	Depth of purse string suture should be in submucosa. Before firing, axial alignment of stapler should be parallel to anal canal all around.	Resuscitation, antibiotics, anterior resection and ileostomy or end colostomy
		Hartmann's type
Retroperitoneal sepsis	Depth of purse-string suture should not take muscles.	Resuscitation
		Antibiotics, rule out perforation in rectum and drainage of pus

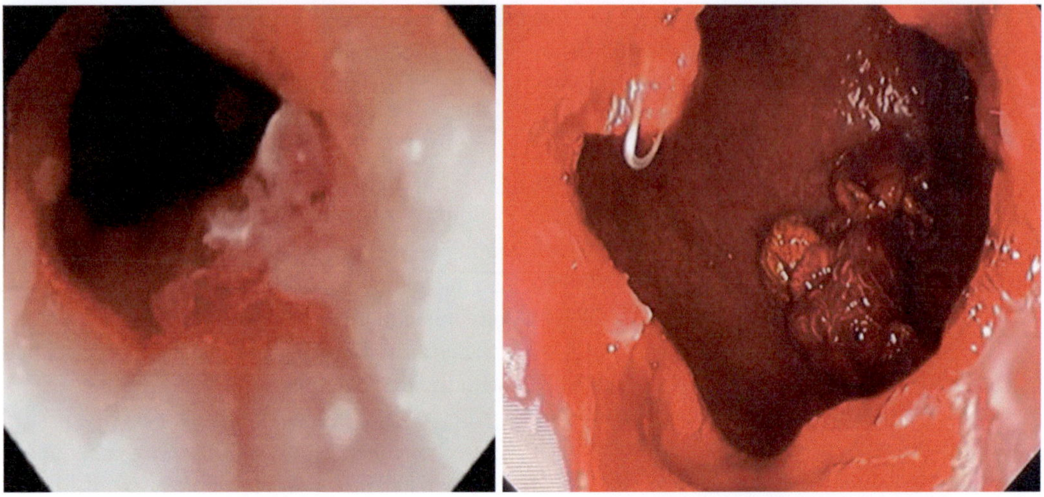

Anal stenosis after MIPH. diaphragm type

Diaphragm incised posterior midline
Stapler pins can be seen

Fig. 6.11 Anal stenosis after stapler haemorrhoidopexy

Algorithm for MIPH Clinical Assessment

History, clinical examination and DRE

Indication/contra indications

Best reserved for circumferential haemorrhoids/grade 3 haemorrhoids

Spinal anaesthesia/GA

Lithotomy/prone jack knife

DRE and lubrication

Put the obturator to dilate the anal canal

Remove the obturator

Pass circular anal dilator (CAD) with obturator inside the anal canal

Fix the CAD to perianal skin

Replace obturator with half speculum or purse string suture anoscope through the cad

Start taking purse string suture, say from 3'o taking mucosa and submucosa at least 3 cm proximal to dentate line

Verify circumferential pick up of mucosa and submucosa in purse string by putting finger through the suture and pulling the threads of purse string

Rule out suture taking any component of posterior vaginal wall

Open the stapler fully and pass anvil of stapler beyond purse string and ensure it

Tighten purse string around rod of stapler below the anvil by double knot

Loose threads of this knot are pulled with suture threader through the slits on side of the stapler

Make a loop of free threads with a loose knot

Align the stapler axis with axis of the anal canal and lower rectum

Assistant pulls the loop with bent finger-like a hook firmly

Surgeon keeps the stapler aligned with left hand and rotates the distal knob to close the stapler with other hand

Check optimal closure of the device by orange marker in the green range

Again check to rule out any engagement of vaginal tissue in stapler head

Keep the stapler in closed position for 45 seconds to one minute, to milk out the tissue fluid from proposed staple line

Remove the safety guard

(continued)

Press the handle of the stapler in one fluid motion to get specific short cracking sound "*Cadauch*"
Keep the stapler in closed position for 20 seconds
Derotate the distal knob to disengage the stapler from tissue
Remove the stapler with slight tilt and rotation motion out of the anal canal
Ensure haemostasis
Clean the rectum and anal canal
Remove circular anal dilator (CAD)
Putting a small gauge ribbon wick is personal choice
Remove any wick or catheter from anal canal before patient gathers sense in the area

References

1. Hawkins AT, Davis BR, Bhama AR, Fang SH, Dawes AJ, Feingold DL, Lightner AL, Paquette IM, On behalf of the Clinical Practice Guidelines Committee of the American Society of Colon and Rectal Surgeons. The American Society of Colon and Rectal Surgeons clinical practice guidelines for the management of hemorrhoids. Dis Colon Rectum. 2024;67(5):614–23. https://doi.org/10.1097/DCR.0000000000003276.
2. Pescatori M, Gagliardi G. Postoperative complications after procedure for prolapsed hemorrhoids (PPH) and stapled transanal rectal resection (STARR) procedures. Tech Coloproctol. 2008;12:7–19. https://doi.org/10.1007/s10151-008-0391-0.
3. Pescatori M, Gagliardi G. Agraffectomy after low rectal stapling procedures for hemorrhoids and rectocele. Tech Coloproctol. 2011;15:265–6. https://doi.org/10.1007/s10151-011-0717-1.
4. del Mar Aguilar Martínez M, Moya P, Arroyo A. Stapled hemorrhoidopexy: techniques and results. In: Ratto C, Parello A, Litta F, editors. Hemorrhoids, Coloproctology, vol. 2. Cham: Springer; 2018. https://doi.org/10.1007/978-3-319-53357-5_27.

Suggested Readings

del Mar Aguilar Martínez M, Moya P, Arroyo A. Stapled hemorrhoidopexy: techniques and results. In: Ratto C, Parello A, Litta F, editors. Hemorrhoids, Coloproctology, vol. 2. Cham: Springer; 2018. https://doi.org/10.1007/978-3-319-53357-5_27.

Lenisa L. Why and when I do prefer the stapled hemorrhoidopexy. In: Ratto C, et al., editors. Hemorrhoids, Coloproctology, vol. 2. Cham: Springer; 2018. https://doi.org/10.1007/978-3-319-53357-5_28.

Naldini G, Martellucci J, Talento P, Caviglia A, Moraldi L, Rossi M. New approach to large haemorrhoidal prolapse: double stapled haemorrhoidopexy. Int J Color Dis. 2009;24(12):1383–7.

Stuto A, Favero A, Cerullo G, Braini A, Narisetty P, Tosolini G. Double stapled haemorrhoidopexy for haemorrhoidal prolapse: indications, feasibility and safety. Colorectal Dis. 2012;14:e386. https://doi.org/10.1111/j.1463-1318.2012.02965.x.

Suggested Viewing

PPH procedure animation Link for SV 6.1 https://youtu.be/lyN2JbS_O1E?si=TFOPADOWFhExDri4

7 Haemorrhoids: Chivate's Procedure Suture Haemorrhoidopexy

Abstract

- Suture Haemorrhoidopexy is a non-excisional method to treat haemorrhoidal disease.
- Procedure requires a special proctoscope designed by Dr. Chivate and being marketed in his name, other than that it does not require any special and costly gadgets.
- How two major components of the disease, i.e., increased vascularity and prolapse of redundant mucosa, submucosa and associated sliding of haemorrhoids are taken care by this procedure is well explained by sketches and clinical photographs.
- To make the steps of the procedure clear, operative video with narration is also included.
- Link for another video, published in a paper, reported by the inventor of the procedure is provided.
- Procedure has few and minor complications, which have been presented in tabulated form for easy access and reference.
- "Tips and Tricks" section provides some pearls of wisdom to improve outcomes.
- For further insights, one can refer to "References" and "Suggested Reading" sections.
- Algorithm to refresh operative steps on way to operation room (OR) is included at the end of the chapter.

Supplementary Information The online version contains supplementary material available at https://doi.org/10.1007/978-981-96-6190-9_7. The videos can be accessed individually by clicking the DOI link in the accompanying figure caption or by scanning this link with the SN More Media App.

7.1 What One Should Know Before the Procedure

- This procedure entails fixing of distal rectal mucosa and submucosa to circular muscle of the rectum by 0.5–1 cm double-locking stitches along the complete circumference at 2 and 4 cm proximal to dentate line in haemorrhoids of grade II, III and IV.
- The procedure got invented while trying to control bleeding in a case of open ligation and excision of haemorrhoids.
- Dr Chivate from Thane, India, applied double-locking stitches in whole circumference proximal to bleeding haemorrhoids and wound. Next day it was observed that not only bleeding stopped but prolapsing tissue also decreased considerably.

7.2 Basis of the Procedure

First, reduce the prolapsing haemorrhoids by gentle massage and steep Trendelenburg position. It takes haemorrhoids back in position above the dentate line. Fix the prolapsing rectal mucosa and submucosa to underlying circular muscle by two rows for circumferential double-locking sutures taken 2 and 4 cm proximal to dentate line. It reduces prolapsing haemorrhoids and ligates feeding vessels and thereby reduces vascularity and prolapse.

S. K. Singla, K. Mital, *Operative Manual of Minimally Invasive and LASER Ano-proctology*,
https://doi.org/10.1007/978-981-96-6190-9_7

7.3 Indications

- Failed office procedure treatment in second-degree haemorrhoids.
- Grade 3 and grade 4 haemorrhoids especially circumferential haemorrhoids.

7.4 Contra-indications

- Any infections in the area.
- Technical difficulty in putting Chivate's proctoscope in narrow android pelvis, anal stenosis.
- Already strangulated or necrosed haemorrhoids.

7.5 Equipment

- Operation table with stirrups for lithotomy.
- For prone position, rolled sheets and cushions with tapes for strapping (optional).
- Sterilised drapes and gowns.
- Povidine iodine solution.
- Xylocaine jelly, surgical gloves, saline-soaked gauge pieces.
- Chivate's proctoscope with light fountain (Fig. 7.1).
- Proctoscope has wide circumference to make mucosa completely flat all around without any loose frills of mucosa.
- Operative proctoscope has wide slit, made in a way that only mucosa proximal to haemorrhoids is visible.
- Area harbouring submucosal cushions is well covered by the plastic body of the scope.
- Light fountain provided with the scope is good enough to light up the operative area as one can see in the operative clinical photographs.
- 2.0 polyglactin biodegradable suture on 1/2 circle 30 mm round body needle.
- Long needle holder 9″.

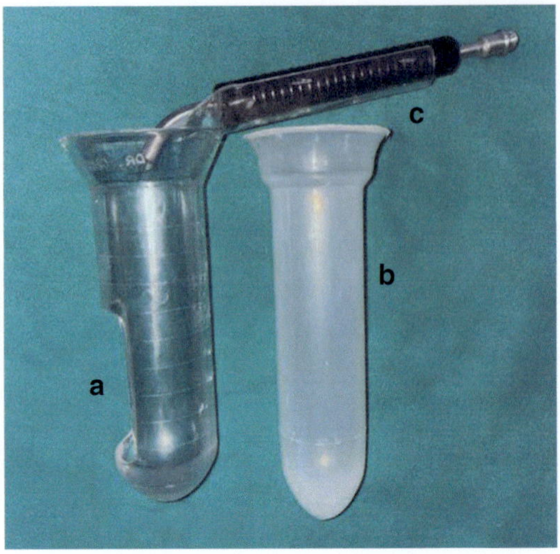

Fig. 7.1 Chivate's operative proctoscope with operating window (**a**), obturator (**b**) and light fountain (**c**)

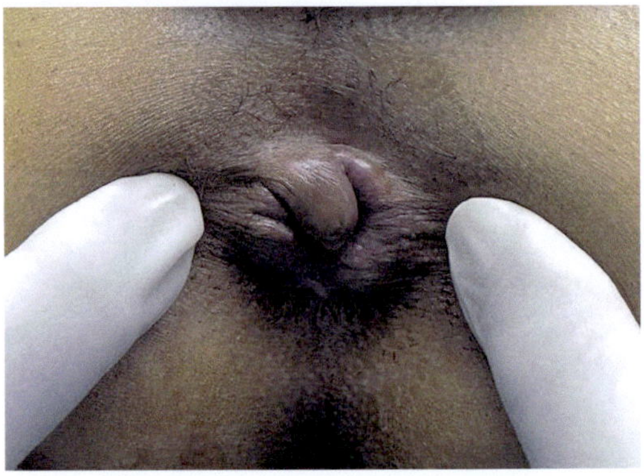

Fig. 7.2 Preoperative assessment for grade of protrusion Grade 3 haemorrhoids

7.6 Pre-operative Preparation

- Pre-operative assessment for grade of protrusion (Fig. 7.2).
- Proctoclysis enema 2 hours before the procedure and ask the patient to evacuate.
- Prophylactic antibiotics ofloxacin and metronidazole with induction of anaesthesia.

7.7 Position

- Lithotomy deep Trendelenburg.

7.8 Procedure [1]

- Gentle massage and reduction of haemorrhoids after lubrication (Fig. 7.3).
- Insertion of specialised proctoscope will further reduce the prolapsing tissue.
- Start first suture at any position circumferentially 2 cm proximal to dentate line. We usually start at 5 0′ position through the window provided in the proctoscope for the purpose (Fig. 7.4).
- Knot the first suture and pull it to tent the tissue, then take bite for running suture, enter needle perpendicular to mucosa 2 mm prior to exit point of previous suture and double lock it passing twice through its loop and press it tight. 1/2 circle 30-mm needle when rotated as described takes smooth muscle of the rectum so that redundant mucosa and submucosa get fixed to smooth muscle. Caution not to push needle beyond the full thickness of rectal muscle (Figs. 7.4 and 7.5).
- Go on rotating the scope so that operating window moves radially. Large diameter of the proctoscope ensures that mucosa remains flat and does not get twisted spirally.
- Complete first suture line by coming back to starting point and secure it with a knot after double lock so that there is no string effect (Fig. 7.6).

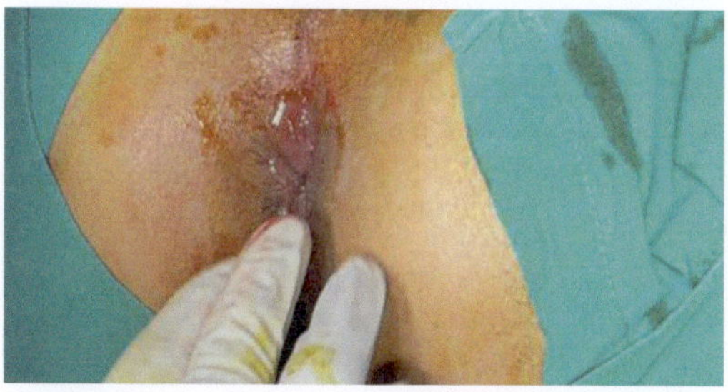

Fig. 7.3 Patient in deep Trendelenburg position, reduction of haemorrhoids after lubrication and gentle massage

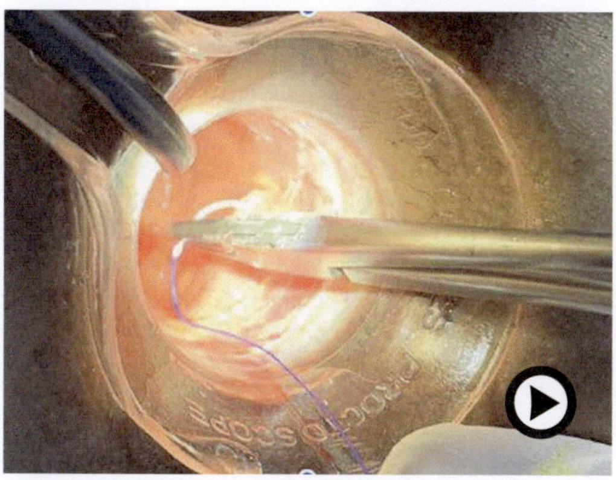

Fig. 7.4 Bite for the first suture 2 cm proximal to dentate line, note how the needle tip is kept perpendicular to mucosa for easy passage through appropriate depth. Video 7.1 Chivate Procedure (▶ https://doi.org/10.1007/000-hpw)

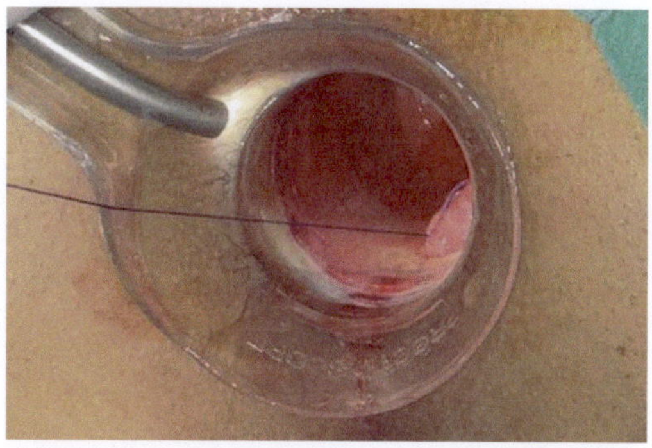

Fig. 7.5 Every bite of continuous suture is double locked for effective ligation and prevention of purse-string effect of running suture

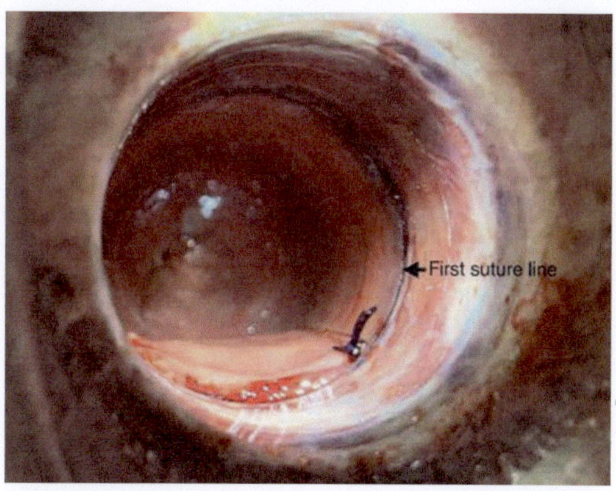

Fig. 7.6 First suture line 2 cm proximal to dentate line

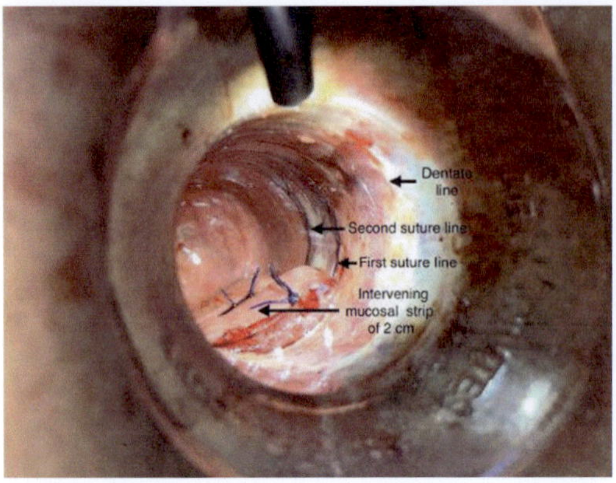

Fig. 7.7 All land marks for suturing in Chivate's procedure

- Apply second suture line 2 cm proximal to first line (Fig. 7.7).
  Intervening strip of mucosa never gets ischaemic (Fig. 7.7).
- Inventor of the procedure hypothesised that second suture line decreases chances of development of collaterals after one suture line blocks the vascular pedicles [2].
- Put the obturator back in the proctoscope. Now pull out proctoscope with obturator otherwise margins of window can abrade large haemorrhoids while withdrawing.
- Check for any ooze which can be controlled with saline-soaked gauze.
- Any bleeding from puncture site if it enters a vessel is automatically taken care by proceeding suture which is taken 2 mm prior to exit-point of preceding suture (see suggested Video SV 7.2).
- Always fully reduce the prolapsing tissue before one starts suturing by keeping patient in deep trendelenburg position.
- Use 2.0 polyglactin suture on 1/2 circle 30-mm taper cut or round body needle. Large circle needle a.c.t 27 mm 5/8 needle used for haemorrhoid artery ligation (HAL) is required, to go deeper and take more tissue to fix mucosa and submucosa to circular muscle.
- Double-locking is must to avoid purse-string effect.
- While withdrawing Chivate's proctoscope, always put obturator in and then remove the assembly otherwise margins of the operative window can abrade large haemorrhoidal cushions.
- Always do check proctoscopy with routine proctoscopes so that any ooze which was not visible due to pressure of large size proctoscope, should become apparent on table before one leaves the patient.

7.9 Complications

Complications after trans-anal suture mucopexy are very minimal and minor (Table 7.1).

Table 7.1 Complications in Chivate's procedure

Complications	Prevention	Management
Urinary retention	I/V Fluid restriction during surgery	One time catheterisation
Bleeding	Very minimal check proctoscopy on table Press with gauge piece or figure-of-8 suture to ligate bleeding point with a small needle and fine suture	Very low incidence resolves itself, do proctoscopy and decide
Pain	Remain proximal to dentate line and good amount of lubrication as diameter of proctoscope is large	Oral analgesics usually suffice
Pruritis	Mechanical irritation of the procedure or because of threads	Antihistaminics
Constipation	Good hydration and control of pain if any	Oral laxatives

Algorithm for Chivate's Procedure

Clinical assessment
Spinal anaesthesia
Deep Trendelenburg position
Reduction of all prolapsed tissue
Gentle massage lubrication and anal dilation with fingers and obturator
No forceful stretching
Put Chivate's proctoscope in anal canal
Take first layer of continuous double locking sutures 2 cm proximal to dentate line
Take second layer of continuous double locking suture 2 cm proximal to first layer leaving 2 cm strip of intervening mucosa
Put obturator back in and withdraw whole assembly out
Do check proctoscopy with routine proctoscope
Any ooze control with wet gauge pressure
Or
Take figure of 8 suture

References

1. Chivate SD, Ladukar L, Ayyar M, Mahajan V, Kavathe S. Transanal suture rectopexy for haemorrhoids: Chivate's painless cure for piles. Indian J Surg. 2012;74(5):412–7. https://doi.org/10.1007/s12262-012-0461-4. Epub 2012 Mar 22. PMID: 24082598; PMCID: PMC3477406.
2. Chivate SD, Killedar MM, Ladukar LD, Vardhani GS, Kavathe SK, Kanekar SR. Transanal suture mucopexy for hemorrhoids. Dis Colon Rectum. 2022;65(5):742–9. https://doi.org/10.1097/DCR.0000000000002191. PMID: 34958048; PMCID: PMC8985695.

Suggested Viewing

Dr Chivate's personal views on the procedure Video Abstract at http://links.lww.com/DCR/B841. (SV 7.1) Chivate SD, Killedar MM, Ladukar LD, Vardhani GS, Kavathe SK, Kanekar SR. Transanal suture mucopexy for hemorrhoids. Dis Colon Rectum. 2022;65(5):742–9. https://doi.org/10.1097/DCR.0000000000002191. PMID: 34958048; PMCID: PMC8985695.

Link for video (SV 7.2) published in Colorectal Disease journal https://www.youtube.com/watch?v=g28akcpcWoQ

8 Fissure in Ano: Office Procedure Botulinum Toxin Injection

Abstract

- Anal fissure induces pain, which leads to spasm of involuntary muscle called as internal anal sphincter. How this traumatic ulcer in distal anal region changes to ischaemic ulcer and refuses to heal, has been explained.
- When medicinal therapy so-called chemical sphincterotomy in the form of calcium channel blockers or nitric oxide donors fail and permanent damage to part of internal sphincter is not justified in the form of lateral internal sphincterotomy, there comes the role of temporary paralysis of internal sphincter.
- How to do that effectively by use of botulinum toxin is explained well.
- Different formulations of botulinum toxin, dosage and how to reconstitute the drug safely and efficiently are described.
- Indications and possible contraindications are enumerated.
- Where and how to inject the prescribed dosage of toxin has been explained step-wise.
- To further make the point, a video of the procedure is also shown and can be viewed on the web-link provided in the chapter.
- As a norm, complications, their prevention and management are grouped in a table for easy reference.
- "Tips and Tricks" will make the reader wiser.
- Some more details can be searched in "References" and "Suggested Reading" sections.

Supplementary Information The online version contains supplementary material available at https://doi.org/10.1007/978-981-96-6190-9_8. The videos can be accessed individually by clicking the DOI link in the accompanying figure caption or by scanning this link with the SN More Media App.

8.1 What One Should Know Before the Procedure

- Fissure leads to increased tone of internal sphincter due to spasm induced by pain, in turn it leads to local ischaemia and non-healing ulcer in lower anal canal called fissure. Traumatic ulcer becomes an ischaemic ulcer.
- Local wound conditions like fibrosed and rolled margins of fissure also delay healing.
- So the treatment is tailored to decrease the tone of internal sphincter to normal and improve local condition of the wound.
- Botox paralyses the sphincter temporarily, thereby normalising tone for some months which allows time for healing of fissure by restoring perfusion [1].
- What is the optimal site for injection of BOTOX? Whether internal sphincter, intersphincteric space or external sphincter is not known but most of the clinicians including us, inject in internal sphincter.

8.2 Indications [2]

- Failed medical therapy.
- Patient at risk for incontinence. Botulinum toxin has been used to treat chronic but

S. K. Singla, K. Mital, *Operative Manual of Minimally Invasive and LASER Ano-proctology*,
https://doi.org/10.1007/978-981-96-6190-9_8

uncomplicated anal fissure while averting the risk of permanent injury of the internal anal sphincter.
- Patient not ready for surgery.

8.3 Contra-indications

- Patients with acute or chronic anal fissure associated with other conditions like chronic inflammatory bowel disease, HIV infection, tuberculosis, sexually transmitted diseases, immunosuppression, anorectal or perianal cancer.
- Patient with complicated chronic anal fissure like fissure fistula complex or associated abscess, should be submitted for surgery.
- Patients with Down syndrome and Alzheimer's disease due to altered cholinergic transmission.
- Pregnancy and lactation.
- Hypersensitivity to the components of the toxin formulations.

8.4 Equipment

- The botulinum toxin type A has two type of formulations.
  1. American formulation (Botox®; Allergan, Irvine, California, USA), the vials contained 100 IU of type A botulinum toxin stored at a temperature of −20 °C and diluted with saline solution at 50 IU/ml, at the time of use
  2. European formulation (Dysport®; Spywood Biopharm, Wrexham, UK), the vials contained 500 freeze-dried IU of type A botulinum toxin diluted in saline solution at 150 IU/ml. A conversion factor of 1 to 3 (1 IU Botox = 3 IU Dysport) is adopted [3]. This conversion factor is due to the different potency of the two toxin preparations.
- Syringes 1 ml and fine needle 27 no.
- Numbing agents and local anaesthetic agents (optional if procedure is planned under local anaesthesia).

8.5 How to Reconstitute the Botulinum Toxin

- Botulinum toxin is available in our country as Botox.
- One vial contains 100 units but we use only 50 units in one case. It is a good idea to post two cases in same sitting to avoid wastage as we need freshly reconstituted solution for every case.
- Use 5 ml normal saline to reconstitute 100 units of BOTOX.
- Inject saline very slowly into the vial to make the solution.
- Do not shake the vial otherwise toxin molecules get destroyed.
- Only roll the vial (Fig. 8.1).
- Similarly, while withdrawing the drug from the vial, do slowly.
- Always use eye-protection glasses while handling botulinum toxin to avoid accidental spillage of toxin on to the conjunctiva, which can cause diplopia.

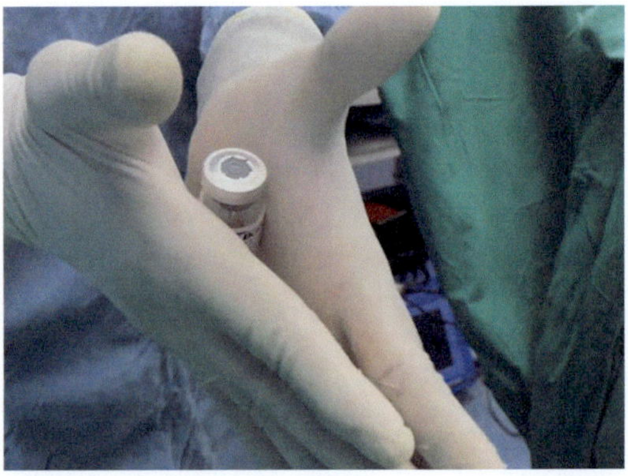

Fig. 8.1 To reconstitute the Botox only roll the vial in palm never shake vigorously

8.6 Pre-procedure Consideration

- No specific preparation is required.
- Its use in healing of fissure and prevention of permanent damage to part of the internal sphincter is explained to the patient.
- But counselling pertaining to inferior results of BOTOX as compared to surgery and possibility of some temporary incontinence at times, is also talked about.
- Concurrent use of medication capable of interfering with the action of the botulinum toxin (aminoglycosides, baclofen, dantrolene, or diazepam) should be avoided.

8.7 Position of the Patient

- Left lateral/Sim's position or lithotomy.

8.8 Anaesthesia

- Short general anaesthesia (GA)/sedation.

8.9 Procedure (Video 8.1)

- Clean and drape as in any intervention.
- Identify intersphincteric space and internal sphincter.
- Use eye-protection glasses.
- Take 1 ml of Botox constituted solution (100 units in 5 ml saline), i.e., 20 units in 1 ml syringe. Inject in internal sphincter on left side of the fissure (Fig. 8.2).
- Again take 1 ml constituted solution (20 units) in 1 ml syringe, and inject 20 units on right side of the fissure (Fig. 8.3). Always use fresh needle-syringe while withdrawing drug from the vial as it may be used in two patients.
- Take 0.5 ml of constituted solution, i.e., 10 units in a fresh 1 ml syringe and inject 10 units in the bed of the fissure (Fig. 8.4).
- Press the puncture site for 2–3 min to prevent any haematoma formation (Video 8.1).

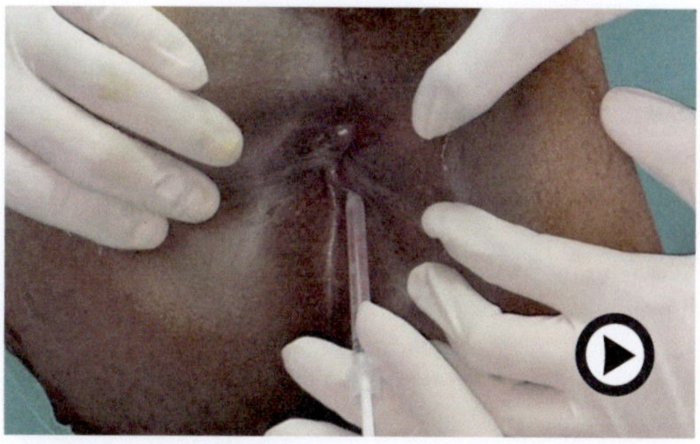

Fig. 8.2 Inject 20 units in internal sphincter (IS) on left of the fissure. Video 8.1 BOTOX application for fissure in ano (▶ https://doi.org/10.1007/000-hpx)

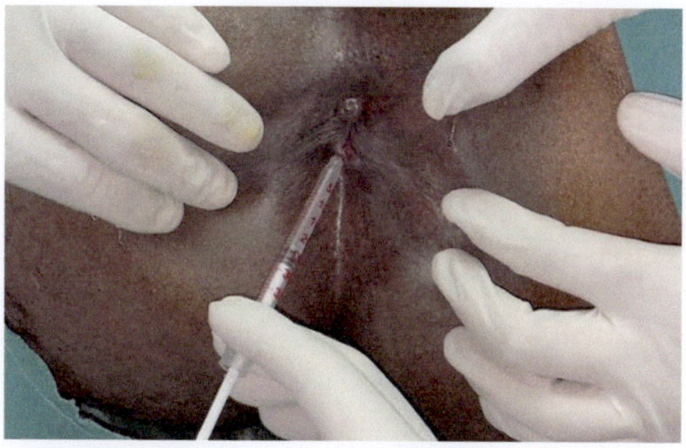

Fig. 8.3 Inject 20 units in IS on right of the fissure

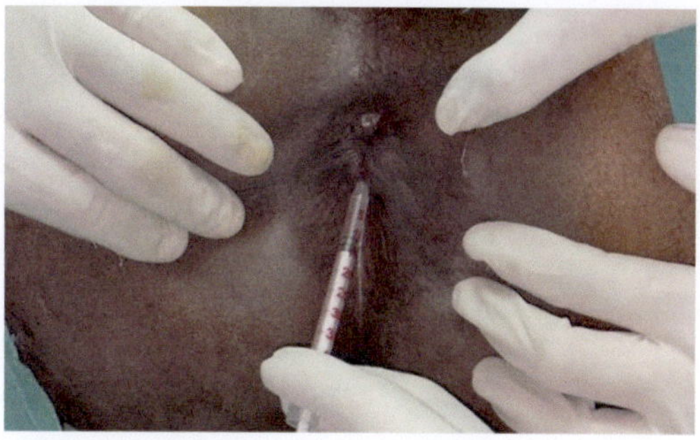

Fig. 8.4 Inject 10 units in fissure bed

8.10 Complication of Botox (Table 8.1)

Table 8.1 Complication of BOTOX prevention and management

Complication	Prevention	Management
Relatively common complication		
Skin rash		Topical steroids
Rare complications		
Peri-anal haematoma and thrombosis [4]	Keep the puncture site pressed for 3 min	Resolves with time. If painful then non steroidal anti inflammatory drugs (NSAID)
Temporary faecal incontinence [4]	Cannot prevent counselling	Self limited after a week counselling
Permanent incontinence [5]	Cannot prevent counselling	Counselling

Algorithm for Botulinum Toxin Injection for Treatment of Anal Fissure

Clinical assessment

Indication/contraindications

Counselling and consent

Lithotomy/left lateral position

Sedation/block/short GA

Reconstitute the toxin preparation in saline

Palpate the internal sphincter and define intersphincteric space

Take 20 units in 1 ml syringe with 27 gauge needle and inject in the internal sphincter on left side of the fissure

Repeat 20 units in 1 ml solution on right side of the fissure in internal sphincter

10 units to be given in internal sphincter in bed of the fissure

Press the puncture sites for 2–3 minutes

References

1. Jost WH, Schimrigk K. Therapy of anal fissure using botulin toxin. Dis Colon Rectum. 1994;37(12):1321–4. https://doi.org/10.1007/BF02257805.
2. Boland PA, Kelly ME, Donlon NE, et al. Management options for chronic anal fissure: a systematic review of randomised controlled trials. Int J Color Dis. 2020;35:1807–15. https://doi.org/10.1007/s00384-020-03699-4.
3. Brisinda G, Albanese A, Cadeddu F, Bentivoglio AR, Mabisombi A, Marniga G, et al. Botulinum neurotoxin to treat chronic anal fissure: results of a randomized "Botox vs. Dysport" controlled trial. Aliment Pharmacol Ther. 2004;19:695–701.
4. Jost WH, Schanne S, Mlitz H, Schimrigk K. Perianal thrombosis following injection therapy into the external anal sphincter using botulin toxin. Dis Colon Rectum. 1995;38(7):781. https://doi.org/10.1007/BF02048044.
5. Peeroo S, Rajagopalan A, Arachchi A, Penfold S, Roschach B, Nguyen TC, Teoh W. Outcomes following intrasphincteric injection of botulinum toxin for treatment of anal fissures. Cureus. 2024;16(2):e53668. https://doi.org/10.7759/cureus.53668. PMID: 38327720; PMCID: PMC10847891.

Suggested Readings

Bobkiewicz A, Francuzik W, Krokowicz L, Studniarek A, Ledwosiński W, Paszkowski J, Drews M, Banasiewicz T. Botulinum toxin injection for treatment of chronic anal fissure: is there any dose-dependent efficiency? A meta-analysis: original scientifc report. World J Surg. 2016. https://doi.org/10.1007/s00268-016-3693-9.

Glover PH, Tang SJ, Whatley JZ, Davis ED, Jex KT, Wu R, Lahr CJ. High-dose circumferential chemodenervation of the internal anal sphincter: a new treatment modality for uncomplicated chronic anal fissure: a retrospective cohort study (with video). Int J Surg. 2015;23(Pt A):1–4. https://doi.org/10.1016/j.ijsu.2015.08.076. Epub 2015 Sep 11. PMID: 26365430.

Shearer J, Gurland B. Anal examination under anesthesia and Botox injection for chronic anal fissures. J Med Insight. 2023;2023(371). https://doi.org/10.24296/jomi/371.

9 Fissure in Ano: Lateral Partial Internal Sphincterotomy (LIS)

Abstract

- Journey of the fissures from rhagades to acute fissures, chronic non-healing fissures and later developing complications like associated sepsis and fistulae is presented in clinical pictures.
- Anal fissures, which do not heal with conservative methods or show signs of chronicity, are best managed by lateral internal sphincterotomy (LIS).
- Indications and contraindications of LIS are explained with clinical photographs.
- Procedure of closed internal sphincterotomy using number 15 surgical blade is demonstrated by clinical photographs and video.
- Complications though very few, are presented in table-form for ready reference.
- "References" and "Suggested Reading" sections will make reader aware about recommendations by surgical society and other advancements in surgical management of this painful condition.

Supplementary Information The online version contains supplementary material available at https://doi.org/10.1007/978-981-96-6190-9_9. The videos can be accessed individually by clicking the DOI link in the accompanying figure caption or by scanning this link with the SN More Media App.

9.1 What One Should Know Before the Procedure

- Local trauma in anal canal (due to hard constipated stools or recurrent stress due to an episode of diarrhoea or may be during child birth) (Fig. 9.1) leads to increased tone of internal sphincter due to spasm of pain. In turn, it leads to local ischaemia at the site of initial trauma and development of a non-healing ulcer in lower anal canal called fissure. Traumatic ulcer becomes an ischaemic ulcer (Fig. 9.2).
- Local-wound condition like fibrosed and rolled margins of fissure also delay healing.

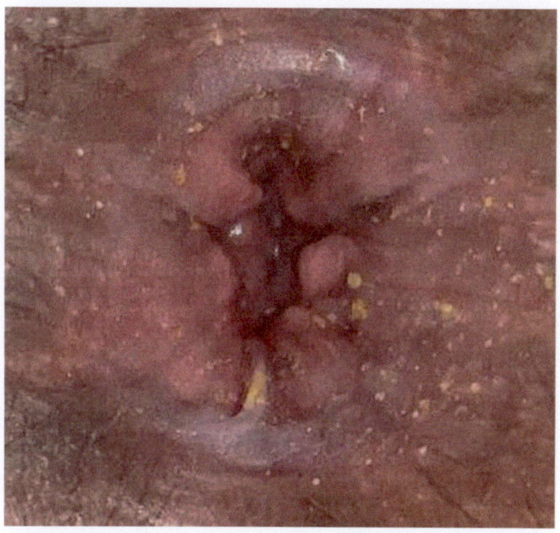

Fig. 9.1 How fissures start, as traumatic ulcer as seen at 6′ 0 usually labelled as rhagades, should be managed by medical therapy

S. K. Singla, K. Mital, *Operative Manual of Minimally Invasive and LASER Ano-proctology*,
https://doi.org/10.1007/978-981-96-6190-9_9

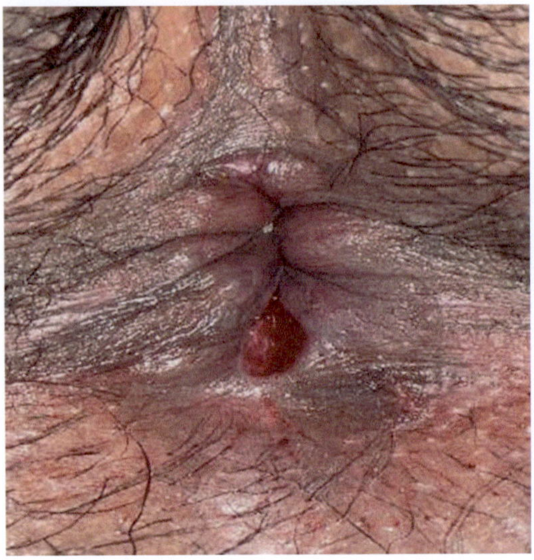

Fig. 9.2 Well-formed acute fissure Without anal tag 42% need surgery

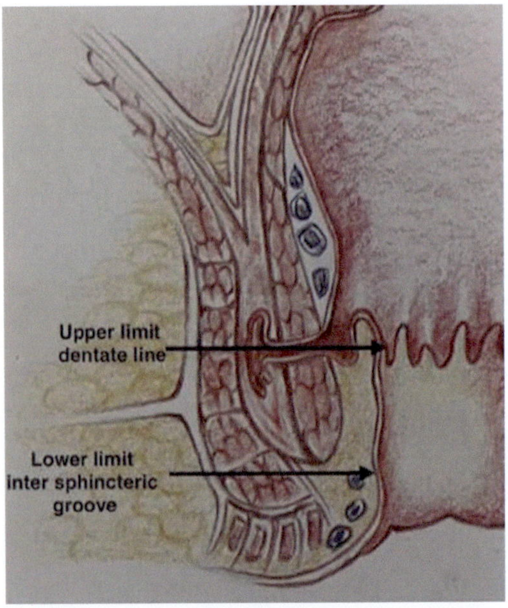

Fig. 9.3 Sketch showing boundaries of classical anal fissure White line of Hilton corresponds to inter-sphincteric groove

- So the treatment is tailored to decrease the tone of internal sphincter to normal and improve local condition of the wound.

  Surface anatomy of fissure (Figs. 9.3, 9.4, and 9.5).

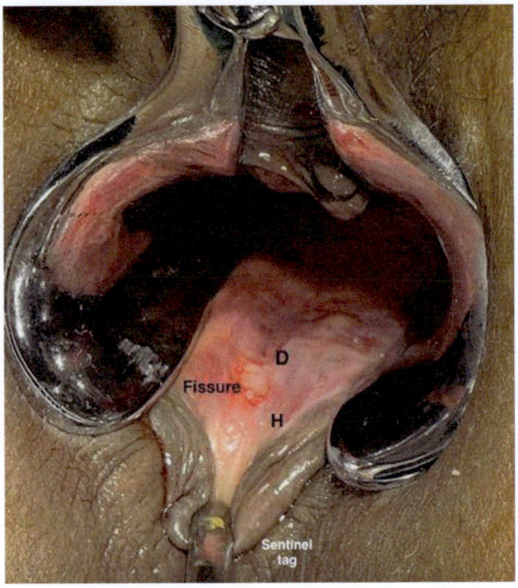

Fig. 9.4 Clinical photograph to show limits of fissure in posterior mid-line (D), dentate line (H), white line of Hilton, note sentinel tag and internal sphincter fibres in bed of the fissure

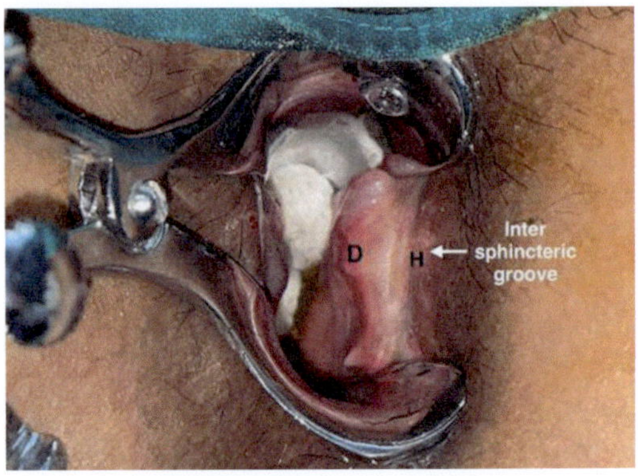

Fig. 9.5 Anal opening. Park's speculum opened to show left lateral sector, (D) dentate line (H). White line of Hilton which corresponds to inter-sphincteric groove

- Classical fissure extends superiorly up to dentate line and limits itself up to white line of Hilton inferiorly, which corresponds to inter-sphincteric groove (Fig. 9.4).
- Inter-sphincteric groove is the surface-marking to enter blade or LASER fibre in the inter-sphincteric space for performing partial lateral internal sphincterotomy (LIS) (Fig. 9.5).

9.2 Indications

- Fissures with intense pain and spasm not managed by appropriate medical therapy and so-called chemical sphincterotomy (Fig. 9.2).
- Chronic anal fissure with stigmata of chronicity
  - Sentinel tag (Fig. 9.6).
  - Hypertrophied anal papilla.
  - Rolled and/or fibrosed fissure margins.
  - Fibres of internal sphincter visible at the base of fissure.
- Patient with complicated chronic anal fissure like associated abscess or fissure fistula complex (Figs. 9.7 and 9.8)

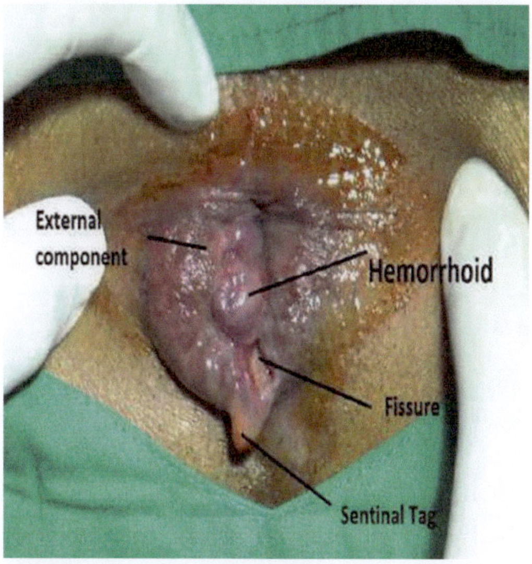

Fig. 9.6 Ch. anal fissure associated anal tag, 72% need surgery

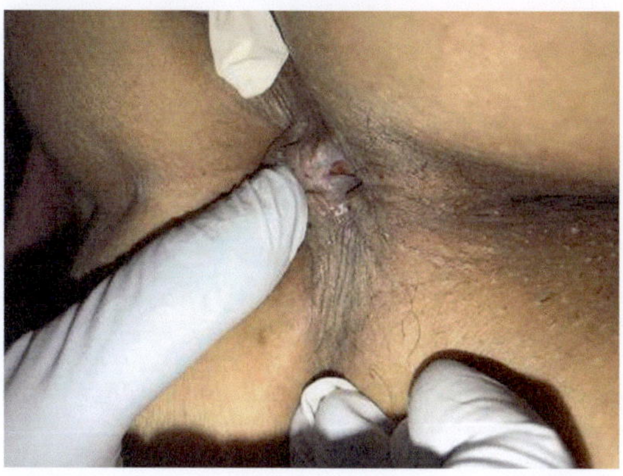

Fig. 9.7 Fissure with associated abscess in Post. midline. Patient in left lateral position

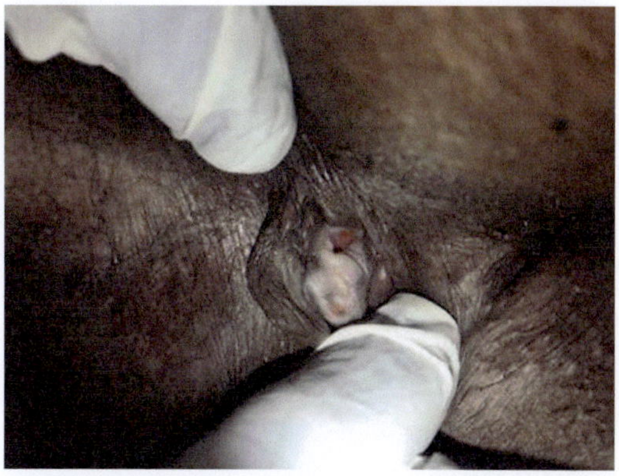

Fig. 9.8 Fissure fistula complex in posterior mid line. Patient in left lateral position

9.3 Contra-indications

- LIS may be excluded as first-line therapy, in women with prior obstetrical injuries, patients with IBD, patients who have undergone previous anorectal operations, and patients with a documented anal sphincter injury [1].
- Patients with acute or chronic anal fissure associated with other conditions like chronic inflammatory bowel disease, HIV infection, tuberculosis, sexually transmitted diseases, immunosuppression, anorectal or perianal cancer.

9.4 Equipment

- Operation table with stirrups for lithotomy
- For prone-position rolled-sheets and cushions with tapes for strapping (optional)
- Sterilized drapes and gowns
- Povidine iodine solution
- Xylocaine jelly, surgical gloves, saline-soaked gauge pieces
- Syringes
- Normal saline and lignocaine 2%
- Park's speculum
- Surgical blade number 15 or Von Graefe's cataract-knife (Fig. 9.9)

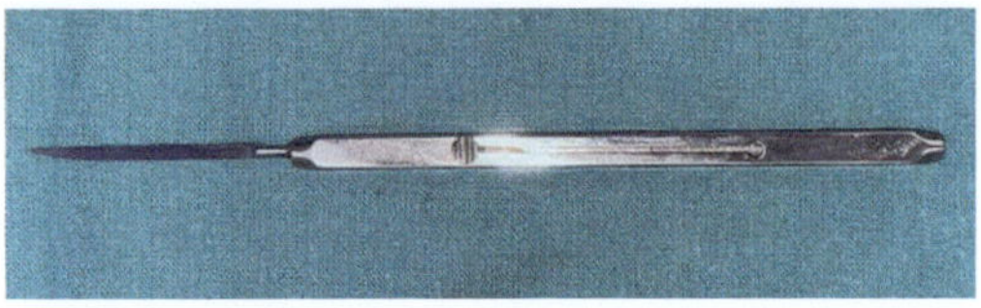

Fig. 9.9 Von Graefe's cataract knife

9.5 Procedure

- Lithotomy position.
- Short GA/pudendal block.
- Lubricate the anal canal with xylocaine jelly 2%.
- Gentle anoscopy.
- Insert Park's speculum in anterior posterior direction/or insert vaginal speculum.
- Inspect fissure (Fig. 9.4).
- Rotate Park's speculum by 90°.
- Open speculum to slightly stretch the anal canal to make sphincter prominent and visible at 1 ′0 to 5 ′0 position (Fig. 9.5).
- Feel the inter-sphincteric groove (Fig. 9.5).
- Insert number 15 blade in the groove by keeping it flat to internal sphincter and lateral to it (Fig. 9.10).
- One can use Von Graefe's cataract knife (Fig. 9.9).
- Go up to dentate line.
- Rotate the blade so that sharp end touches the lateral side of internal sphincter.
- Cut the internal sphincter from out to in, i.e., lateral to medial while protecting the anoderm (Fig. 9.11).
- Remove the blade.
- Remove the speculum.
- Feel the defect caused by lateral partial internal sphincterotomy.
- Pinch the area to stop any bleeding (Fig. 9.12).
- Bleeding from cut muscle stops as soon as patient comes out of anaesthesia and muscle contracts.
- Associated sentinel-tag is excised and margins of the fissure excised to freshen the margins.
- Any associated abscess or fistula (which usually is very superficial) is laid open and margins excised.

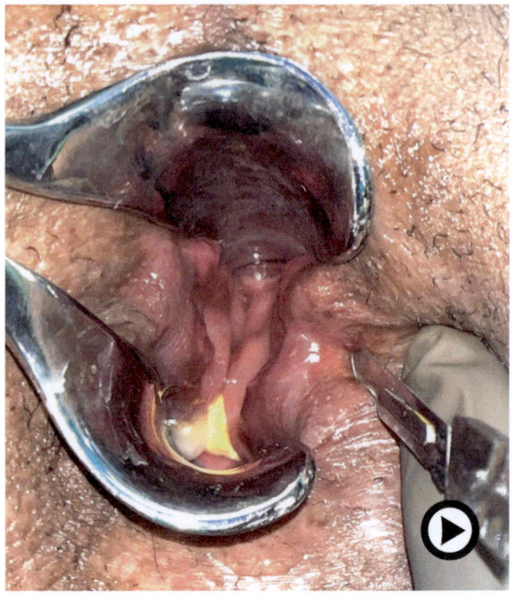

Fig. 9.10 Insertion of number 15 blade in the groove. Note: blade is flat to internal sphincter and lateral to it. Video 9.1 Closed partial lateral internal sphinctrotomy (▶ https://doi.org/10.1007/000-hpy)

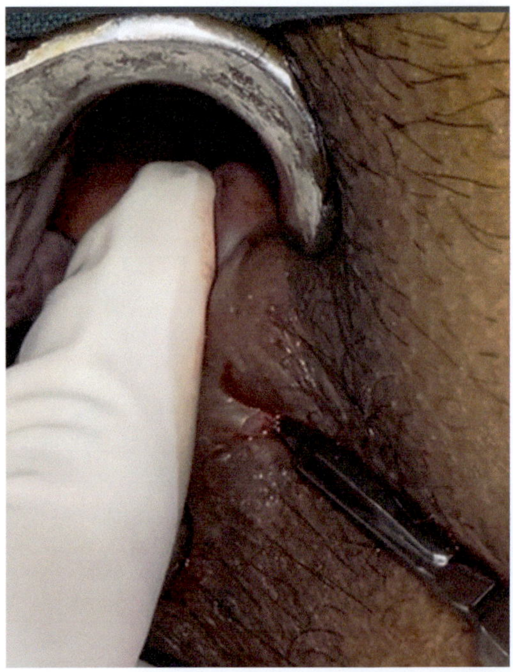

Fig. 9.11 Incise the distal internal sphincter from out to in and guard anoderm by left-hand index finger

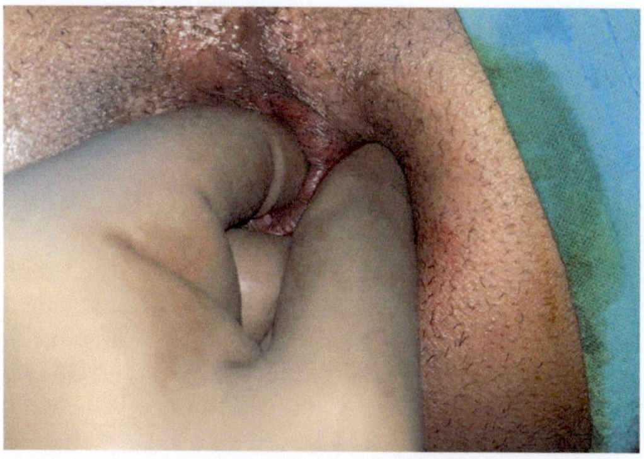

Fig. 9.12 Pinch with thumb and index finger of left hand to stop bleeding

- 5 to 10 cc solution of methylene blue 1% mixed with bupivicaine 0.25% in 1:5 ratio is injected intra-dermal around the wound below the dentate line (Video 9.1).

9.6 Tips and Tricks

- Opening of Park's speculum in lateral position brings sphincter on stretch which, in turn, felicitates identification of inter sphincteric groove.
- Do not use number 11 blade as its tip has more chances of damaging anoderm. Instead use number 15 surgical blade. Be careful when using Von Graefe's knife for the same reason.
- Bleeding from cut sphincter stops, once effect of anaesthesia is over and muscle contracts.
- Pinch the area for 3 min to stop bleeding otherwise next day, at times, one finds echymosis in the area.
- 2022 Updated recommendations by ASCRS [1].

Lateral internal sphincterotomy tailored to the length of the fissure yields similar healing-rates but decreased faecal incontinence rates compared with traditional lateral internal sphincterotomy extending to the dentate line. Grade of recommendation: strong recommendation based on high-quality evidence, 1A.

9.7 Complications of LIS (Table 9.1)

Table 9.1 Complications of LIS

Complications	Prevention	Management
Bleeding from stab site	Avoid external vascular channel while inserting blade	Press for 3 min or bipolar coagulation
Damage to anoderm	Avoid number 11 blade	Stitch with 3.0 suture
Flatus incontinence	Do tailored sphincterotomy, only up to the length of fissure [1].	Kegel's exercise to increase anal tone as external sphincter also contributes towards resting tone
Submucous fistula	Avoid damage to anoderm and mucosa	Lay it open

Algorithm for LIS

Clinical assessment
Fissure with increased tone
Not relieved by conservative means
Fissure with signs of chronicity and increased anal tone
Complex anal fissure with associated fistula or abscess
Saddle block/short GA/with or without pudendal block
Put the anal speculum to slightly stretch the internal sphincter(IS)
Stab 15 no blade in the intersphincteric space and advance till dentate line, keeping blade flat to internal sphincter
Rotate the sharp end of blade towards IS and keep left hand index finger as guard
Cut the distal internal sphincter
Pinch the area for at least 3 minutes to stop bleeding

References

1. Davids JS, Alexander MD, Hawkins T, Bhama AR, Feinberg AE, Grieco MJ, Lightner AL, Feingold DL, Paquette IM. The American Society of colon and rectal surgeons clinical practice guidelines for the management of anal fissures. Dis Colon Rectum. 2022;66:190–9. https://doi.org/10.1097/DCR.0000000000002664.

Suggested Readings

Alawady M, Emile SH, Abdelnaby M, Elbanna H, Farid M. Posterolateral versus lateral internal anal sphincterotomy in the treatment of chronic anal fissure: a randomized controlled trial. Int J Color Dis. 2018;33(10):1461–7.

Lee KH, Hyun K, Yoon SG, Lee JK. Minimal lateral internal sphincterotomy (LIS): is it enough to cut less than the conventional tailored LIS? Ann Coloproctol. 2021;37(5):275–80. https://doi.org/10.3393/ac.2020.00976.0139. Epub 2021 Jul 9. PMID: 34246204; PMCID: PMC8566144.

Liang J, Church JM. Lateral internal sphincterotomy for surgically recurrent chronic anal fissure. Am J Surg. 2015;210(4):715–9. https://doi.org/10.1016/j.amjsurg.2015.05.005. Epub 2015 Jun 27. PMID: 26231724.

Salati S. Anal fissure – an extensive update. Pol J Surg. 2021;93(4):46–56. https://doi.org/10.5604/01.3001.0014.7879.

10 LIS and LASERS

Abstract

- How a traumatic ulcer in the anus changes to ischaemic ulcer called as fissure is well explained.
- When medical ways to decrease intra-anal pressure fail and ulcer refuses to heal, one resorts to surgical ways to modulate intra-anal pressure by incising distal part of internal anal sphincter called as internal sphincerotomy. Why to do it laterally is explained.
- One can use mechanical energy in the form of surgical blade to execute lateral internal sphinctrotomy (LIS) or one can use light amplification by stimulated emission of radiation (LASER) energy to exhibit LIS, with an advantage of minimal bleeding even when external vascular channels are prominent at 3 0′ position.
- Different ways to do LIS with LASER are explained fully by clinical photographs and videos.
- Possible complications, their prevention and management are presented in tabulated form for ready reference.
- Further in-depth information about precise role of LASER can be found in "Suggested Reading" section.

Supplementary Information The online version contains supplementary material available at https://doi.org/10.1007/978-981-96-6190-9_10. The videos can be accessed individually by clicking the DOI link in the accompanying figure caption or by scanning this link with the SN More Media App.

10.1 What One Should Know Before the Procedure

- Fissure leads to increased tone of internal sphincter due to spasm of pain, in turn, it leads to local ischaemia and non-healing ulcer in lower anal canal called "fissure".

  Traumatic ulcer becomes an ischaemic ulcer.
- Local wound conditions like fibrosed and rolled margins of fissure also delay healing.
- So the treatment is tailored to decrease the tone of internal sphincter to normal and improve local condition of the wound.
- Midline posterior sphincterotomy leads to key-hole deformity, that is why distal internal sphincter is incised at a lateral site (3′0) or posterolateral site (4′0).

10.2 Indications

- Fissures with intense pain and spasm not managed by appropriate medical therapy or so-called chemical sphincterotomy.
- Chronic anal fissure with stigmata of chronicity
  - Sentinel tag
  - Hypertrophied anal papilla
  - Rolled and/or fibrosed fissure margins
  - Fibres of internal sphincter visible at the base of fissure
- Patients with complicated chronic anal fissure like fissure—fistula complex or associated abscess.

S. K. Singla, K. Mital, *Operative Manual of Minimally Invasive and LASER Ano-proctology*,
https://doi.org/10.1007/978-981-96-6190-9_10

10.3 Contra-indications

- Patients with acute or chronic anal fissure associated with other conditions like chronic inflammatory bowel disease, HIV infection, tuberculosis, sexually transmitted diseases, immunosuppression, anorectal or perianal cancer.

10.4 Equipment (Fig. 10.1a, b)

- Operation table with stirrups for lithotomy
- For prone position, rolled sheets and cushions with tapes for strapping (optional)
- Sterilized drapes and gowns
- Povidine iodine solution
- Xylocaine jelly, surgical gloves, saline-soaked gauge pieces

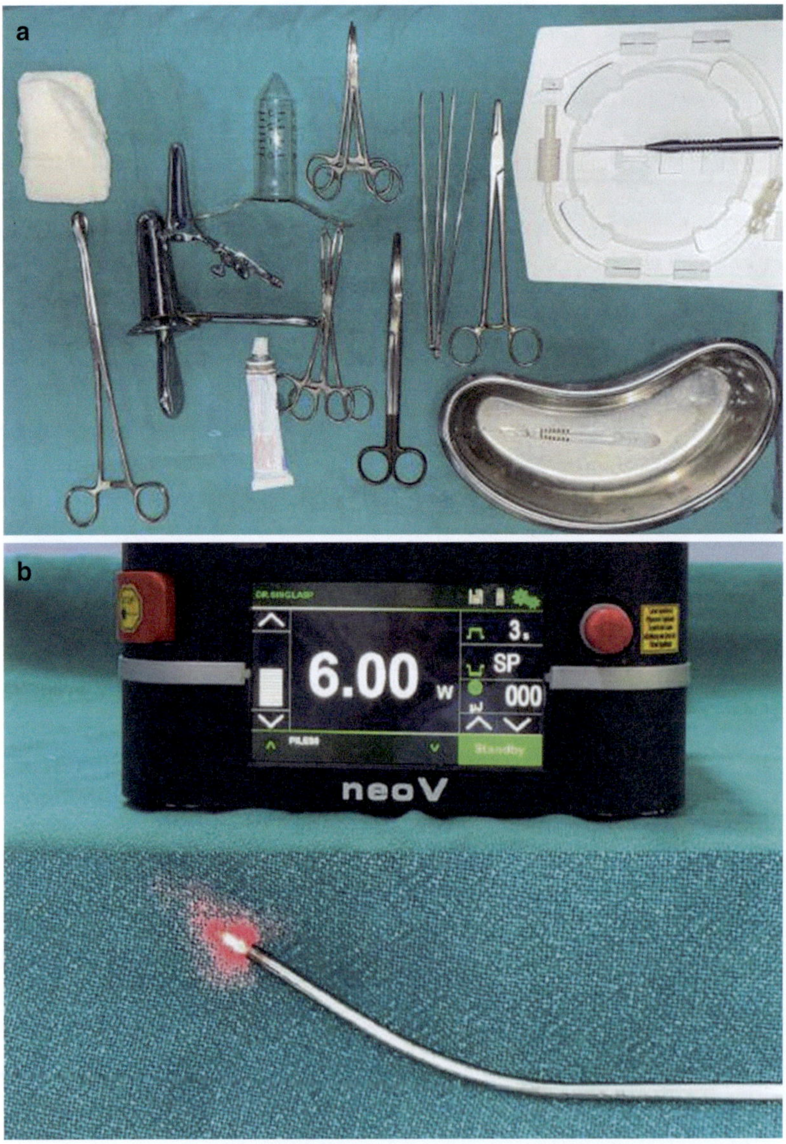

Fig. 10.1 (**a**) Trolley for surgery for fissure in ano with LASER fibre. (**b**) LASER machine 1470 nm diode LASER and bare LASER fibre

- Syringes
- Normal saline and lignocaine 2%
- Park's speculum
- LASER machine diode 1470 nm and bare fibre (Fig. 10.1a, b)

10.5 Procedure (Video 10.1)

- Lithotomy position.
- Short GA/pudendal block.
- Lubricate the anal canal.
- Do anoscopy.
- Insert Park's speculum in antero-posterior direction.
- Inspect fissure.
- Rotate park speculum by 90°.
- Open speculum to stretch the anal canal to make sphincter prominent and visible at 1 0′ to 5 0′ position (Fig. 10.2).
- Feel the inter-sphincteric groove.
- Inject some saline at 3 o′ position over inter-sphincteric groove (Fig. 10.3).
- Give small incision over inter-sphincteric groove with bare fibre using 7 Watts energy of 1470 diode LASER in continuous mode (Fig. 10.4).
- Put small mosquito forceps lateral-to-internal sphincter and slightly open it (Fig. 10.5).
- Hook up fibres of distal internal sphincter over it, which can be recognised by comparative white colour (Fig. 10.6).

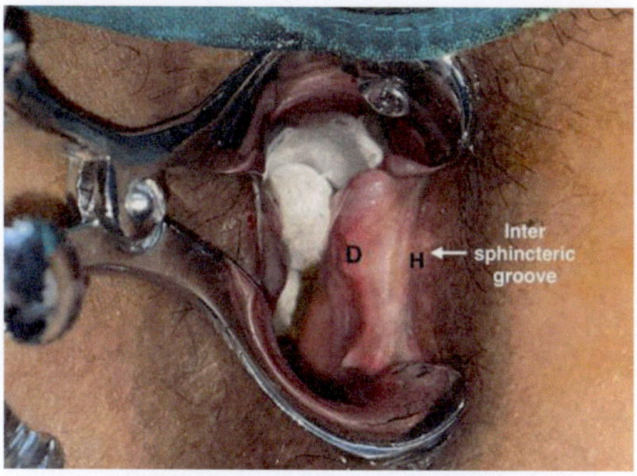

Fig. 10.2 Anal opening. Park's speculum opened to show left lateral sector, (D) dentate line (H) White line of Hilton which corresponds to inter-sphincteric groove

- Incise fibres of internal sphincter with bare fibre giving 7 Watts continuous wave LASER energy (Fig. 10.7).
- Feel the defect created by sphincterotomy up to dentate line.
- Usually there is no bleeding of consequence.

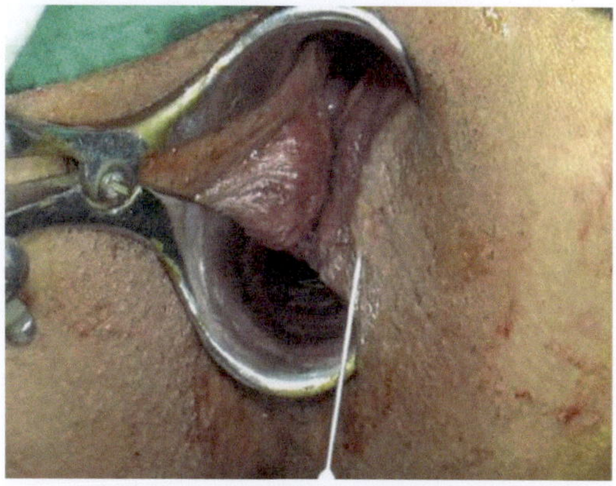

Fig. 10.3 Saline injected to provide tumescence and to prevent burn of the skin by LASER energy

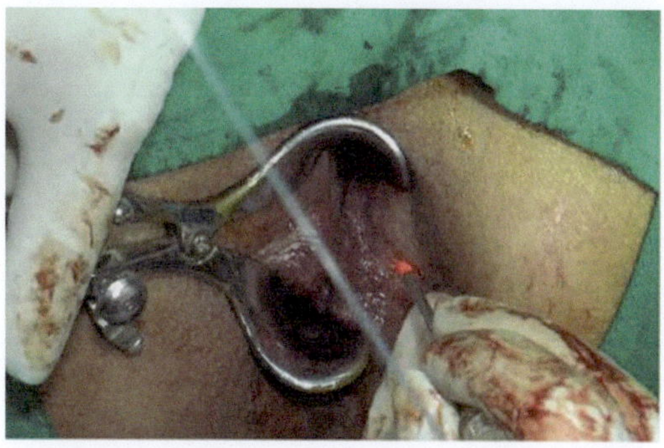

Fig. 10.4 Incision at 3′0 with bare LASER fibre 7 Watts continuous wave energy

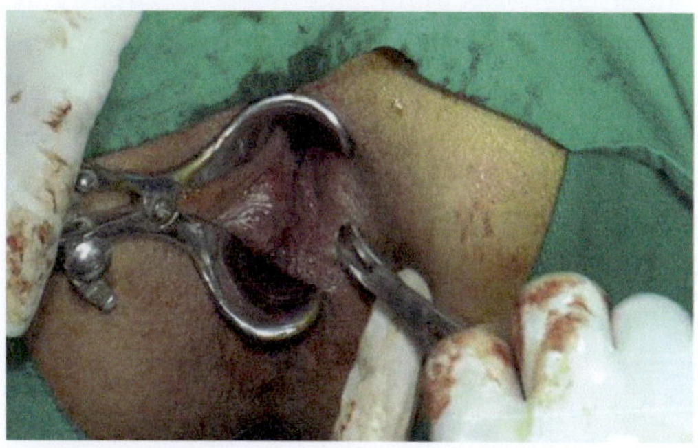

Fig. 10.5 Curved mosquito to create small space lateral to internal sphincter

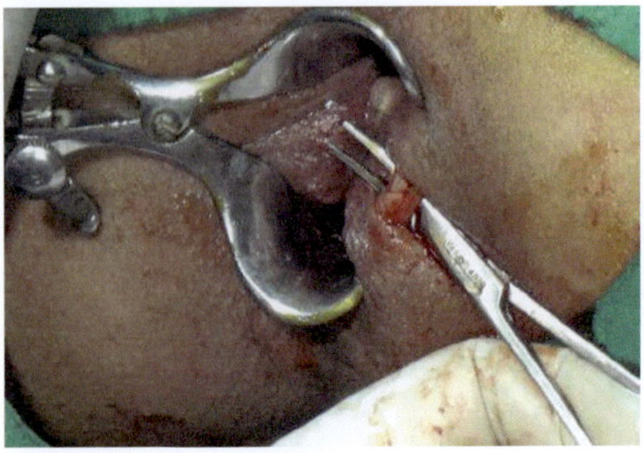

Fig. 10.6 Lift fibres of distal internal sphincter on curved artery forceps. Note: Whitish fibres are of IAS and reddish fibres are of subcutaneous EAS

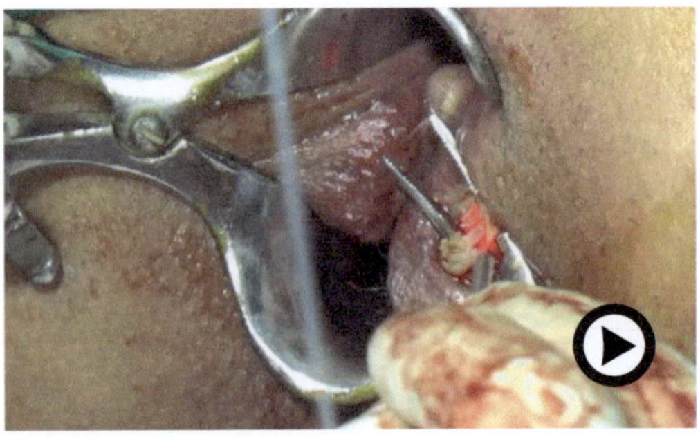

Fig. 10.7 Fibres of IAS incised with bare LASER fibre 7 Watts energy continuous wave. Video 10.1 LIS by LASERS (▶ https://doi.org/10.1007/000-hq0)

10.6 Alternative Way to Use LASER Fibre for LIS Under Vision Through Smaller Incision

- Put anal speculum and open it slightly to stretch anal sphincters mildly.
- Inject saline between anoderm and internal sphincter (IS).
- Make a small incision over inter-sphincteric groove (Fig. 10.8).
- Put curved mosquito forceps lateral to IS as a guard.
- Use forceps to handle the anoderm.
- Put LASER probe, between the mosquito forceps and forceps and incise IS fibres up to dentate line with 7 Watts continuous pulse energy (Figs. 10.9 and 10.10).
- Feel the defect created by LIS.
- Excise skin-tag by bare fibre LASER continuous wave (Fig. 10.11).

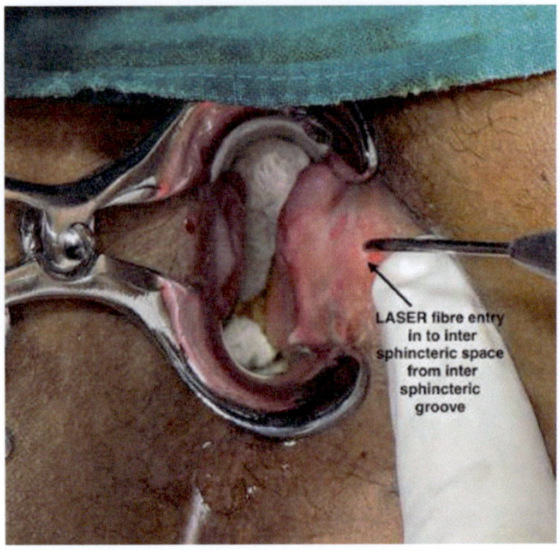

Fig. 10.8 Small incision over the inter-sphincteric groove by LASER

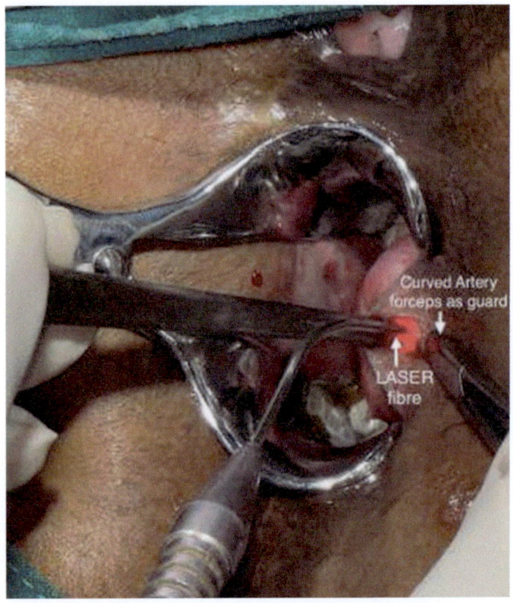

Fig. 10.9 LASER fibre between forceps and mosquito forceps as guard for anoderm and ES, respectively

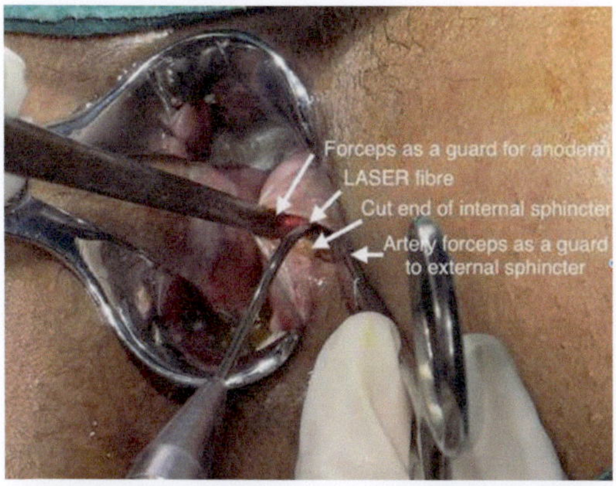

Fig. 10.10 LIS under vision, showing cut end of internal sphincter

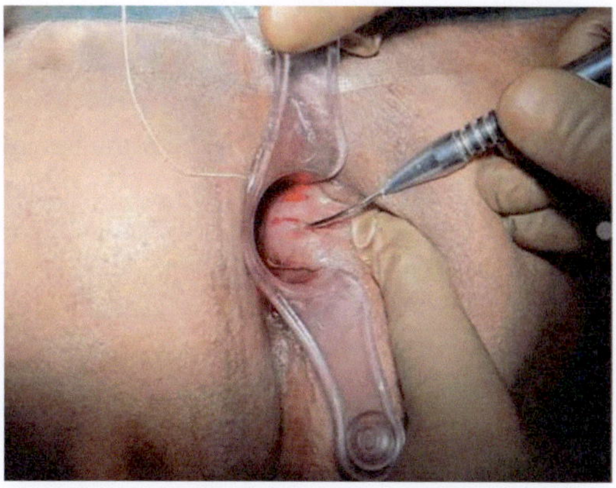

Fig. 10.12 LASER fibre negotiated up to dentate line in the space between anoderm and internal sphincter

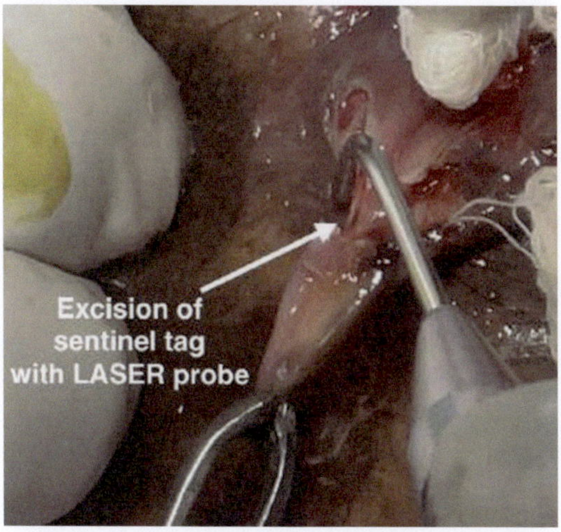

Fig. 10.11 Sentinel tag incision with LASER

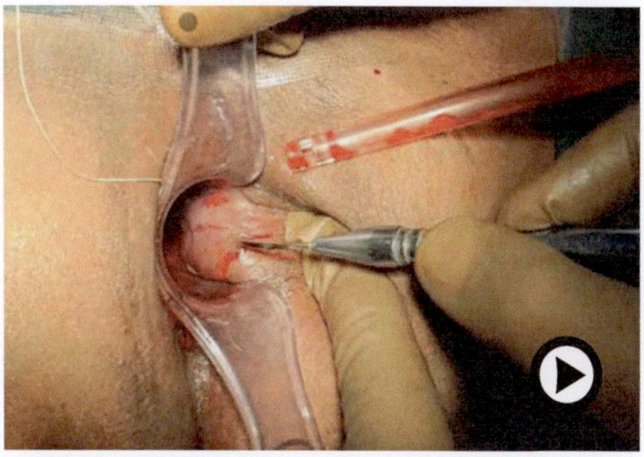

Fig. 10.13 Activated LASER fibre withdrawn to cut distal internal sphincter. Video 10.2 Closed LIS by LASER (▶ https://doi.org/10.1007/000-hpz)

10.7 Closed LIS by LASER (Video 10.2)

- Inspect and palpate the inter-sphincteric groove.
- Inject saline between anoderm and internal sphincter to create space between anoderm and sphincter.
- Wear eye-protective glasses.
- Ready the bare fibre.
- Put the fibre in the space between anoderm and internal sphincter with a press on the foot-pedal to deliver a burst of energy 7 Watts and negotiate fibre till the dentate line (Fig. 10.12).
- Rotate the angled handle so that tip of bare fibre touches medial side of internal sphincter.
- Start delivering energy in continuous mode and withdraw the fibre there by cutting distal internal sphincter (Fig. 10.13).

10.8 Fissure Local-Wound Management

- Rotate the Parks speculum to check the fissure bed.
- With bare LASER fibre, rolled margins of fissure and fissure bed are sprayed, and latter curetted with fine curette (Figs.10.14 and 10.15).
- It freshens the margin and removes dirty granulation tissue without enlarging the wound (Fig. 10.16).
- Skin-tag or hypertrophied anal papilla is excised with LASER energy by bare fibre.

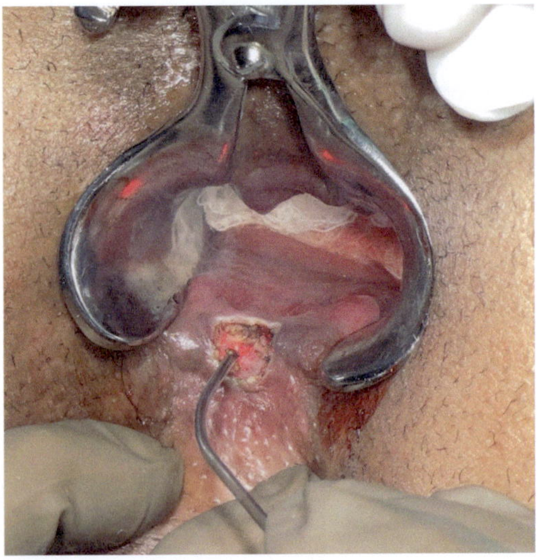

Fig. 10.14 Rolled margins and bed of fissure sprayed with LASER

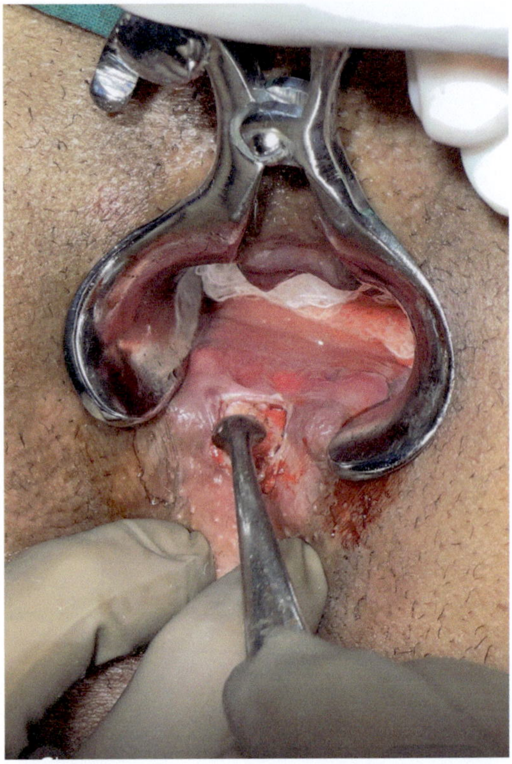

Fig. 10.15 Curette fissure bed and margins after LASER

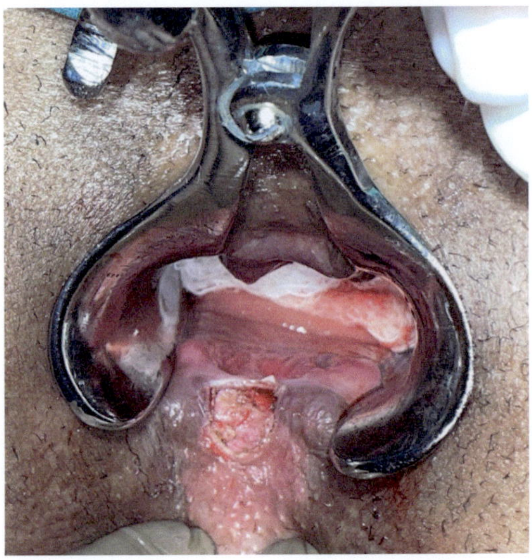

Fig. 10.16 Clean bed of fissure, flat margins after LASER and curettage

10.9 Injecting Methylene Blue for Prolonged Analgesia

- We inject 1% methylene blue solution with 0.25% bupivicane in 1:5 ratio in intra-dermal plain, in any dissection below the dentate line.
- Fine 27 gauge needle is used for the purpose.
- 5 to 10 cc solution is sufficient for most of the surgeries.
- It keeps the area numb for 3–4 days.
- Caution the patient for violet tinge in urine after methylene blue injection.

10.10 Complication of LIS (Table 10.1)

Passive soiling
Do limited sphincterotomy up to the height of fissure
Clean twice after passing stools with an interval of 5 min. Kegel's exercise to increase anal tone as external sphincter also contributes towards resting tone

Table 10.1 Complications of LIS, prevention and management

Complication	Prevention	Management
Injury to anoderm	Inject saline between anoderm and internal sphincter. Do not go close to Anoderm	Stitch with 3.0 biodegradable suture
Bleeding	Move LASER fibre slow	Press for 3 min LASER spray or bipolar coagulation
Late complications Incontinence to flatus	Do limited sphincterotomy up to the height of fissure	Kegel's exercise to increase anal tone as external sphincter also contributes towards resting tone

Algorithm for LIS Lasers

Indications/contraindications
Position lithotomy and anaesthesia same as for LIS with blade
Put anal speculum to stretch the anal sphincter slightly
Define intersphincteric groove
Give a small incision with LASER 7 watt continuous wave energy
Put curved mosquito in intersphincteric space and hook fibres of IS below the dentate line on the curved part of the mosquito artery forceps
Cut IS fibres with bare fibre 7 watts energy continuous wave
No bleeding of consequence
Feel the defect in IS
Alternate way
Inject saline between the anoderm and IS to create a space and to keep anoderm lifted away
Put LASER fibre in this space using same energy burst and negotiate fibre up to dentate line
Bend the tip of fibre towards IS
Activate LASER fibre and withdraw while cutting the IS
Feel the defect caused by distal sphincterotomy

Suggested Reading

Ambe PC. Laser interventions in coloproctology. A plea for standardized treatment protocols. Tech Coloproctol. 2023;27(10):953–5. https://doi.org/10.1007/s10151-023-02859-2.

Perianal Abscess Minimal Invasive Approach

11

Abstract

- Anatomy of perianal spaces is explained by sketches and hand-drawings.
- Pathological basis of crypto glandular infections and pathological anatomy of perianal abscess is explained by board-drawings from authors, class-room teachings.
- Minimally invasive ways to handle perianal abscesses by fistuloscope and traditional minimal invasive ways are explained fully by clinical photographs and videos.
- Why drain a perianal abscess close to anal opening? Do we really need a cruciate incision to drain a perianal abscess? Why not to swipe finger vigorously in draining an ischiorectal abscess? have been answered.
- Emphasis has been made to locate internal opening and management of associated fistula without cutting external sphincter in one go in inflamed tissues, or managing trans-sphincteric fistula by slowly cutting seton.
- Reader may feel confident to manage associated fistula, if one does not need to cut external sphincter.
- Drainage of abscess is important in emergency, if surgeon is not sure of internal opening or not confident of operating on associated fistula better leave fistula management, for specialist care later.
- Role of imaging (magnetic resonance imaging (MRI)) in emergency-setting of managing perianal abscess has been defined.
- Complication of the procedures, their prevention and management are arranged in table form for ready reference.
- Tips and Tricks will prepare the reader to improve outcomes in difficult situations.
- "References" and "Suggested Reading" sections are to provide information about the basis of our understanding and the ways other authors deal these cases. This information will make readers further wise.

Supplementary Information The online version contains supplementary material available at https://doi.org/10.1007/978-981-96-6190-9_11. The videos can be accessed individually by clicking the DOI link in the accompanying figure caption or by scanning this link with the SN More Media App.

S. K. Singla, K. Mital, *Operative Manual of Minimally Invasive and LASER Ano-proctology*,
https://doi.org/10.1007/978-981-96-6190-9_11

11.1 What One Should Know Before the Procedure

11.1.1 Anatomy of Perianal Spaces (Figs. 11.1, 11.2, and 11.3) [1]

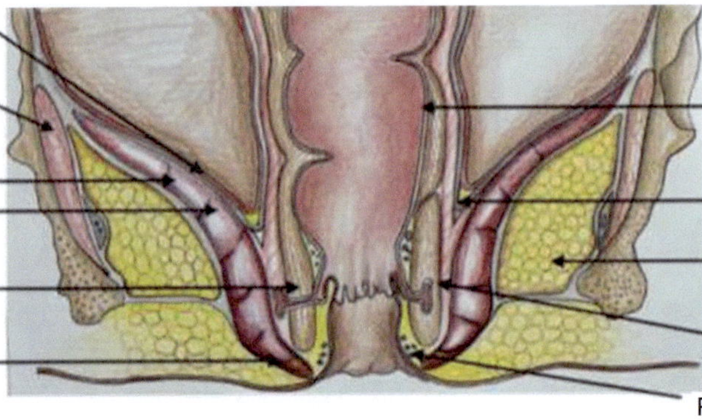

Fig. 11.1 Perianal and perirectal spaces, coronal view

Fig. 11.2 Perianal and perirectal spaces, saggital view

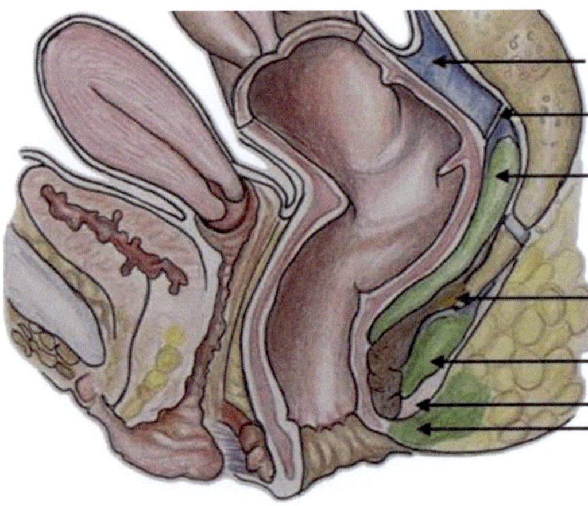

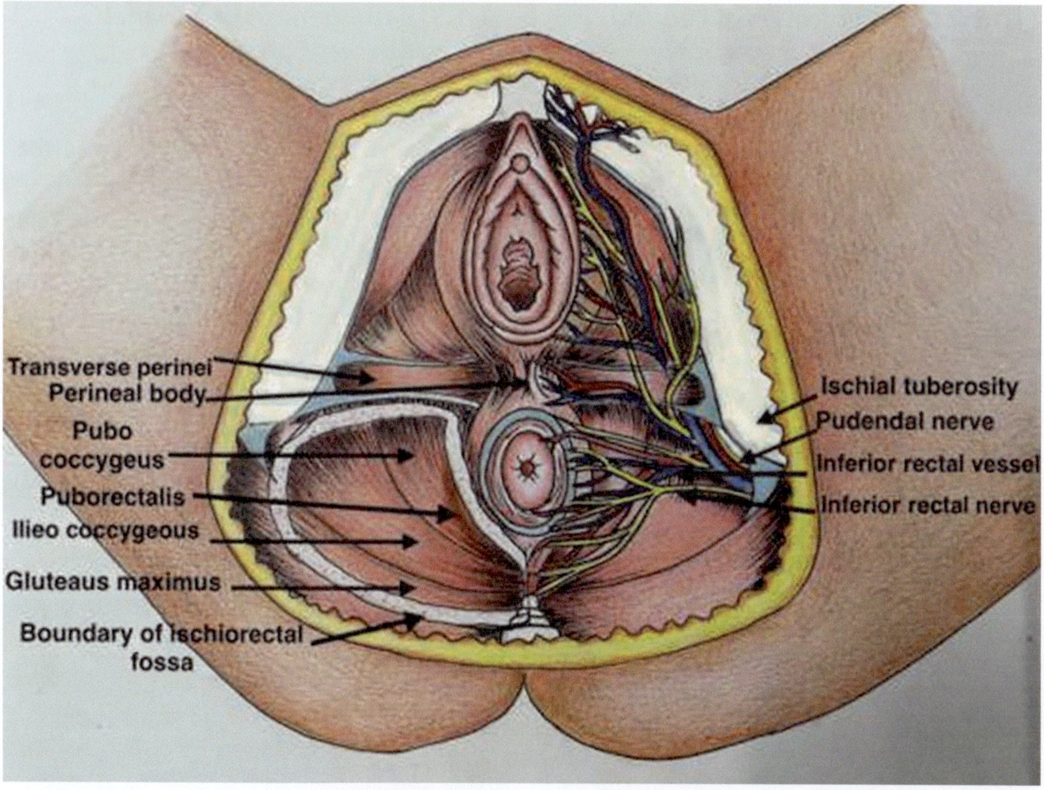

Fig. 11.3 Anatomy—boundaries and contents of ischiorectal fossa

11.1.2 Contents of Perianal Spaces Relevant for Perianal Abscess Formation and Management (Fig. 11.4)

Submucous space contains submucous glands.

11.1.2.1 Anal Glands

There are 6–8 anal glands in midanal canal at the level of dentate line.

Two-third penetrate internal sphincter and half of them go up to inter-sphincteric space. But none of them enter the external sphincter.

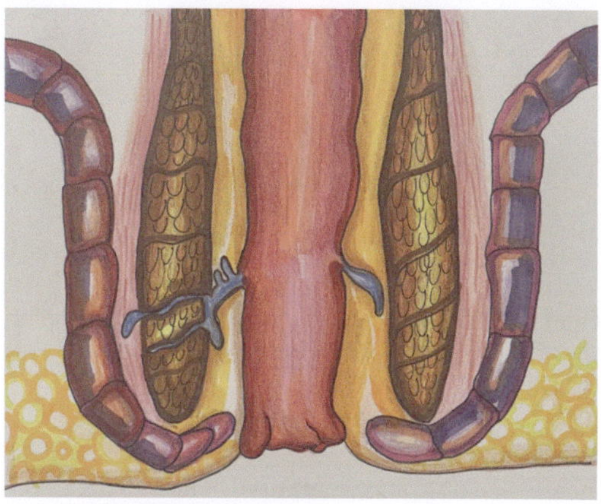

Fig. 11.4 Contents of submucous space—anal glands which penetrate up to inter sphincteric space

11.1.2.2 Communication of Perianal Spaces Occurs vertically as Well as Horizontally (Figs. 11.5 and 11.6)

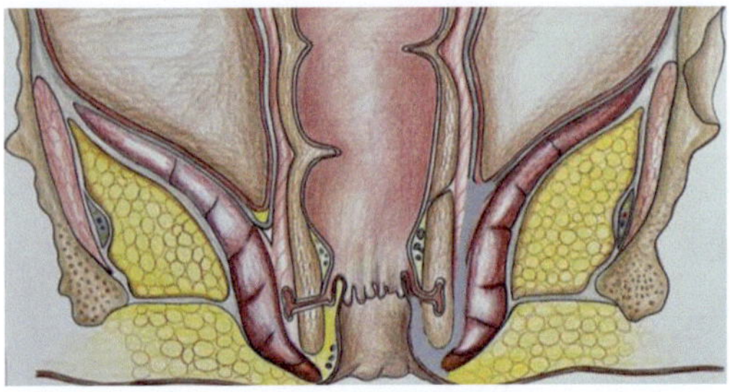

Fig. 11.5 Communication of perianal spaces vertically, inter-sphincteric space communicates with perianal and supralevator space shown in grey colour

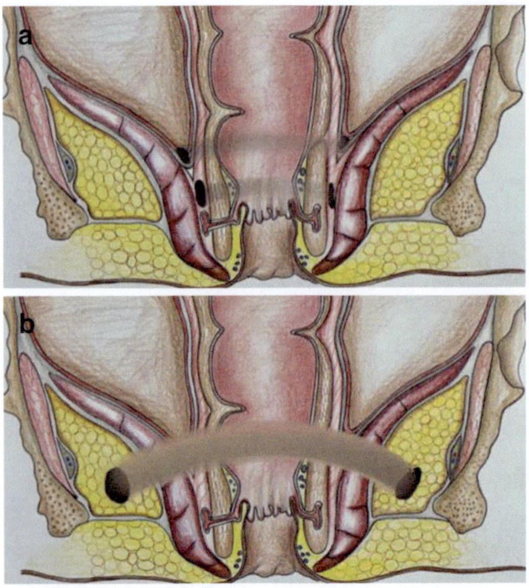

Fig. 11.6 Communication of perianal spaces, circumferentially. (**a**) Intersphincteric and supralevator. (**b**) Ischiorectal

11.1.3 Pathogenesis of Perianal Abscess Formation and Spread

Ducts of anal glands gets blocked leading to dilatation of glands which get infected (Fig. 11.7).

Infected enlarged and cystic glands when rupture in confined space lead to abscess formation.

There is a communication between perianal spaces, along these routes pus can spread around the anal canal.

A potential space between external sphincter, levator ani and their supporting fascia inferiolaterlly has been identified as a route of spread for pus recently, based on MRI studies on patients with fistula in ano [2] (Fig. 11.8).

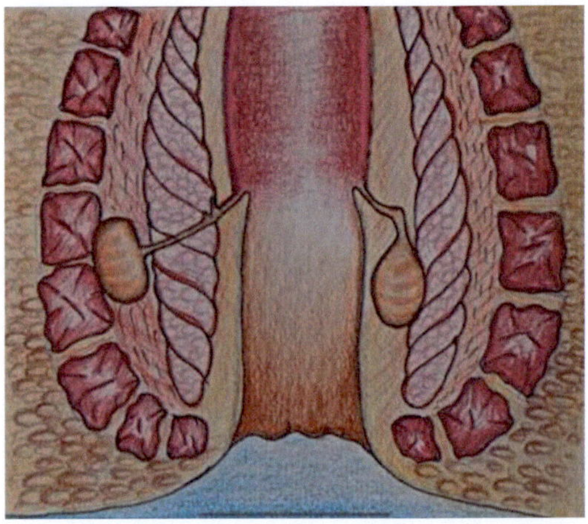

Fig. 11.7 Blocked anal glands in submucous and intersphincteric space, get enlarged and cystic

11.1.4 Pathological Anatomy of Perianal Abscesses

Abscess around the anal canal is named after the space they occupy (Figs. 11.9, 11.10, 11.11, 11.12, 11.13, 11.14, and 11.15).

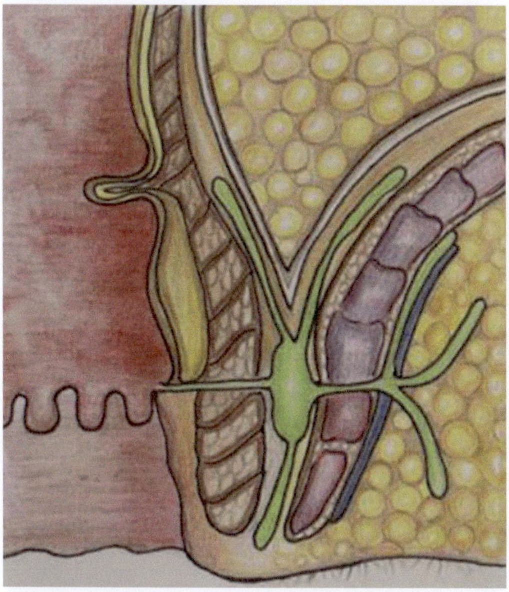

Fig. 11.8 Routes of spread of infection from ruptured intersphincteric space gland, in perianal spaces

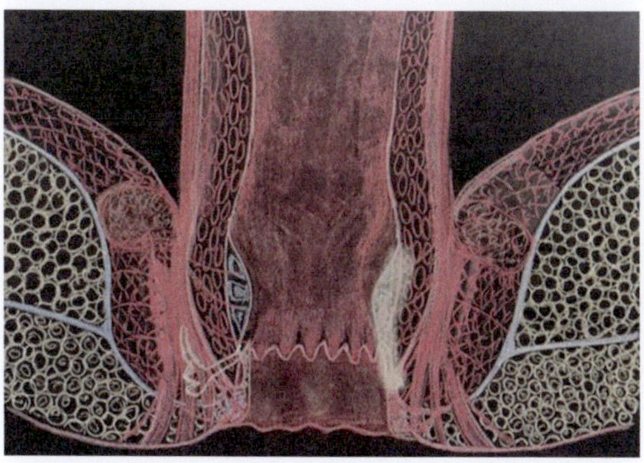

Fig. 11.9 Submucous abscess, when anal gland confined to submucous space gets blocked, infected and ruptures

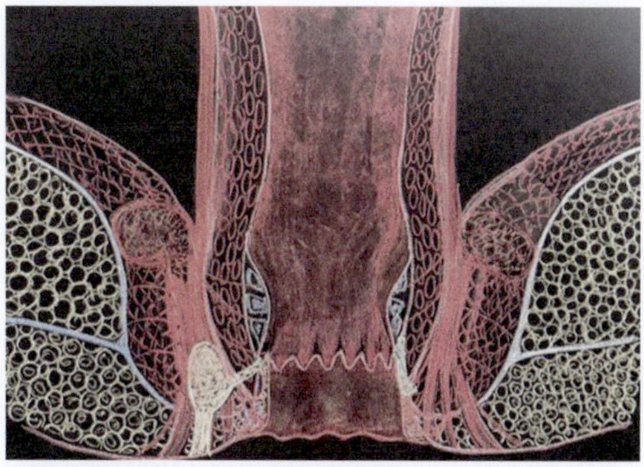

Fig. 11.10 Intersphincteric abscess

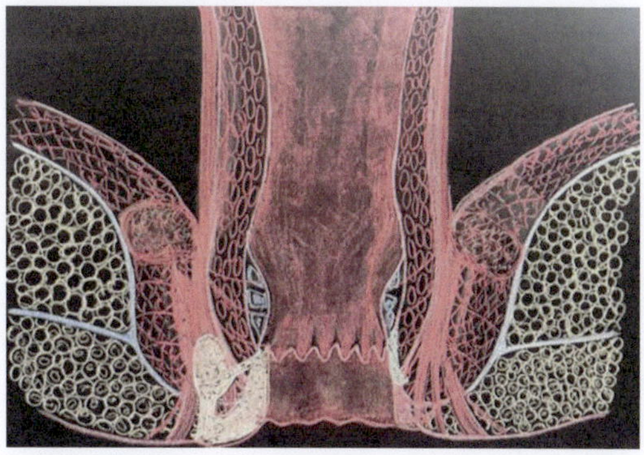

Fig. 11.11 Spread of pus from intersphicteric space to perianal space called as perianal abscess

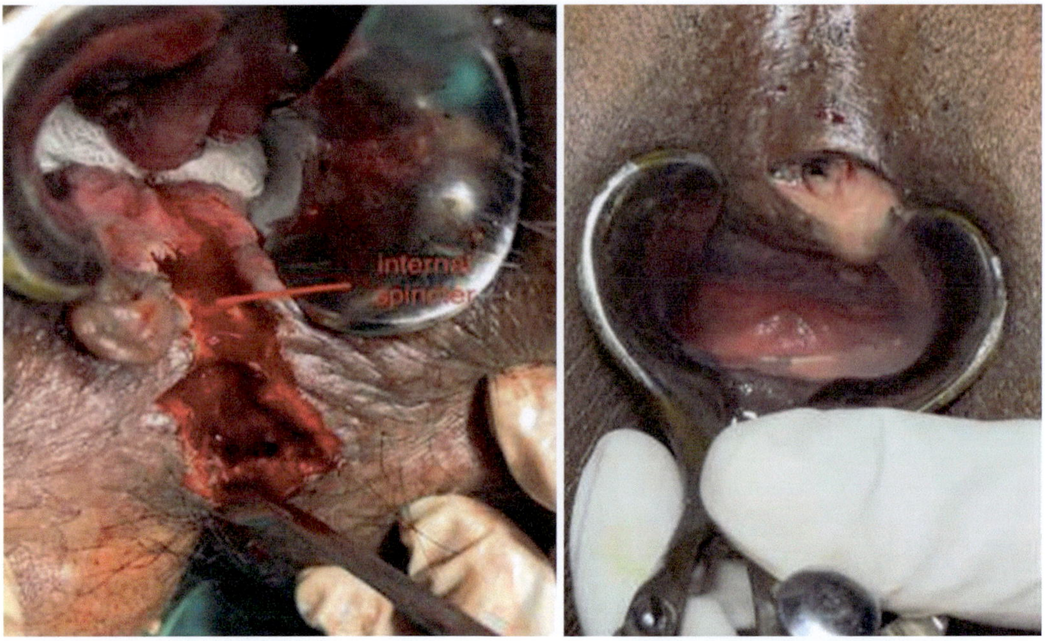

Fig. 11.12 Clinical photographs of intersphincteric abscess spread to perianal space known as perianal abscess

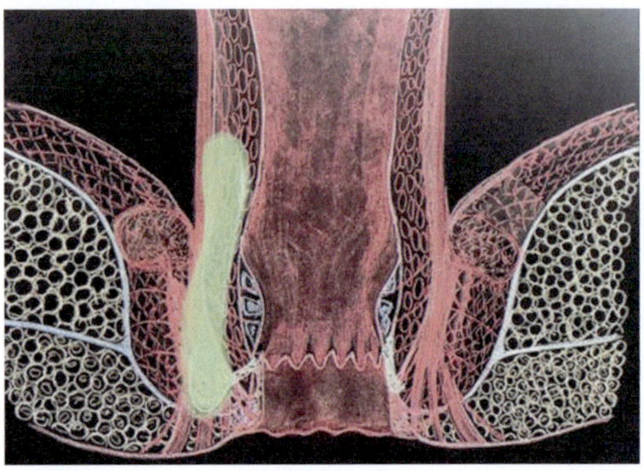

Fig. 11.13 Intersphincteric pus instead of coming down, going high in deep space and confined within rectal wall between circular muscle (internal sphincter) and longitudinal muscle (conjoint longitudinal muscle)

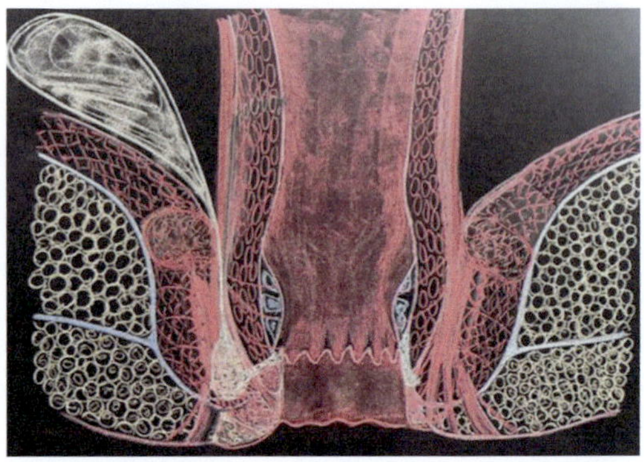

Fig. 11.14 Intersphincteric pus going deep over the levator muscle. For other routes for supralevator collection from pelvic or retro peritoneal pathology and translevator from infra levator collection in ischiorectal fossa, check Fig. 11.71

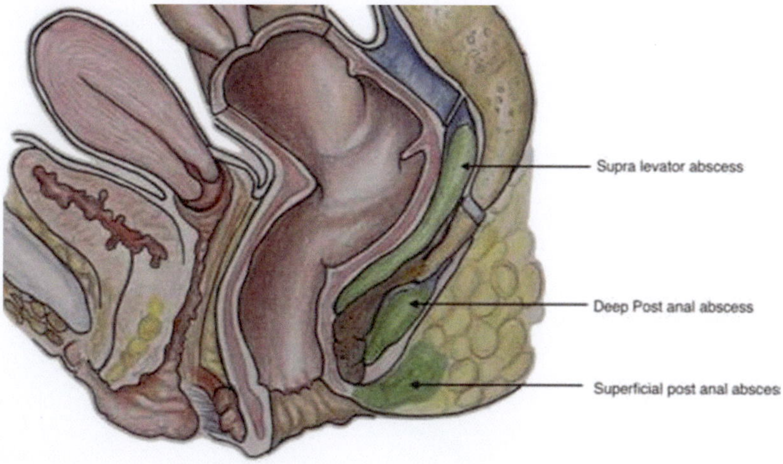

Fig. 11.15 Sagittal section showing relationship between various postanal abscesses

11.1.5 Clinical and Radiological Correlation of Intersphincteric Collection Going Deep in Supralevator Space (Fig. 11.16)

11.1.6 Ischiorectal Abscess, Internal Communication and Spread

Once infection spreads from intersphincteric space through external sphincter into ischiorectal space, fat in ischiorectal fossa gets necrosed easily and abscess may attain large size before patient seeks medical attention (Fig. 11.17).

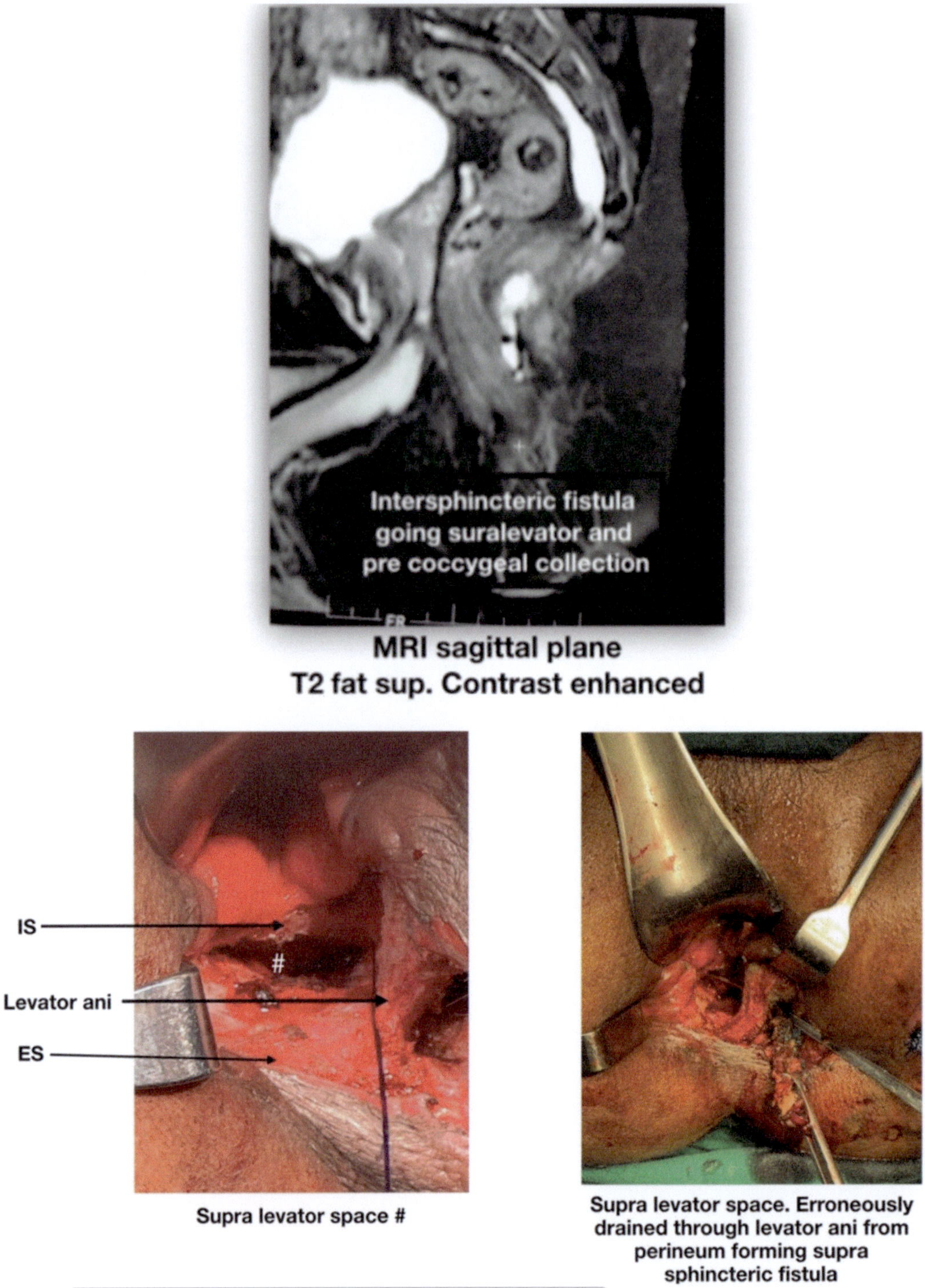

Fig. 11.16 Compare between 11.15 sketch and MRI in sagittal section and clinical photograph in lithotomy

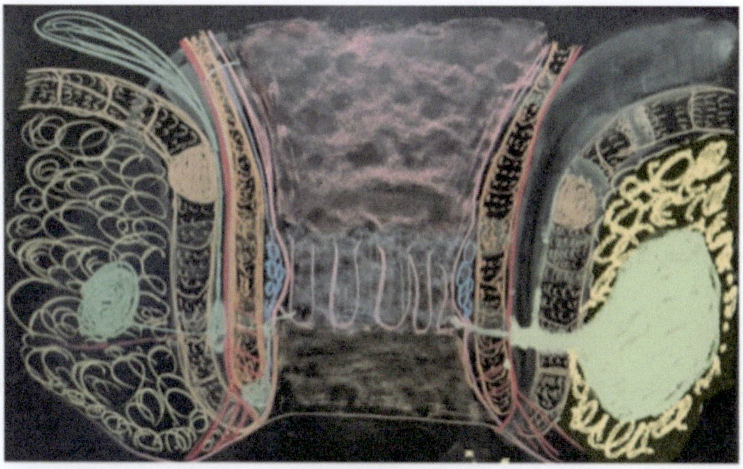

Ischiorectal abscess

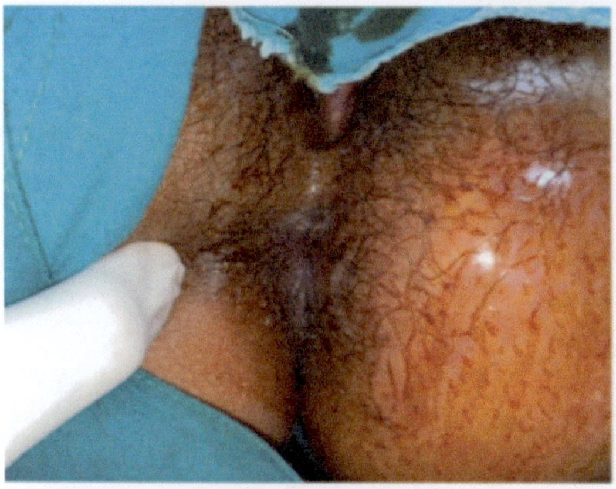

Ischiorectal abscess

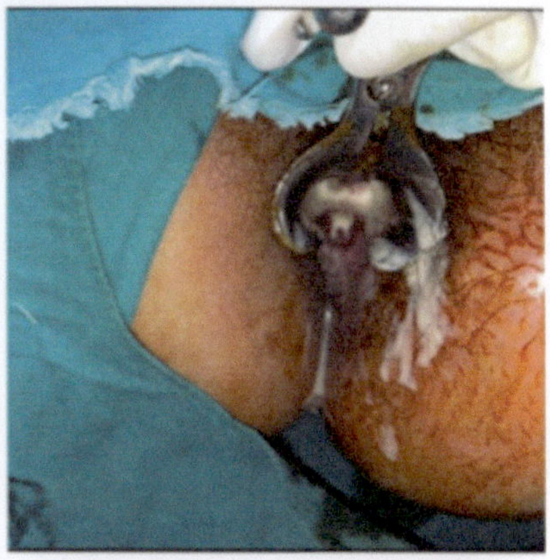

Internal opening posterior midline

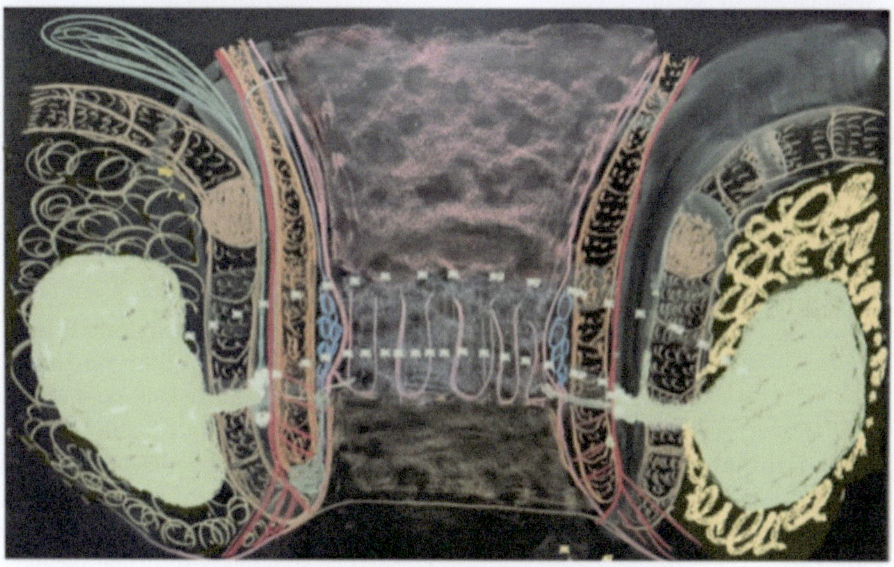

Ischiorectal abscess both fossae (Horse shoe type)

Fig. 11.17 Ischiorectal abscess may attain large size and can present on both sides termed as horse-shoe-shaped abscess

11.2 Minimal Invasive Surgery for Management of Perianal Abscesses

11.2.1 Indications

- All perianal infections and abscess without gangrene.

11.2.2 Contra-Indications

- Necrotising infections, Fournier's gangrene need extensive debridement and should not be managed by minimal invasive methods.

11.2.3 Equipment

- Operation table with stirrups for lithotomy.
- For prone position, rolled sheets and cushions with tapes for strapping (optional).
- Sterile drapes and gowns.
- Povidine iodine solution.
- Xylocaine jelly, surgical gloves, saline-soaked gauge pieces.
- Syringes.
- Normal saline and lignocaine 2%.
- Park's speculum and vaginal speculum of various size.
- Fistuloscope.
- Volkmann's scoupe of various sizes.
- Drains. Tube drains.
- Sutures—nylon, polyglactin and PDS on needle (2.0 suture on half circle 30 mm and 5/8 circle needle 27 mm).
- Adult diaper.
- Sanitary napkins.

11.2.4 Inter-Sphincteric Abscess

11.2.4.1 Anaesthesia

Short general anaesthesia (GA)/Spinal.

11.2.4.2 Position

Lithotomy

11.2.4.3 Procedure

- Put lubricated Park's speculum.
- Rotate and open to stretch the appropriate segment of anal canal based on clinical examination and MRI findings.
- Press the abscess, at times pus seeps from internal opening (Fig. 11.18).
- Aspirate with 18 gauge needle to confirm the presence of pus in the inter-sphincteric space.
- Separate the syringe from the needle and inject small amount of diluted methylene blue to find any fistulous tract.
- Stroke the egress point of dye with monopolar cautery.
- Give a small nick at aspiration point. Push sinus forceps to enter in to abscess cavity and drain the abscess (Fig. 11.19).
- Evacuate the pus, curette out the cavity and do thorough lavage with saline mixed with few drops of hydrogen peroxide.
- Enlarge the lower end of incision by incising internal sphincter and anoderm below the dentate line up to internal opening, if noticed (Fig. 11.20a, b).
- Debride the margins and marsupialise to prevent any premature closure. For suturing, we replace Park's speculum with vaginal speculum (Fig. 11.21).
- For marsupialisation, polyglactin 2.0 suture on needle is used in interrupted manner to fix the margins of the wound with base of the wound. It keeps the cavity shallow and flat (Fig. 11.22).

11.2.4.4 Injecting Methylene Blue for Prolonged Analgesia

- We inject 1% methylene blue solution with 0.25% bupivicane in 1:5 ratio in intra-dermal plain, in any dissection below the dentate line (Fig. 11.23).
- Fine 27 gauge needle is used for the purpose.
- 5–10 cc solution is sufficient for most of the surgeries.

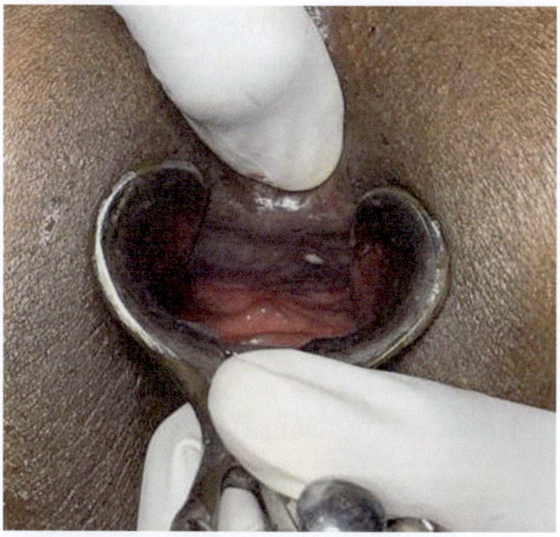

Fig. 11.18 Inter-sphincteric abscess presenting as anterior perianal abscess, on pressure pus seeps through the internal opening

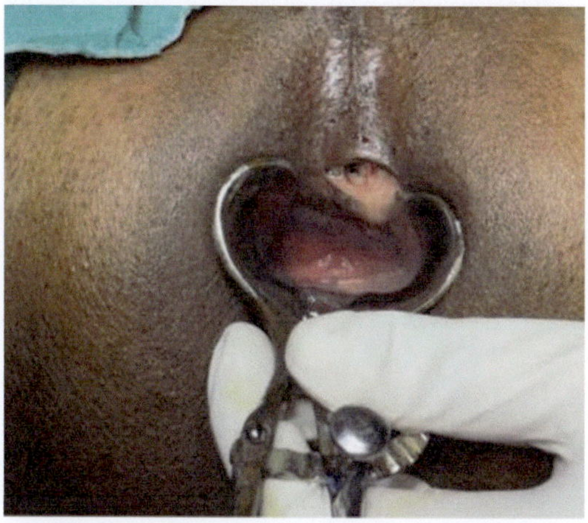

Fig. 11.19 Incision over inter-sphincteric space to drain the abscess

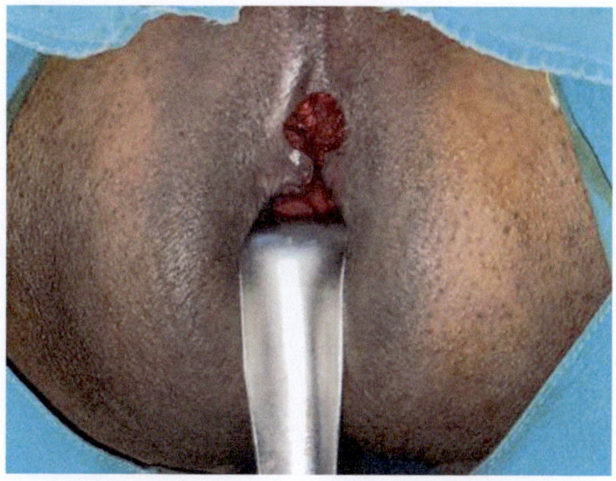

Fig. 11.21 Marsupialisation of the cavity after debridement, change the Park's speculum with vaginal speculum, it facilitates suturing

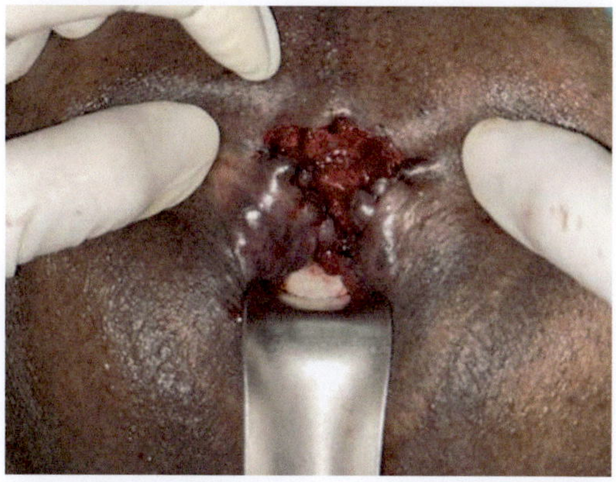

Fig. 11.22 Marsupialisation makes the cavity shallow and flat

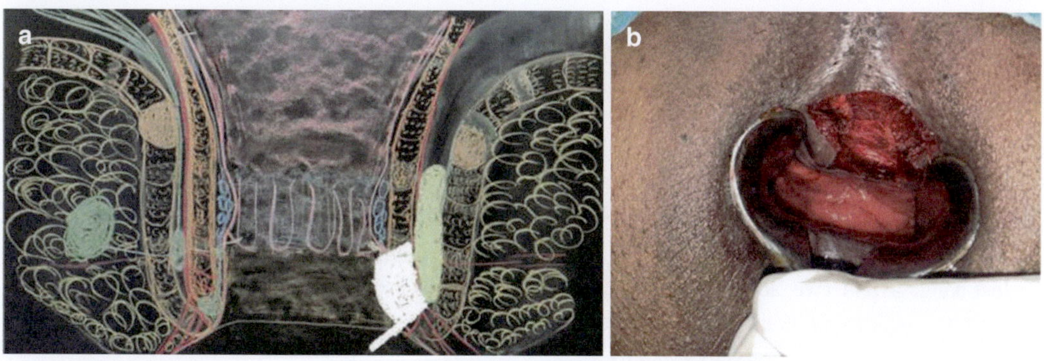

Fig. 11.20 (**a**) Inter-sphincteric abscess drainage inside the anal canal shown by white marker, incising internal sphincter and anoderm below the dentate line. (**b**) Laid open anterior inter-sphincteric abscess cavity after incision of internal sphincter and anoderm

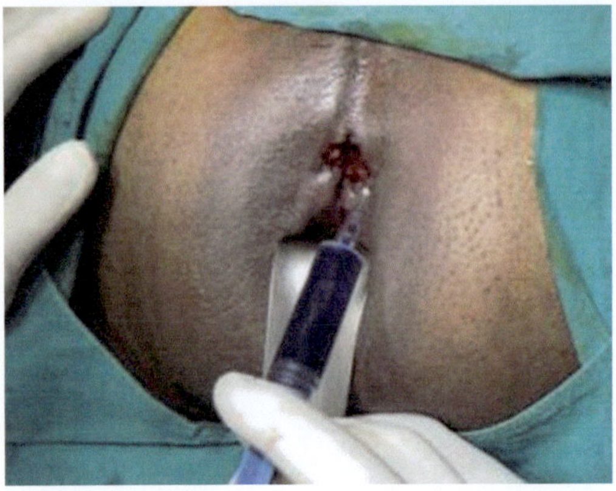

Fig. 11.23 Injection of 1% methylene blue solution with 0.25% bupivicane in 1:5 ratio in intra-dermal plain with 27 gauge needle

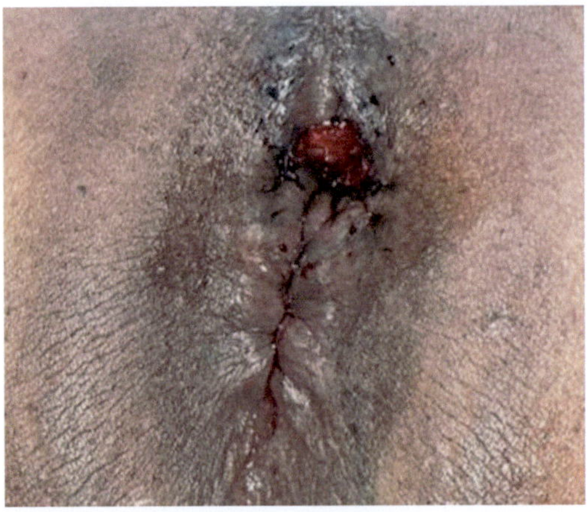

Fig. 11.24 Tattooing with methylene blue below the dentate line decreases pain for 3–4 days

- It keeps the area numb for 3–4 days (Fig. 11.24) [3].
- Caution the patient for violet tinge in urine after methylene blue injection.

11.2.4.5 Post-procedure Advise

- Patients are instructed to flush clean the cavity with saline or clean water, after every act of defecation.
- No packing is required.
- Just keep a pad (we advocate using female sanitary napkins or adult diapers depending on the amount of secretions) to soak any secretion from the wound, it helps prevent maceration of the surrounding skin.

11.2.4.6 Antibiotics

- Ofloxacin and metronidazole are started intravenously (I/V) with induction of anaesthesia and three doses are given to every patient.
- Antibiotics are continued for patients having cellulitis or showing systemic signs of sepsis or immunocompromised patients.

11.3 Management of Anal Abscess by Fistuloscope

- One of the authors (K.M.) often uses Meinero's scope to drain and debride the abscess cavity under vision, using very small incision to accommodate the scope and latter put the drain.
- The drainage of anal abscess can be done from inside the anal canal or from the perineum (Fig. 11.25).
- Even though the fistuloscope is rigid, it can easily manoeuvre in the abscess cavity and fistula tracts.

11.3.1 Technique

- The fistuloscope is inserted into the abscess as near as possible to the anal canal and from inside the anal canal.
- There are two stages of video endoscopic management of perianal abscess:
  (a) Diagnostic phase—to locate.
- Internal opening.
- Secondary tracts.
  (b) Operative phase—with the aim to.
- Debride the abscess cavity under vision from inside.
- Thorough cleaning and drainage so that cavity collapses early.
- Management of internal opening.

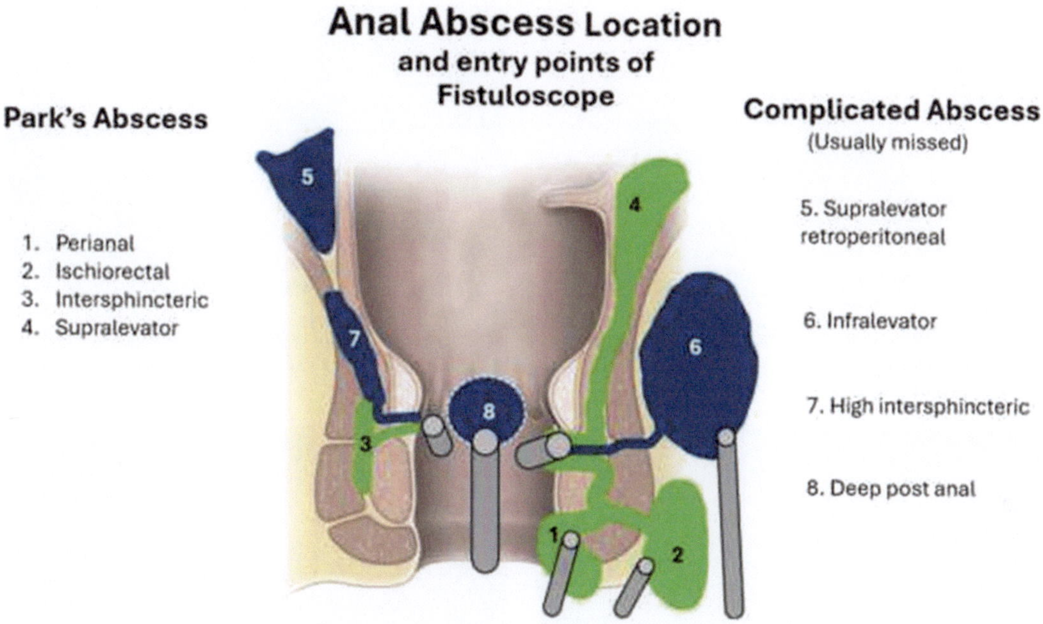

Fig. 11.25 Entry points for fistuloscope based on location of the abscess

11.3.2 Inter-Sphincteric Abscess Drainage by Fistuloscope

11.3.2.1 Anaesthesia

- Spinal/GA.

11.3.2.2 Position

- Lithotomy (Fig. 11.26).

11.3.2.3 Procedure

- Boundaries of abscess cavity on inspection and palpation are marked.
- Wide bore-needle inserted in abscess cavity to confirm presence of pus (Fig. 11.27).
- Through the same needle, put diluted methylene blue mixed with few drops of hydrogen peroxide inside the abscess cavity (Fig. 11.28).
- Put speculum inside the anal canal and check egress of dye and froth of H_2O_2 from inside the anal canal from internal opening (Fig. 11.29).
- Give a stab incision over the abscess in intersphincteric groove and subsequently slightly open with mosquito forceps or sinus forceps (Fig. 11.30).
- Fistuloscope inserted inside the abscess cavity, wait for a minute to get the vision clear by running fluid (Figs. 11.31 and 11.32).
- Insert grasper gently with closed jaws through the operative channel of the scope and debride the cavity (Fig. 11.33).

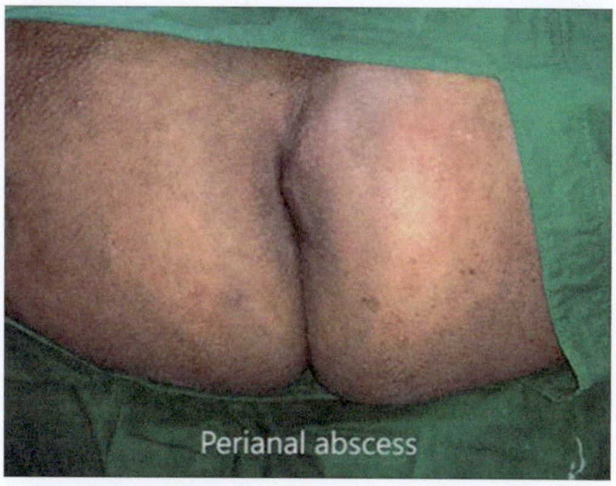

Fig. 11.26 Patient under spinal anaesthesia lithotomy position, left anterior inter-sphincteric abscess

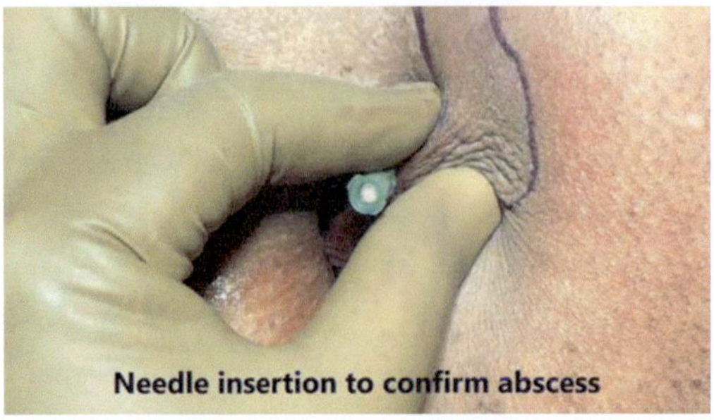

Fig. 11.27 Boundaries of abscess marked and needle inserted to check egress of pus

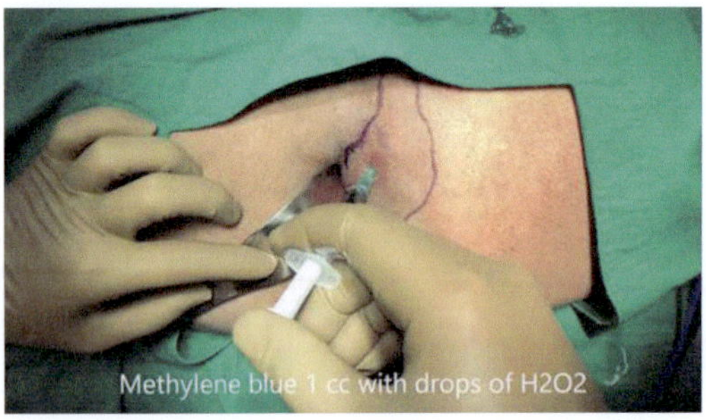

Fig. 11.28 Diluted dye mixed with drops of H_2O_2 instilled in the cavity to locate internal opening

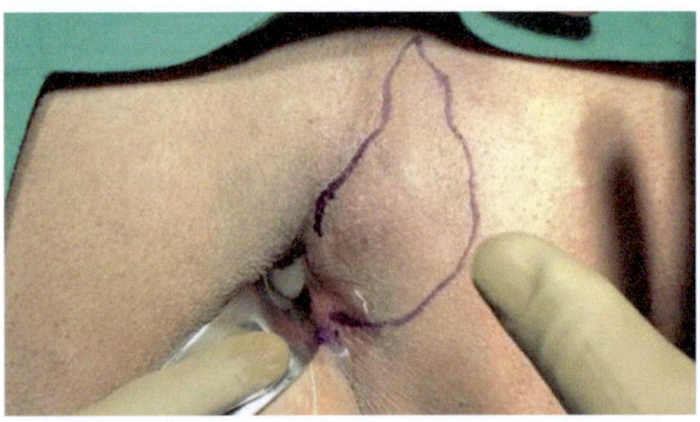

Fig. 11.29 Speculum inside the anal canal and observe egress of the dye and froth of H_2O_2 from internal opening

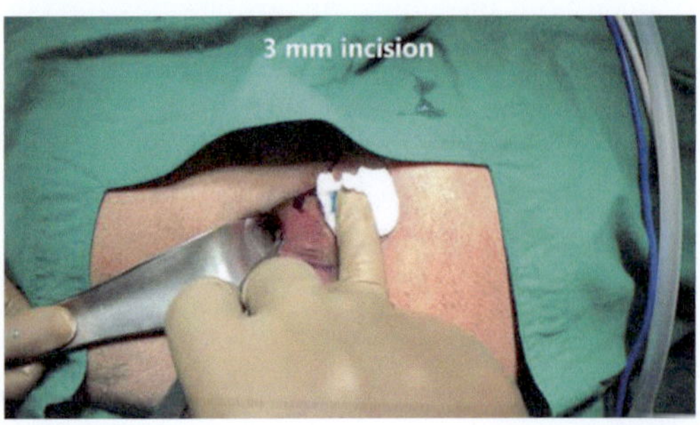

Fig. 11.30 Stab-incision over inter-sphincteric groove in area involved by abscess

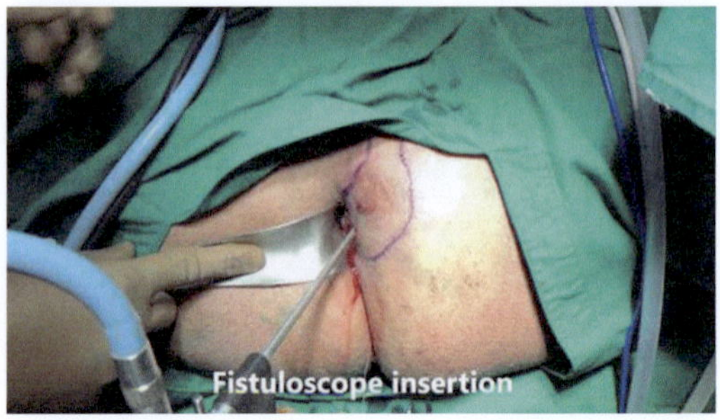

Fig. 11.31 Meinero's scope with running fluid inserted in the cavity from stab site

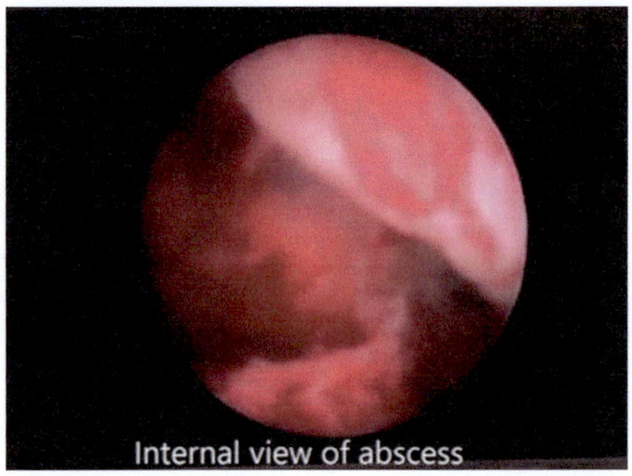

Fig. 11.32 Internal view of the abscess cavity on screen, running fluid clears the vision

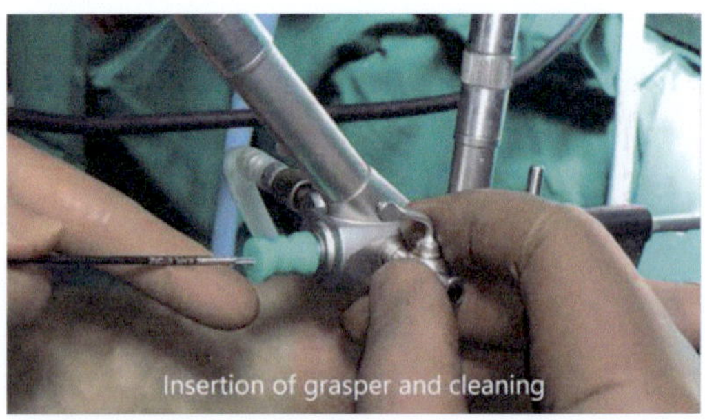

Fig. 11.33 Gently threading the grasper in the operative channel of the scope, note 2-mm instruments are very delicate

- Curette with Volkmann's scoupe without breaking any tissue which resists (Fig. 11.34).
- Flush out the debrided material from the cavity by irrigating the cavity with saline and put a drain for continuous drainage (Figs. 11.35 and 11.36).

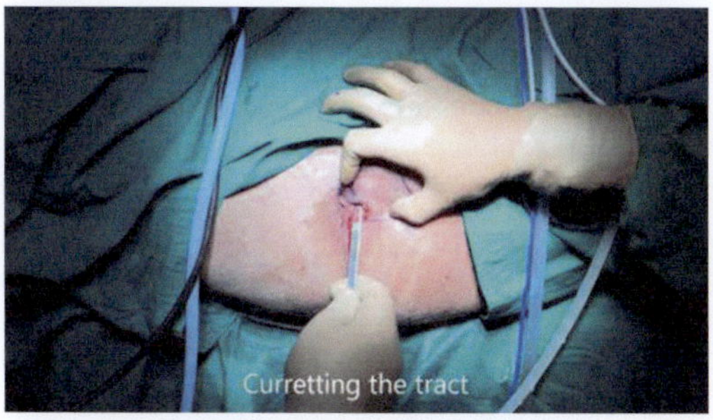

Fig. 11.34 Curette thoroughly the cavity walls

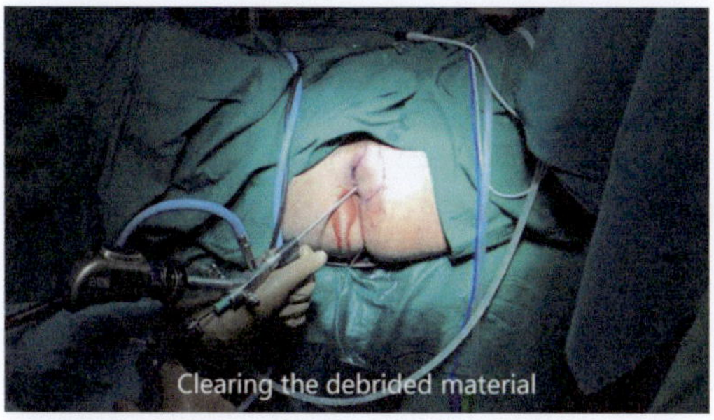

Fig. 11.35 Flushing out the necrotic material and slough from the cavity

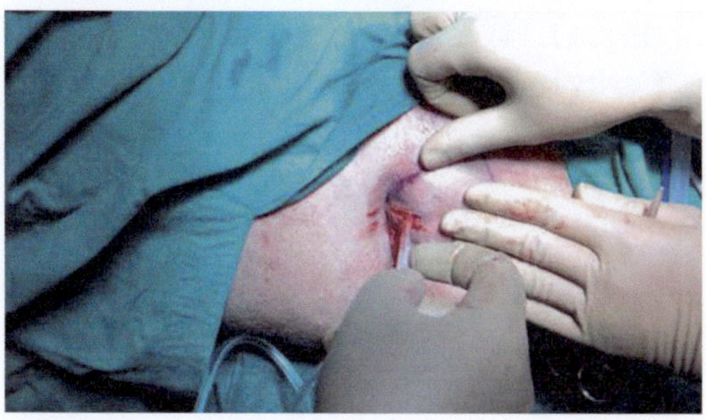

Fig. 11.36 Tube drain inserted and fixed for irrigation and drainage

11.4 Inter-Sphincteric Abscess Going Deep and Supralevator

- MRI defines abscess and its limits (Fig. 11.37).

11.4.1 Extra Equipment

- Fistuloscope and accessories.
- Saline/glycine with mannitol.

11.4.2 Procedure

- Dilate or open the internal opening at dentate line by taking an incision 5 mm around the internal opening, at times pus may start coming out of the opening.
- Put sinus forceps and dilate, more pus will come out.
- Put a fistuloscope inside and check the limits of abscess cavity, which may extend circumferentially in inter-sphincteric space as a horse-shoe-shaped cavity or may simultaneously extend superior in supralevator space posteriorly.
- Fulgrate the whole cavity with monopolar electrode/LASER fibre.
- Do thorough curettage with Volkmann's scoupe.
- Irrigate cavity thoroughly with saline and hydrogen peroxide solution.
- Check-endoscopy can be done to ensure complete debridement.
- Extend the incision at lower-end of the inter-sphincteric cavity for persistent drainage and make the wound at anal verge-saucer shape by incising distal internal sphincter for easy flushing of the remanant cavity.
- Check for any extension through the external sphincter that means trans-sphincteric extension.

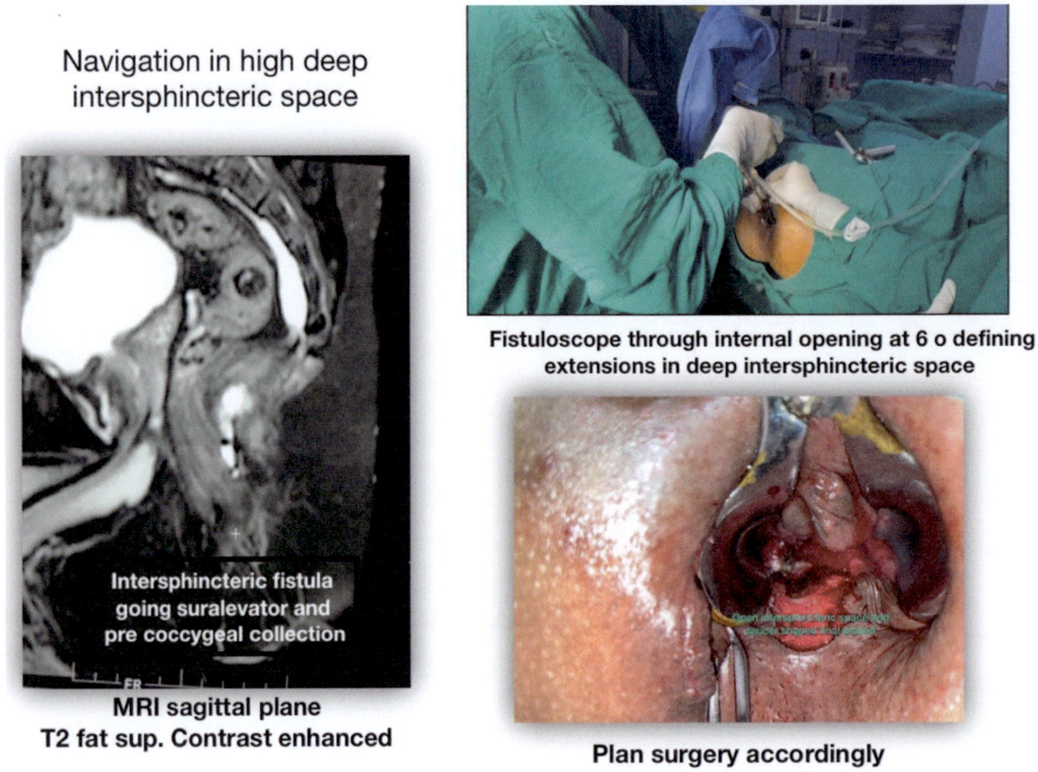

Fig. 11.37 MRI showing inter sphincteric abscess going supralevator in pre-coccygeal area, fistuloscope used to treat this abscess, lower end of the wound made wide and saucer shaped for post-operative irrigation

11.5 Stepwise Explanation of Managing another Case of Deep Inter-Sphincteric Abscess by Fistuloscope

- Get a MRI done to delineate the whole anatomy and make 3D picture of abscess spread in one's cortex diary (Fig. 11.38).
- Put probe from external opening to the internal opening at dentate line and lay it open on the probe (Figs. 11.39, 11.40, and 11.41).
- Put fistuloscope through the internal opening into proximal inter-sphincteric space and supralevator space (Fig. 11.42).

  Visualise and debride the abscess cavity from inside with endo forceps (Fig. 11.43).
- 1470 diode LASER with 10 watts energy continuous wave delivered by radial fibre is used to fulgrate the abscess cavity (Fig. 11.44).
- Cavity is thoroughly curetted with Volkmann's scoupe.
- Foleys catheter with 3 cc distilled water in balloon is kept in the abscess cavity for 5 days for persistent drainage (Fig. 11.45).

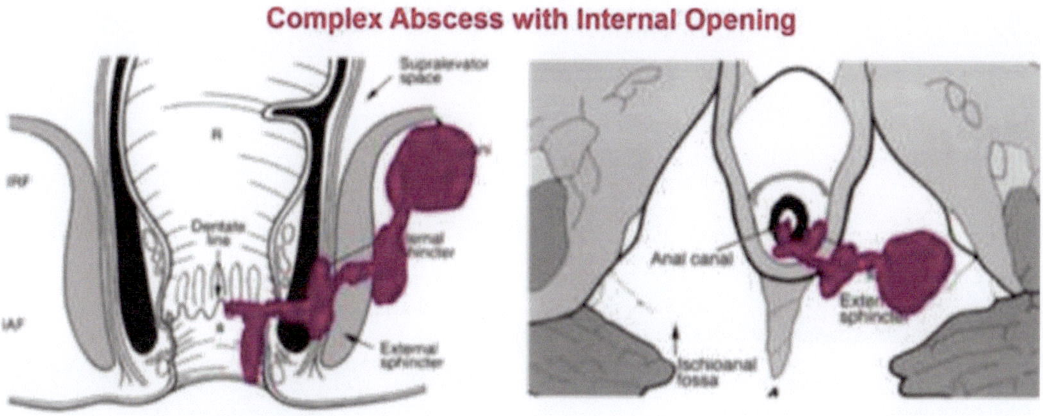

Fig. 11.38 Sketch made from MRI in a case of deep inter-sphincteric abscess with trans-sphincteric extension

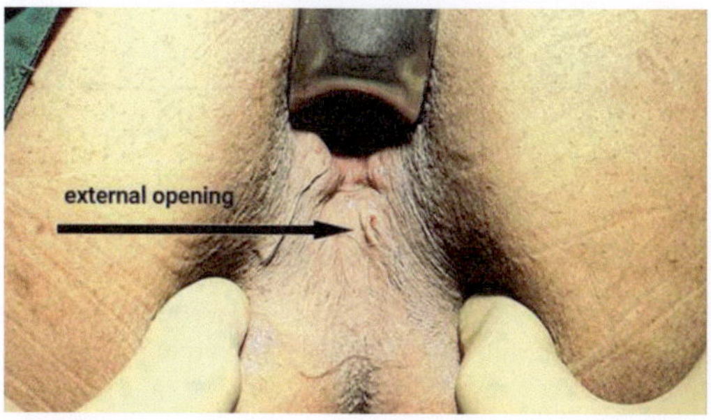

Fig. 11.39 Clinical picture from outside of the same case as shown in Fig. 11.38

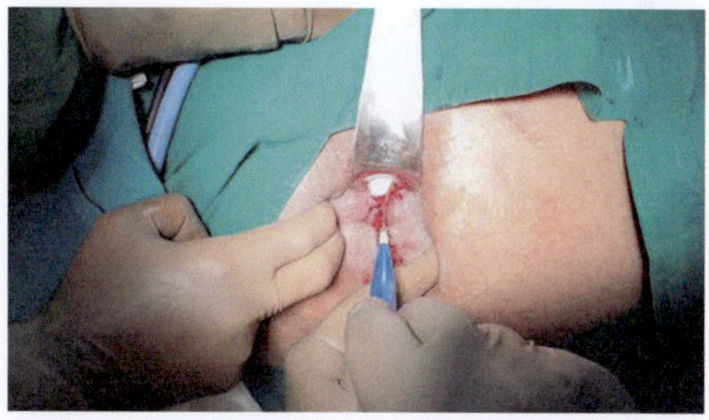

Fig. 11.41 Lay open the distal tract on metal probe

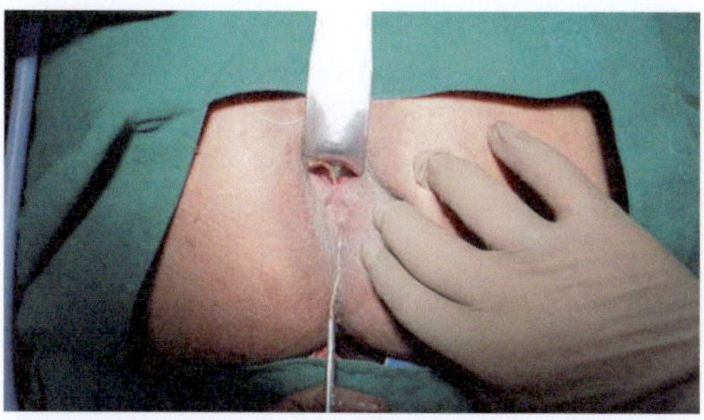

Fig. 11.40 Probing the distal component of fistula through external opening

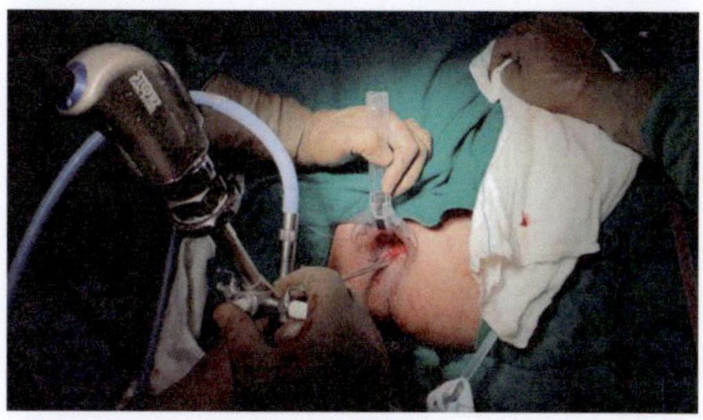

Fig. 11.42 Fistuloscope passed into deep intersphincteric space through the internal opening at dentate line

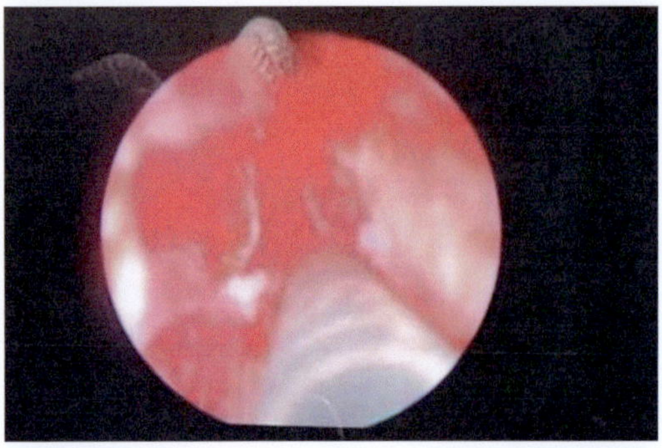

Fig. 11.43 Endoscopic view of the abscess cavity, note endoforceps being used for debridement

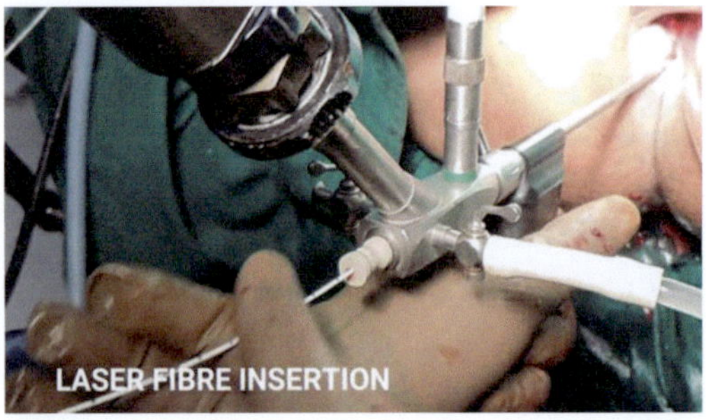

Fig. 11.44 Radial LASER fibre inserted through operative channel of the scope to fulgrate walls of the abscess cavity

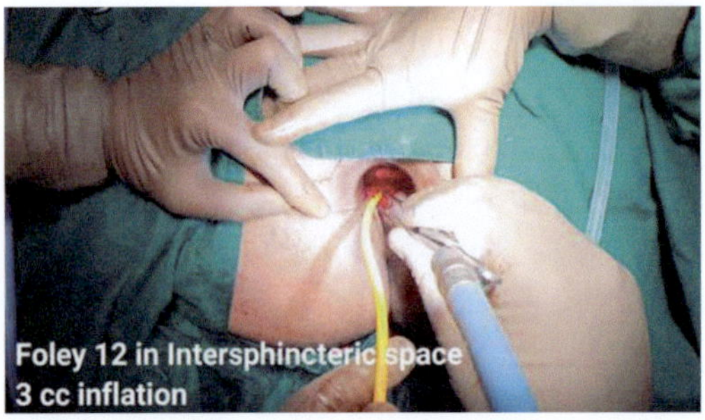

Fig. 11.45 Foley's catheter as drain

11.6 Alternative Minimally Invasive Management of Abscess in Deep Inter-Sphincteric Space Going Supralevator

- Open anal speculum inside anal canal, at times pus under pressure, may start flowing as shown in Fig. 11.46.

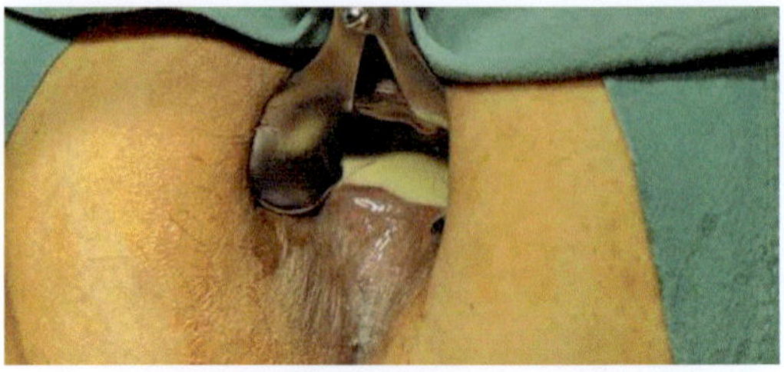

Fig. 11.46 Pus from deep inter-sphincteric space abscess, flowing on opening of Park's speculum

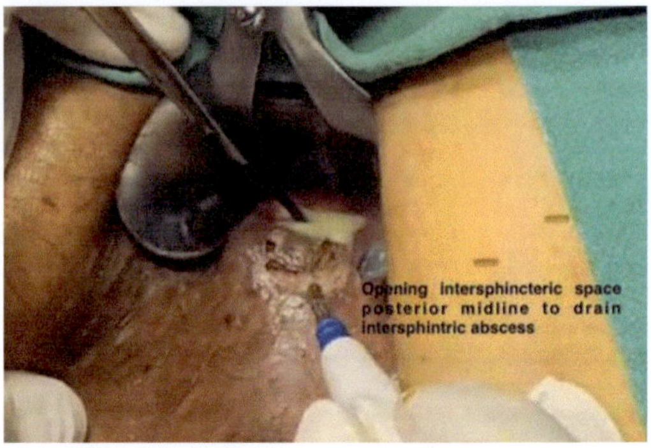

Fig. 11.47 Wide open internal opening by taking incision around the opening and taking fibres of distal internal sphincter over a reverse probe

- Wide open the internal opening, taking incision around the internal opening.
- Excise small portion of internal sphincter in its distal part (Fig. 11.47).
- More pus will flow from deep intersphincteric space.
- For tract going proximal to dentate line, dilate the opening and insert fistuloscope.
- Fulgrate tract and cavity with monopolar electrode or LASER fibre as previously shown.
- Debride and thoroughly wash the proximal tract and cavity which may extend in to supralevator space.
- Curette the cavity well.
- Incise internal sphincter above the dentate line for few millimetres and leave it wide open for flushing (Fig. 11.48).
- One can marsupialise the edges of the opening to avoid pre-mature closure.

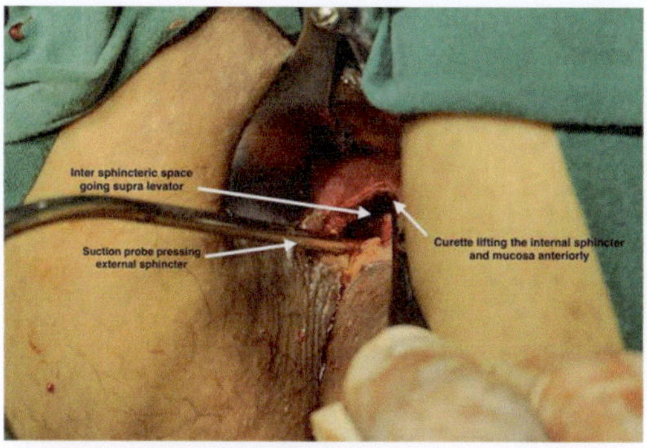

Fig. 11.48 Open deep inter sphincteric space up to supralevator space, after debridement with fistuloscope lower end kept wide open for postoperative irrigation

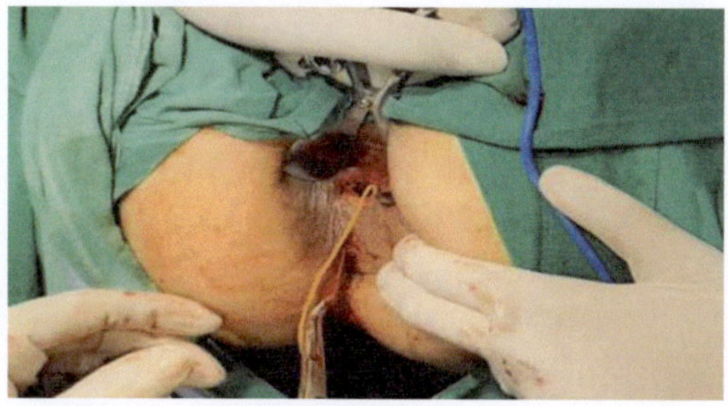

Fig. 11.49 Passing medicated chemical seton (ksharsootra) to drain the posterior trans-sphincteric extension of the abscess

11.7 Management of Associated Trans-Sphincteric Extension of Abscess in Ischiorectal Fossa or Postanal Space

- Make an external opening in post midline or laterally in ischiorectal fossa, but very close to anal-verge over a probe to drain the part of abscess outside the skeletal muscle.
- Debride and curette the abscess cavity with fistuloscope under vision.
- One can put a draining seton around the external sphincter and latter do definite management of trans-sphincteric fistula.
- One of the authors (S.K.S.) puts a chemical seton (ksharsootra *IN SANSKRIT. KSHAR MEANS ALKALIAN- SOOTRA MEANS THREAD*, made by treatment of Ayurvedic herbs on cotton thread) through the trans-sphincteric extension and keep it loose in the beginning as a draining seton [4] (Fig. 11.49).
- Extra length of seton is put in to abscess cavity which further does its chemical debridement.
- Five to seven days later when infected fluid discharge decreases considerably, we tighten the seton around sphincter complex converting it into cutting seton.
- Skin and anoderm are always incised before converting ksharsootra into cutting seton or for that matter before tying any cutting seton around external sphincter.
- We usually change it with new seton every fortnight till it cuts through the tissue slowly.
- Tissue cut proximally by seton heals in the mean time, and this way patient is saved from second surgery for transphincteric fistula, with very low recurrence and almost no incontinence [5].
- Our only indication for chemical-cutting seton is when there is associated abscess with trans-sphincteric extension.

11.8 Ischiorectal Abscess (Figs. 11.50, 11.51, 11.52, 11.53, 11.54, 11.55, 11.56, 11.57, 11.58, 11.59, 11.60, 11.61, 11.62, and 11.63)

- Clinical examination is done to define limits of abscess and locate internal opening under anaesthesia.
- Do all efforts to locate the internal opening:
  - At times pus from internal opening shows itself (Fig. 11.50).
  - Else aspirate the abscess-cavity and instil dilute methylene blue dye with few drops of hydrogen peroxide in the abscess cavity to show at internal opening (Figs. 11.58 and 11.59).
- We usually do definitive management of fistula with drainage of abscess.
- Give incision as close to anal verge as possible so that in case of subsequent fistula development, tract is small (Figs. 11.51 and 11.52).
- Avoid cruciate skin incision as it is not required and leads to more skin necrosis (Fig. 11.51).

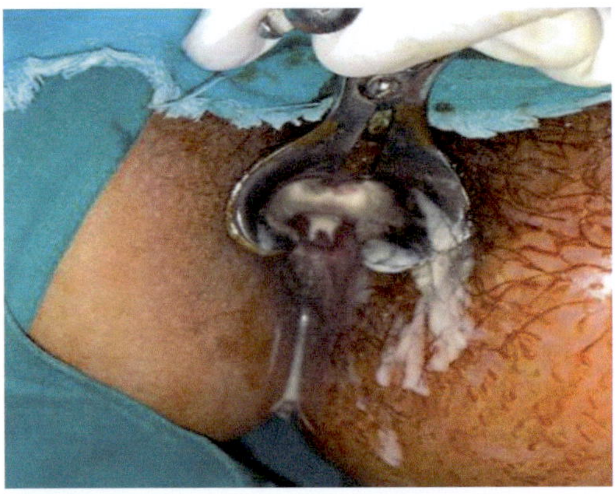

Fig. 11.50 Under anaesthesia, on putting anal speculum pus seen coming from post midline 6 0′ clock position with pressure, in a case of ischiorectal abscess as shown in Fig. 11.52

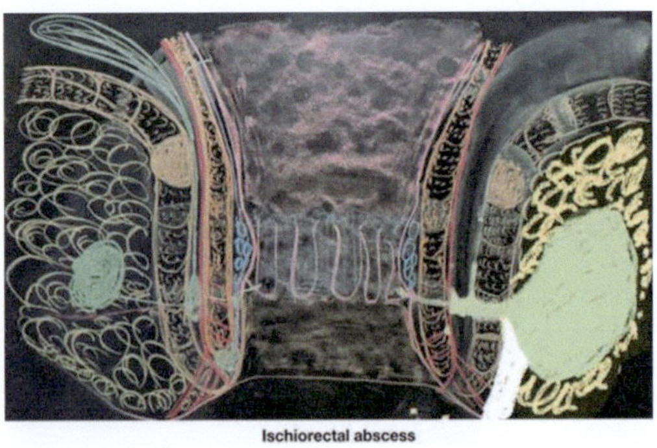

Fig. 11.51 Abscess lateral to external sphincter drained outer to external sphincter through ischiorectal fossa close to anal opening shown by white marker

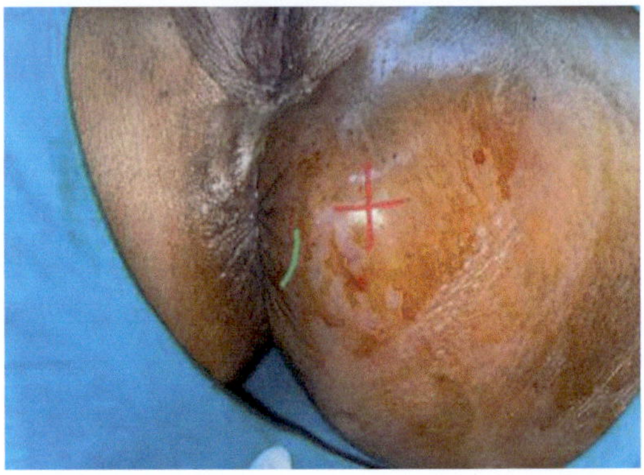

Fig. 11.52 Left ischio rectal fossa abscess, incision shown in red colour should be avoided in favour of incision shown in green colour closer to anal canal to drain the abscess

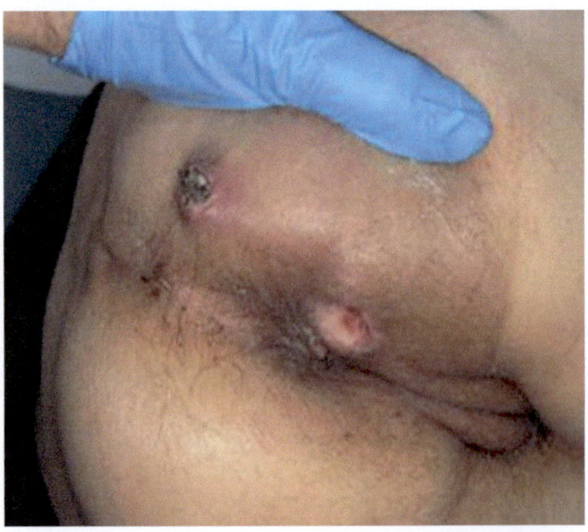

Fig. 11.53 Large necrotising abscess right ischiorectal fossa. Patient in left lateral position note small incision close to anal verge on right side and a counter drain in dependant position fixed flushed to skin with nylon sutures

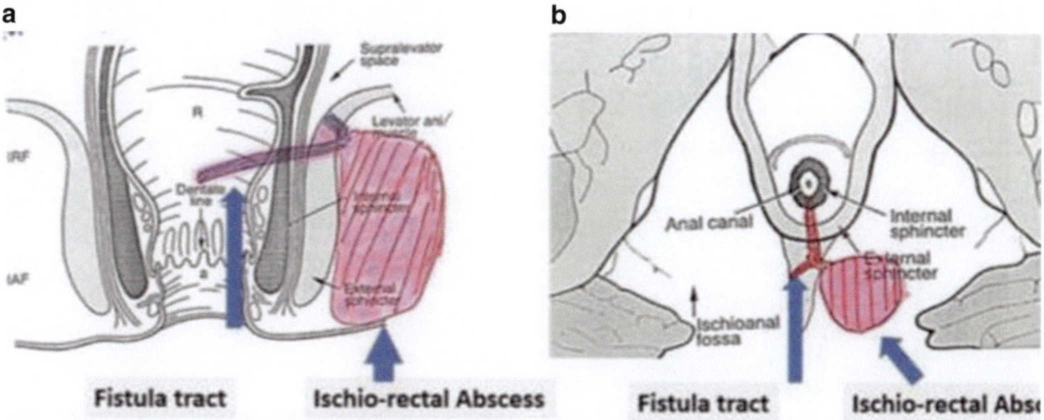

Fig. 11.54 Line diagrams of MRI for fistula in ano Coronal (**a**) and axial (**b**) view

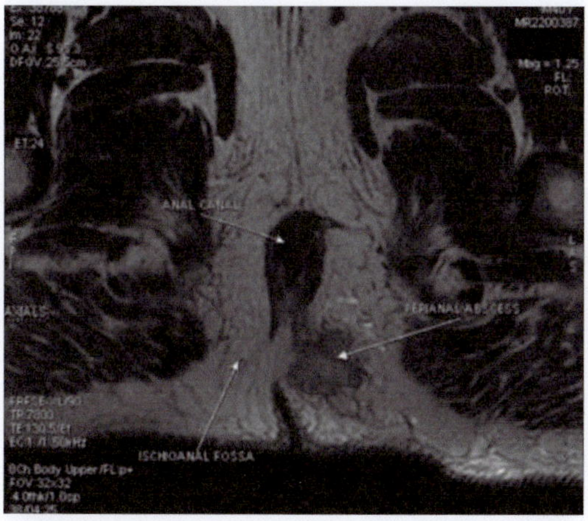

Fig. 11.55 Coronal view MRI showing perianal abscess left side

- In name of breaking loculations, do not damage the nerves and vessels traversing ischiorectal fossa.
- If suppuration comprises of liquid pus, no necrosed solid tissue, one may need very small incision to drain and curette it.
- Use tube drains (Foley's catheter, Mallecot catheter, K90 catheter or abdominal drain) for consistent drainage and irrigation.
- Drains except Foley's catheter are fixed, flushed to skin with 3 radial nylon sutures (Fig. 11.53).

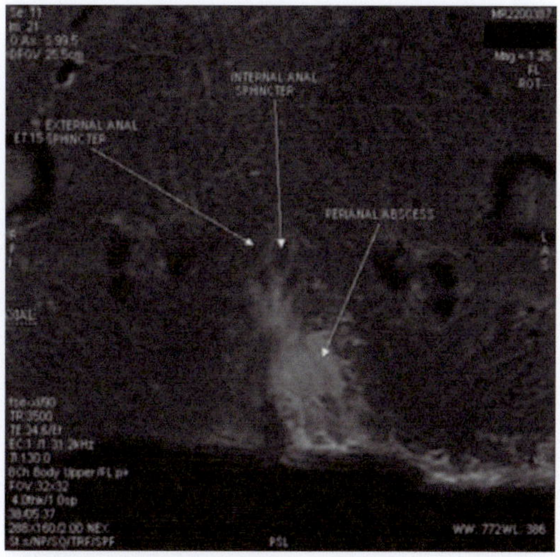

Fig. 11.56 MRI fat suppressed image showing perianal abscess and internal opening

11.8.1 Stepwise Approach in a Case of Ischiorectal Abscess (Infralevator) Drainage with Fistuloscope

- It is good idea to get pre-operative MRI to define the abscess, especially when planning minimal invasion (Figs. 11.54, 11.55, 11.56, and 11.57).

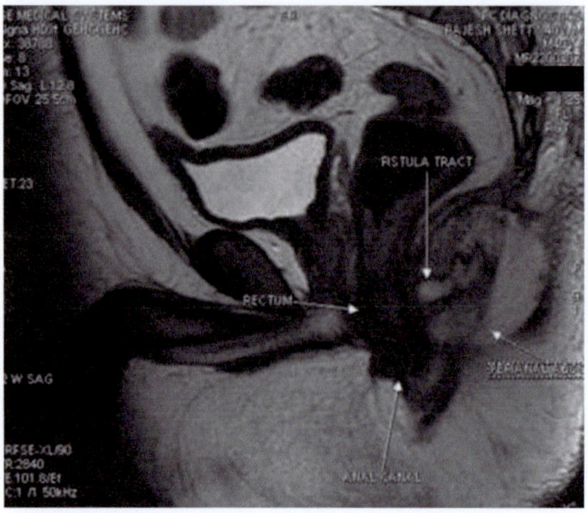

Fig. 11.57 Sagittal view of MRI showing internal opening in posterior midline and infralevator abscess cavity

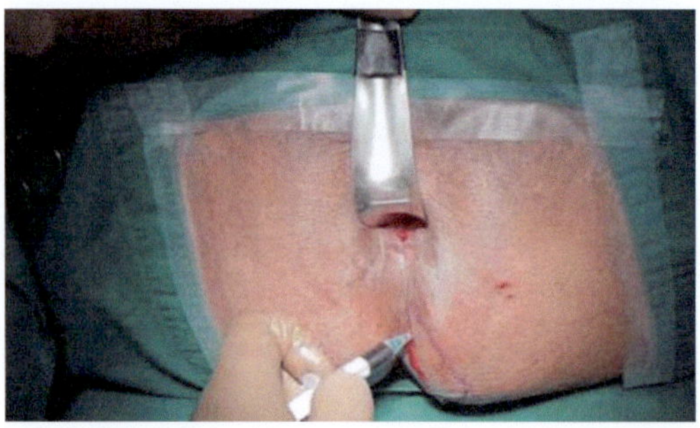

Fig. 11.58 Instilling dye in the abscess cavity

MRIs without suppressing fat give better anatomical details (Fig. 11.55) while fat suppressed images define abscess better (Fig. 11.56).

- Patient under spinal anaesthesia in lithotomy position.
- Mark the abscess cavity on palpation as shown, aspirate pus and inject dye with few drops of hydrogen peroxide (Fig. 11.58).
- Put lubricated speculum in the anal canal to observe the site of egress of dye inside the anal canal (Fig. 11.59).
- Intersphincteric space opened by incising around the internal opening to drain the source of infection (Fig. 11.60).
- Give a stab incision on abscess close to anal opening and fistuloscope inserted in the abscess cavity and debridement done under vision (Fig. 11.61).
- Draining loop passed through the internal opening and around the sphincter (Fig. 11.62).
- Foley's inflated inside the cavity for drainage purpose (Fig. 11.62).

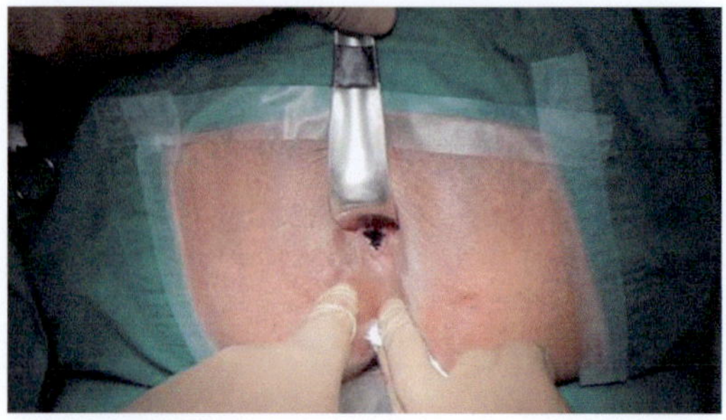

Fig. 11.59 Egress of dye confirms internal opening in posterior midline

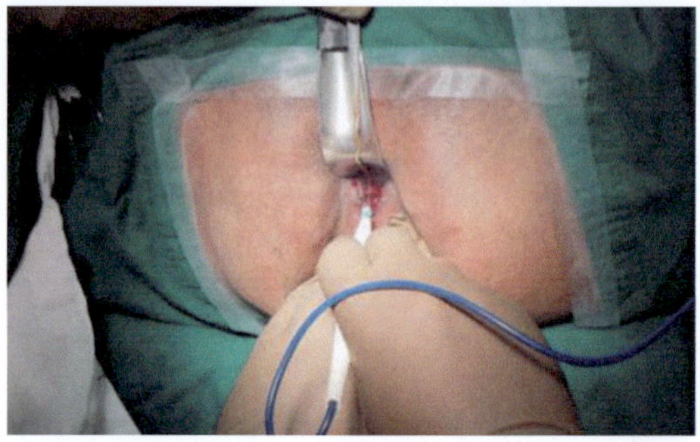

Fig. 11.60 Internal opening excised to enter intersphincteric space to drain the source of infection

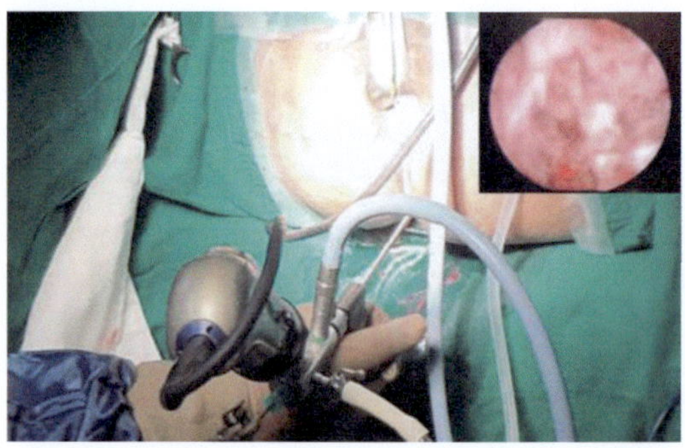

Fig. 11.61 Fistuloscope in the abscess cavity to debride inside lining under vision

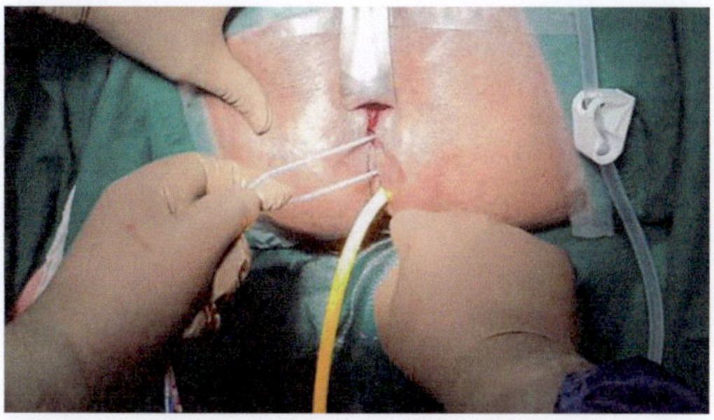

Fig. 11.62 Draining loop through transphincteric component and Foleys in abscess cavity

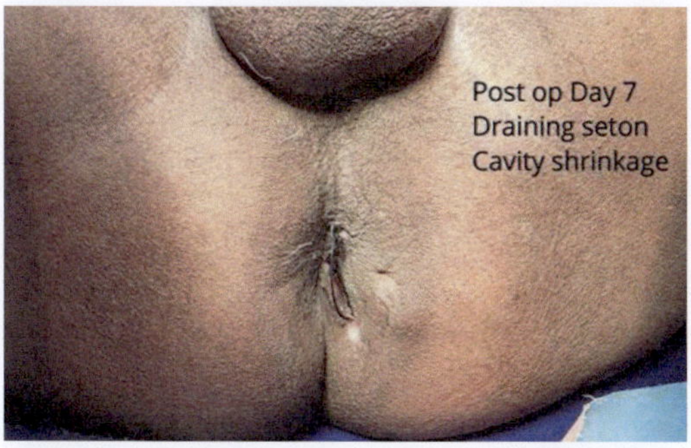

Fig. 11.63 Loose seton through the internal opening around external sphincter

- Later drainage tube is replaced by draining seton and Foley's is removed (Fig. 11.63).

11.8.2 Horse-Shoe and Deep Postanal Abscess

Similarly, minimally invasive surgery can be done for horse shoe and deep postanal abscess, once one localises the limits of abscess cavity and internal communication (Figs. 11.64 and 11.65).

11.8.3 Horse-Shoe Abscess (Fig. 11.64)

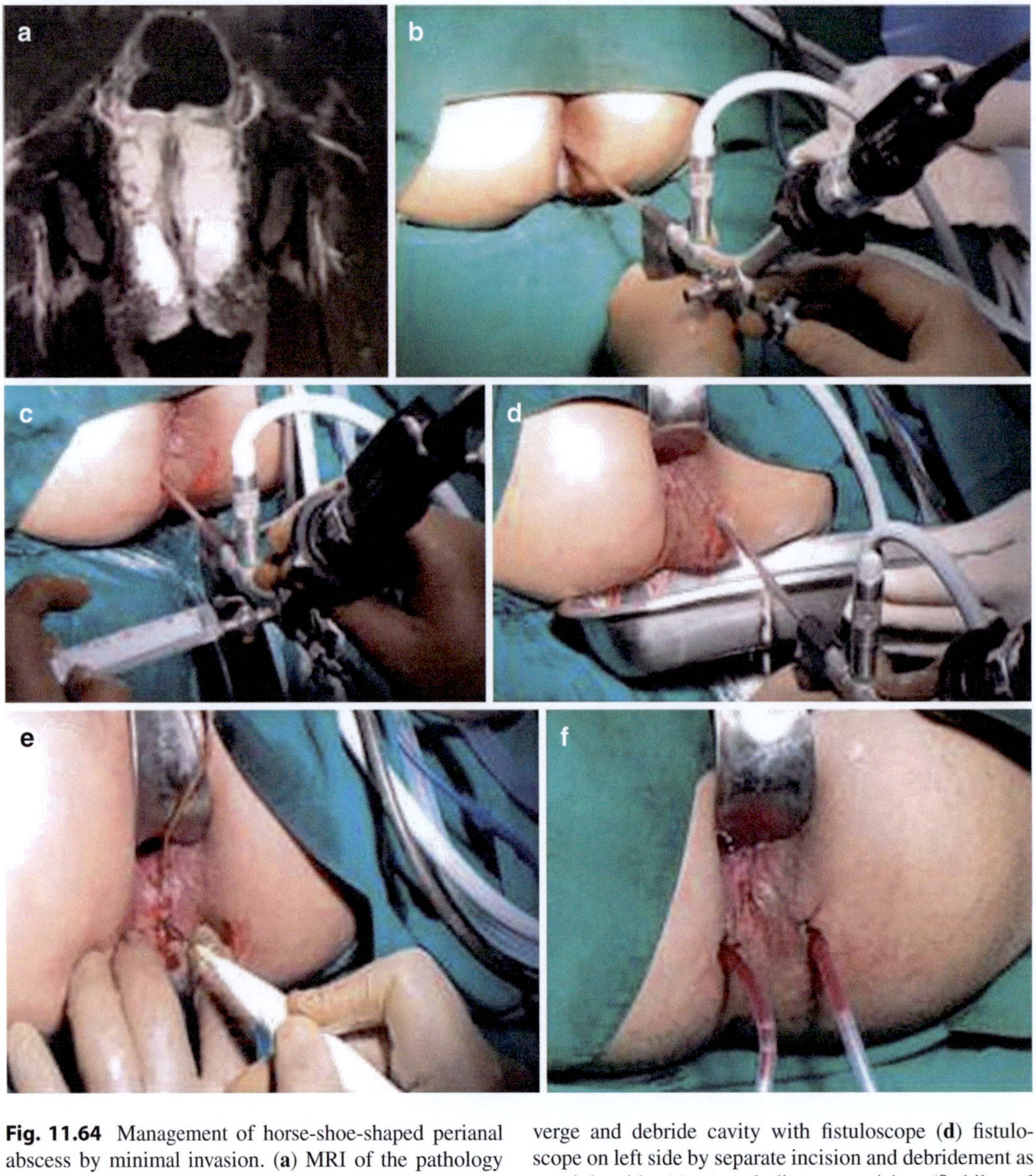

Fig. 11.64 Management of horse-shoe-shaped perianal abscess by minimal invasion. (**a**) MRI of the pathology (**b**) putting scope through the internal opening in posterior midline (**c**) incision over right side cavity close to anal verge and debride cavity with fistuloscope (**d**) fistuloscope on left side by separate incision and debridement as on right side (**e**) central disease excision (**f**) bilateral drains

11.8.4 Deep Postanal Abscess (Fig. 11.65)

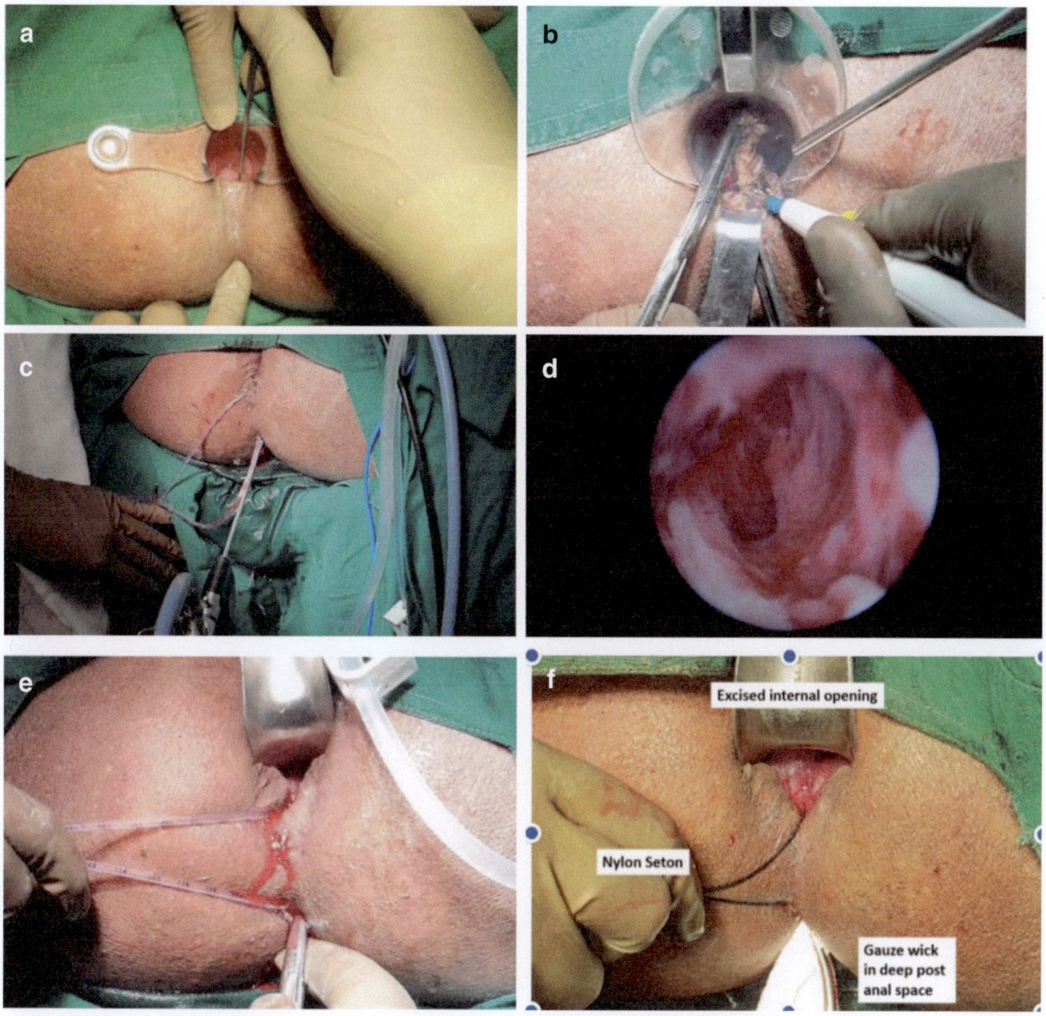

Fig. 11.65 Management of deep postanal abscess by MIS. (**a**) probing internal opening and feeling tip in posterior midline deep, gently under anaesthesia. (**b**) Excise central disease. (**c**) Putting scope in deep post anal space after incision over tip of the probe incising skin and fibres of ano coccygeal ligament longitudinally. (**d**) Inside view of the abscess cavity. (**e**) Curettage of cavity and putting loop around sphincter complex. (**f**) Partly closed internal opening after central disease excision and Draining seton and loose gauge wick

11.9 Definitive Management of Perianal Abscess in Ischiorectal Fossa with Concomitant Trans-Sphincteric Fistula by Hybrid Approach (Fig. 11.66; Video 11.1)

- After confirmation of the abscess, drainage and debridement is done under vision by 1470 nm diode LASER through fistuloscope.
- For definitive management of associated fistula, central disease is excised by excision of internal opening and exploration of inter-sphincteric space.
- Transanal closure of the opening in external sphincter is done with PDS 2.0 suture (Fig. 11.66g).
- Drain is kept in abscess cavity for 5–7 days.

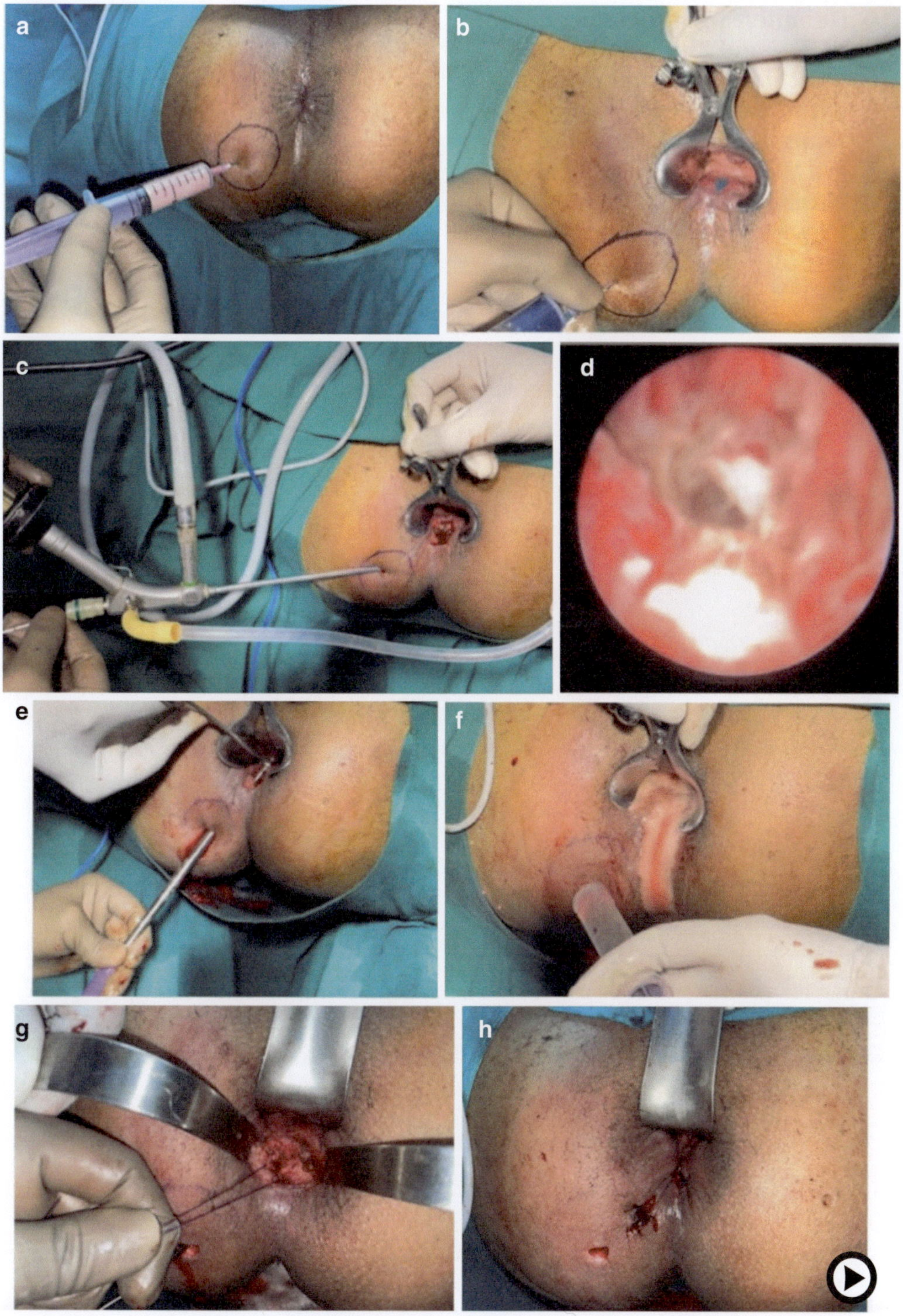

Fig. 11.66 (**a**) Needle aspiration of pus. (**b**) Internal communication at dentate line. (**c**) Central disease excision and fistuloscope insertion with LASER fibre. (**d**) Internal view of abscess cavity—fulgration by LASER. (**e**) FiXicision. (**f**) Lavage with H_2O_2 and saline. (**g**) Closure of internal opening in external sphincter by PDS 2.0. (**h**) Drain in abscess cavity. Video 11.1 Definitive management of perianal abscess in ischiorectal fossa with concomitant transphincteric fistula by hybrid approach (▶ https://doi.org/10.1007/000-hq1)

11.10 Definitive Management of Perianal Abscess in Ischiorectal Fossa with Concomitant Transsphincteric Fistula in a Minimally Invasive Way by Putting a Cutting Seton (Fig. 11.67)

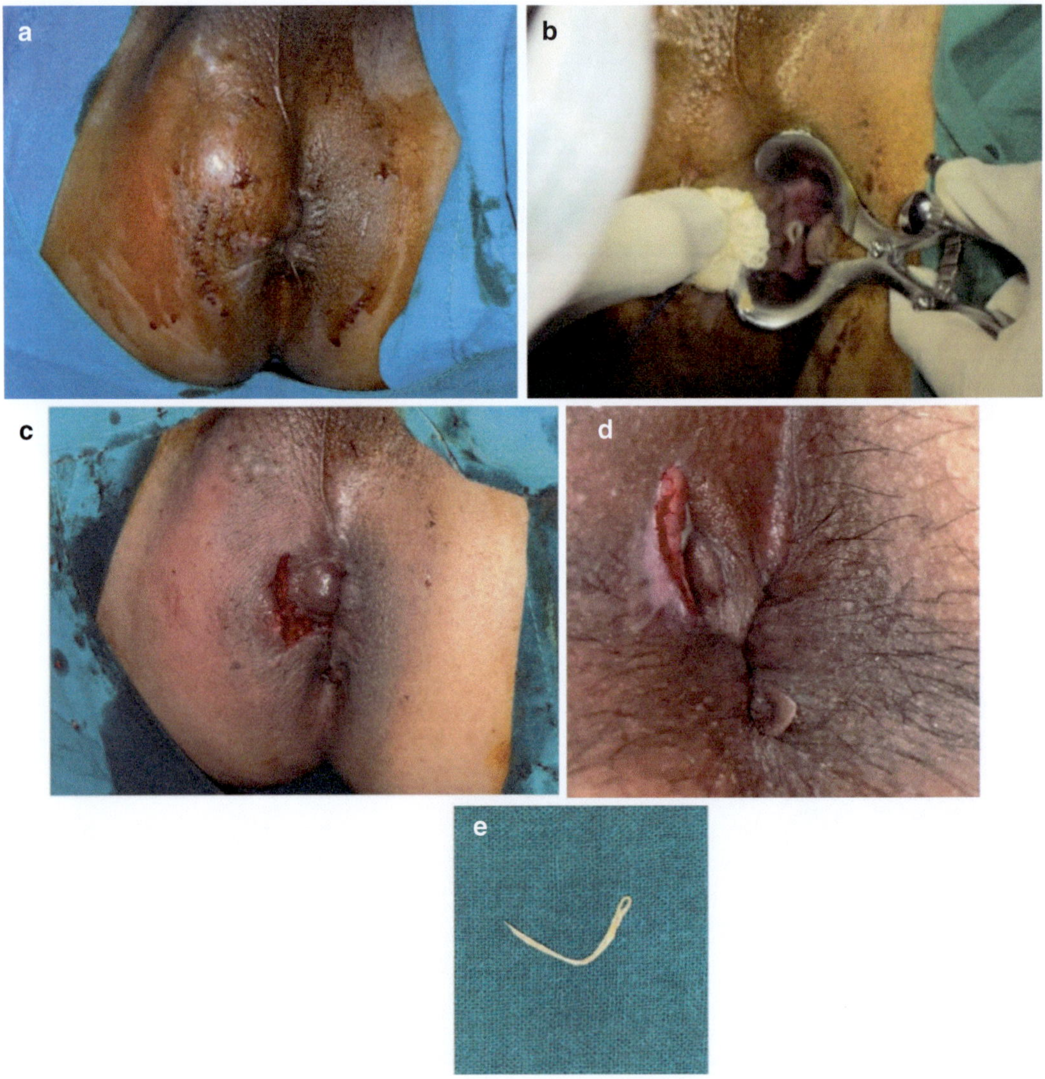

Fig. 11.67 (**a**) Right anterior perianal abscess. (**b**) Internal opening marked with stroke of electric cautery at the site of egress of dye. (**c**) Abscess drained by incision close to anal verge seton (Ksharsootra) passed for associated fistula. (**d**) Wound after seton came out within 3 weeks. (**e**) Seton came out after slowly cutting through the muscle patient brought it from home

11.11 Post-operative Care

- Wash the area with water, two to three times a day or as many times patient goes for evacuation, to keep it clean.
- Except for first post-surgery dressing, no packing is usually required. Post-surgery dressing should also be very loose-pack and sufficient enough to just control any bleed from margins of the wound.
- If tube drain is kept for dependent drainage, one can flush it with saline to keep the cavity clean and empty, for initial five to seven days till cavity collapses.
- After adequate drainage and debridement of abscess, antibiotics are required for local cellulitis, systemic sepsis, necrotising infections, immunocompromised patients and patients on prosthetic valves or other prosthesis.
- Use of pus-culture and antibiotics as per sensitivity is controversial but can be ordered in high-risk patients.
- Usually antibiotics, when required are given to cover whole spectrum of aerobic and anaerobic bacteria with metronidazole.
- Stool softeners are prescribed to avoid constipation, avoid any diarrhoea.
- Sanitary napkins provide good dressing-material to soak any secretions from wound to avoid maceration of skin around. We advise to paste sanitary napkins in rear side of undergarment or one can use adult diapers in early post-operative days if secretions and discharge from the wound is heavy.
- When we use ksharsootra (chemical seton) in a concomitant case of fistula in ano with abscess, initially we tie it loose to act as draining seton.
- Once the infected secretions decrease and cavity collapses, which usually takes place in five to seven days, depending on size of the cavity, we replace it with a fresh seton and tie it snuggly enough to act as slow cutting seton. Never tie it too tight as it causes pain.
- We replace seton with a fresh seton every fortnight till it comes out. Use local block or sedation as per sensitivity level of the patient while changing seton.
- Alkaline pH of ksharsootra is buffered within 24 hours.

11.12 Complications (Table 11.1)

Table 11.1 Complications of MIS to drain perianal abscess

Complications	Preventions	Management
Incomplete drainage	Incision may be small but scope makes it feasible to do complete fulgration, debridement under vision which should be thorough put the drain in dependent position.	Curette and drain again.
Premature closure	Thorough curettage allows early collapse of the cavity, dilate the opening if required.	Re-open the cavity by liberal incision and keep it open till cavity heals completely.
Persistent fistula	Preop. MRI	Manage fistula on its merit.
	Try to locate internal opening and extension in inter sphincteric space.	

11.13 Tips and Tricks

- Detailed knowledge about anatomy of perianal spaces and paths of spread of intersphincteric pus cannot be overemphasised.
- All cases of perianal abscess due to cryptoglandular origin actually have a connection at dentate line due to anatomy of anal gland.
- Although patients with perianal abscess present in emergency, pre-op imaging by MRI helps in complex cases. A detailed anorectal examination under anaesthesia is of paramount value.
- Always give incision over intersphincteric space to drain an intersphincteric abscess.
- For draining intersphincteric abscess going up in supralevator space without any external opening, fistuloscope is of immense value in the management of such cases.
- For draining an abscess in ischiorectal fossa or post-anal space, give incision as close to anal verge as possible to drain the affected area. Do not give cruciate skin incision, instead use drain in dependant area.
- In the name of breaking loculi, do not damage nerves and blood vessels running in ischiorectal fossa by swiping finger blindly in the cavity. Anything which resists to finger or instrument, should not be torn.
- Better do complete debridement under vision with the scope.
- Follow the rule of skeletal muscle while selecting the site of drainage.
  - Pus collection medial or inside the skeletal muscle (external sphincter and levator ani) is drained in the anorectum (Figs. 11.68 and 11.69).
  - Pus lateral or outside the external sphincter or supralevator abscess which has breached the skeletal muscle is drained outside the muscle through ischiorectal fossa (Fig. 11.70).

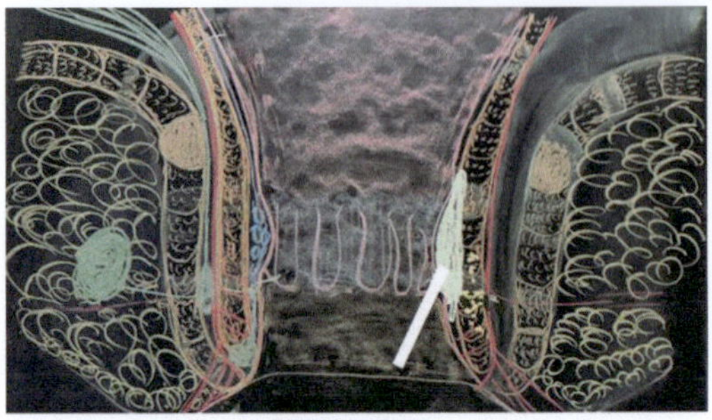

Fig. 11.68 Drainage inside the anal canal shown by white line

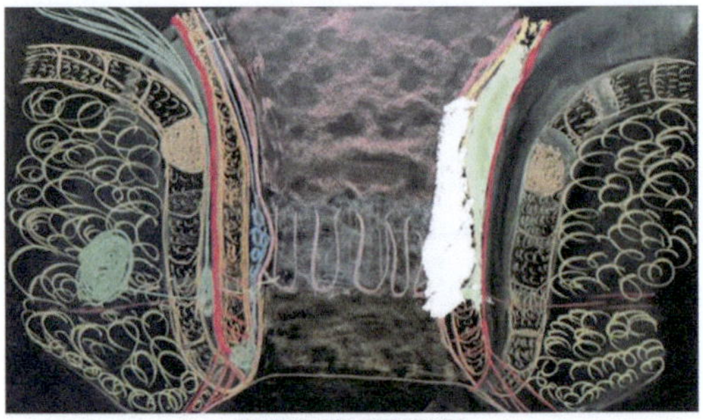

Fig. 11.69 Deep intersphincteric abscess drainage inside the anal canal shown by white marker

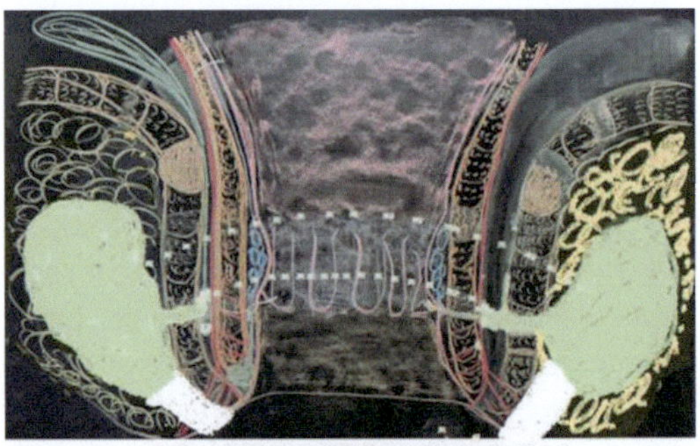

Fig. 11.70 Abscess lateral to external sphincter drained outer to external sphincter through ischiorectal fossa shown by white marker

A supralevator abscess can originate from three sources:

1. Extension of intersphincteric cryptoglandular abscess.
2. Pelvic and abdominal organs, e.g., pus, from ruptured appendix bulging in the rectum.
3. Translevator extension from ischiorectal abscess (Iatrogenic or spontaneous).

Former two are to be drained inside anorectum and latter is to be drained through perineum via ischiorectal fossa [6] (Fig. 11.71).

It is good idea to obtain MRI in such cases to find origin of abscess.

Type 1 which is the commonest of all, if drained through perineum, will lead to formation of suprasphincteric fistula a difficult entity to manage (Fig. 11.72).

- Carefully examine the anal canal for fistula and manage it as described.
- After drainage of the ischiorectal abscess, intersphincteric exploration with ligation of intersphincteric fistula tract (LIFT) can also be done as definitive management of associated fistula with fairly good results [7].

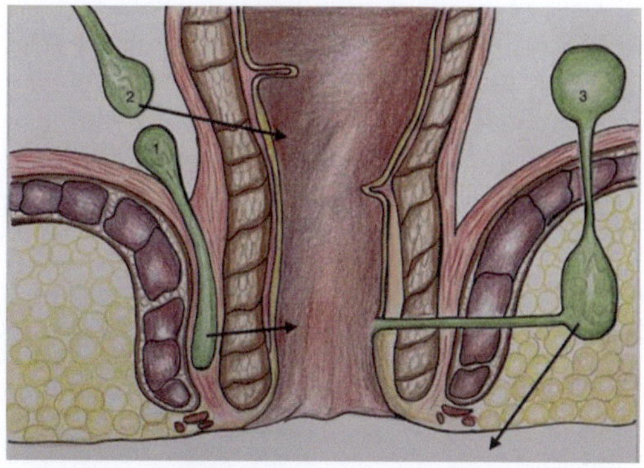

Fig. 11.71 Supra levator abscess (SLA) of intersphincteric origin (1) drained at dentate line, pelvic origin; (2) drained in the rectum, trans-levator extension of ischiorectal abscess; (3) drained through the perineum with definitive management of trans-sphincteric fistula

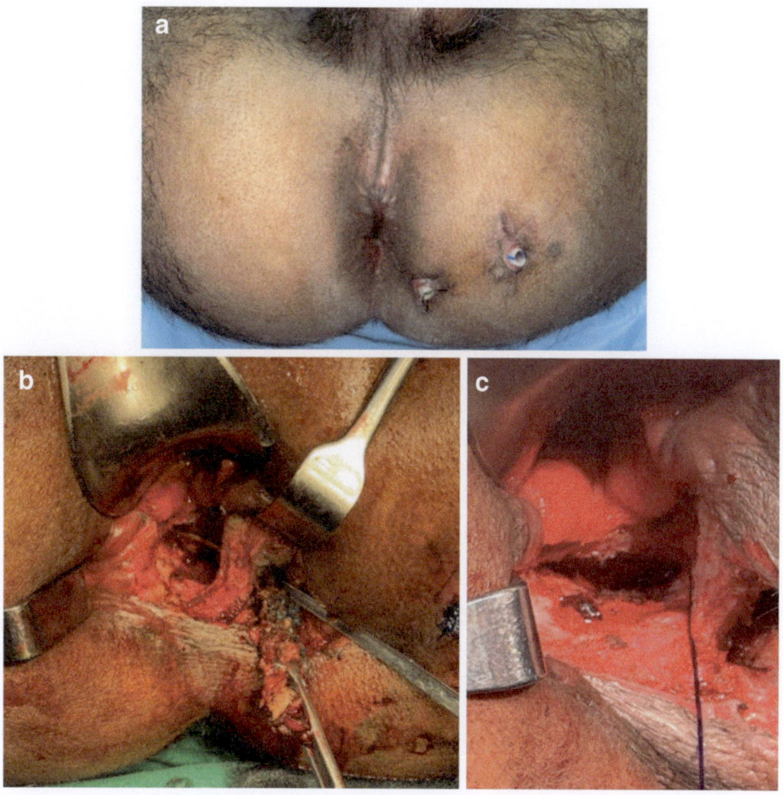

Fig. 11.72 (**a**) Supralevator abscess of inter-sphincteric origin drained through perineum. (**b**) Formation of suprasphincteric fistula which was cored out through levator ani (iliococcygeous). (**c**) Transanal closure of opening in levator through inter sphincteric space, using 2.0 PDS. (Operated by Dr. Parvez Sheikh)

11.14 How to Manage Necrotizing Peri Anal Abscess/Fournier's Gangrene (Figs. 11.73 and 11.74)

In case of necrosis minimally invasive method should not be used instead these patients require extensive debridement of necrosed tissue till vascularity is visible. As sphincters are spared, can be managed without faecal diversion.

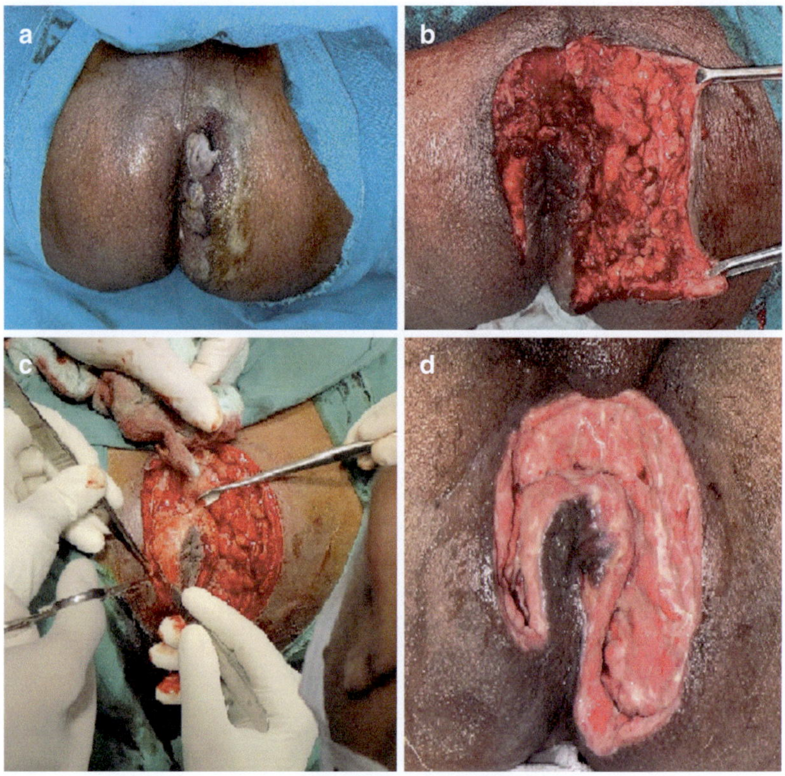

Fig. 11.73 Necrotizing perianal abscess. (**a**) Multiple discharging sinuses with skin necrosed and gangrenous tissue. (**b**) Necrosed tissue debrided till the vascular tissue appears all around. (**c**) Second debridement on the third day. (**d**) Post-operative after 9 days. Necrotizing peri anal abscess needs extensive debridement. Sphincters are spared. Can be managed without faecal diversion

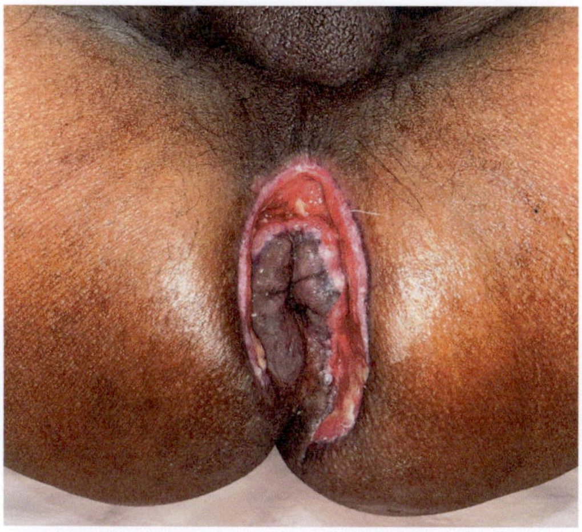

Fig. 11.74 Same patient, 25th postoperative day. Check the contraction of the wound

Algorithm for Perianal Abscess

History and clinical presentation
MRI/perianal ultrasound
Abscess in side skeletal muscle drain-in
Outside the skeletal muscle drain-out
Remain close to anal verge
Don't give cruciate incision
Don't break nerves and blood vessels with finger in ischiorectal fossa, in the name of breaking loculi
Use drains
Locate internal opening
Do definitive management of fistula
If possible by non-excisional method, or use seton, or just drain the abscess and leave fistula for specialist management

References

1. Jorge JMN, Habr-Gama A. Anatomy and embryology of the colon, rectum, and anus. In: Wolff BG, et al., editors. The ASCRS textbook of colon and rectal surgery. New York: Springer; 2007. https://doi.org/10.1007/978-0-387-36374-5_1.
2. Garg P, Dawka S, Yagnik VD, Kaur B, Menon GR. Anal fistula at roof of ischiorectal fossa inside levator-ani muscle (RIFIL): a new highly complex anal fistula diagnosed on MRI. Abdom Radiol (NY). 2021;46(12):5550–63. https://doi.org/10.1007/s00261-021-03261-y. Epub 2021 Aug 29. PMID: 34455464
3. Azhough R, Jalali P, Dashti MR, Taher S, Aghajani A. Intradermal methylene blue analgesic application in posthemorrhoidectomy pain management: a randomized controlled trial. Front Surg. 2024;11:1354328. https://doi.org/10.3389/fsurg.20241354328.
4. ICMR collaborating centers, central bio-statistical monitoring unit, Madras: multicentric randomized clinical trial of Kshara sutra (Ayurvedic medicated thread), in the management of fistula-in ano. Indian J Med Res. 1991;94:77–185.
5. Management of Complex Fistula-in-ano by Interception of Fistula Track with Application of Ksharasutra (IFTAK): s Novel Technique Manoranjan Sahu1 Ashish Sharma1. J Coloproctol. 2022;42(4):2793285.
6. Parks AG, Gordon PH, Hardcastle JD. A classification of fistula-in-ano. Br J Surg. 1976;63(1):1–12. https://doi.org/10.1002/bjs.1800630102. PMID: 1267867.
7. Rojanasakul A, Booning N, Huimin L, Pongpirul K, Sahakitrungruang C. Intersphincteric Exploration With Ligation of Intersphincteric Fistula Tract or Attempted Closure of Internal Opening for Acute Anorectal Abscesses. Dis Colon Rectum. 2021 Apr 1;64(4):438–445. https://doi.org/10.1097/DCR.0000000000001867. PMID: 33394781.

Suggested Reading

Adamina M, Pozza G. How to drain an abscess Springer Nature Switzerland AG 2022 235. In: Ratto C, et al., editors. Anal fistula and abscess, coloproctology. https://doi.org/10.1007/978-3-030-76670-2_17.

Aparício DJ, Leichsenring C, Sobrinho C, Pignatelli N, Geraldes V, Nunes V. Supralevator abscess: new treatment for an uncommon aetiology: case report. Int J Surg Case Rep. 2019;59:128–31. https://doi.org/10.1016/j.ijscr.2019.05.016. Epub 2019 May 13. PMID: 31132611; PMCID: PMC6536772

Kelly ME, Heneghan HM, McDermott FD, et al. The role of loose seton in the management of anal fistula: a multicenter study of 200 patients. Tech Coloproctol. 2014;18:9153919.

Millan M, García-Granero E, Esclápez P, Flor-Lorente B, Espí A, Lledó S. Management of intersphincteric abscesses. Color Dis. 2006;8(9):777–80. https://doi.org/10.1111/j.1463-1318.2006.01035.x. PMID: 17032324

Patton V, Chen CM, Lubowski D. Long-term results of the cutting seton for high anal fistula. ANZ J Surg. 2015;85(10):720–7. https://doi.org/10.1111/ans.13156. Epub 2015 May 21. PMID: 25997475

Rosen DR, Kaiser AM. Definitive seton management for transsphincteric fistula-in-ano: harm or charm? Colorectal Dis. 2016;18:4883495.

Sahu M, Sharma A. A novel technique: management of complex fistula-in-ano by interception of fistula track with application of Ksharasutra (IFTAK). J Coloproctol. 2022;42(04):279–85. https://doi.org/10.1055/s-0042-1756145.

Schiano di Visconte M, Piccoli G, Brusciano L, Docimo L, Veronese M. A mini-invasive procedure for the treatment of supralevator abscess of cryptoglandular origin by extrasphincteric extension: preliminary results at 1-year follow-up. Int J Color Dis. 2019;34(4):763–7. https://doi.org/10.1007/s00384-019-03243-z. Epub 2019 Jan 15. PMID: 30645671

Téoule P, Seyfried S, Joos A, Bussen D, Herold A. Management of retrorectal supralevator abscess-results of a large cohort. Int J Color Dis. 2018;33(11):1589–94. https://doi.org/10.1007/s00384-018-3094-7. Epub 2018 May 29. PMID: 29845388

van Onkelen RS, Gosselink MP, Schouten WR. Treatment of anal fistulas with high intersphincteric extension. Dis Colon Rectum. 2013;56(8):987–91. https://doi.org/10.1097/DCR.0b013e3182908be6. PMID: 23838868

Zinicola R, Cracco N. Draining an anal abscess: the skeletal muscle rule. Color Dis. 2014;16(7):562.

Zinicola R, Cracco N, Rossi G, Giuffrida M, Giacometti M, Nicholls RJ. Acute supralevator abscess: the little we know. Ann R Coll Surg Engl. 2022;104(9):645–9. https://doi.org/10.1308/rcsann.2021.0257.

12 Fistula in Ano: How Relevant It Is to Know the Anatomical Classification of Fistulae in Ano Before Going to Operation Theatre

Abstract

Fistula is a chronic suppuration which starts from infected anal gland in intersphincteric space, gets trapped between the internal and external sphincter and can breach sphincter mechanism at different levels.

- Fistula takes some predictable routes which are categorised as anatomical types by A G Parks. Park's classification is explained by class-room board drawings and video.
- Recently magnetic resonance imaging (MRI) has played a significant role in detection of these tracts and associated abscesses. MRI-based classification of fistula in ano as suggested by Morris and popularly k.a. St. James University classification has been explained by diagrams.
- Suggestions to improve the St. James classification are submitted with a detailed check-list of MRI reporting for fistula in ano.
- Recently Pankaj Garg has come out with another classification published as Garg classification of fistula in ano to improve upon the previous classifications. He recently defined, new fistula variant based on MRI studies and baptised as roof of Ischiorectal fossa inside levator ani (RIFIL), is also mentioned.
- All important classifications are analysed, and their strong and weak points have been explored to find their relevance in the management of this tricky condition.
- Author's own concept of three anatomical parts of a fistula, is also defined in an attempt to standardise fistula management.
- Recent developments should improve the outcomes of fistula surgery.

12.1 What Does One Need to Know for Successful Surgery of Fistula in Ano?

Following essentials are better known to the operator:

- Accurate anatomical knowledge of the area and predictable routes taken by fistulae in various combinations.
- Base-line sphincter function.
- Anatomy of this region is complex with vulnerable physiology.
- Many times some damage to sphincter mechanism is inevitable, keep it to minimum.

Supplementary Information The online version contains supplementary material available at https://doi.org/10.1007/978-981-96-6190-9_12. The videos can be accessed individually by clicking the DOI link in the accompanying figure caption or by scanning this link with the SN More Media App.

S. K. Singla, K. Mital, *Operative Manual of Minimally Invasive and LASER Ano-proctology*,
https://doi.org/10.1007/978-981-96-6190-9_12

12.2 Expectations from a Classification

An idle classification of fistula in ano should.

- Give a detailed road map of routes taken by fistula tracts so that surgeon can make 3D model of diseased anal canal.
- Categorise commonly occurring patterns in groups and in order of complexity.
- Guide about the method of treatment and tells prognosis.
- Be simple and propose a common language for medical fraternity to help in comparing results and development of further research.

12.3 Some Known Classifications of Fistula in Ano

12.3.1 Goodsall's Rule [1]

It was an initial attempt to find internal opening based on location of external opening in a case of fistula in ano. Mark an imaginary transverse line across the middle of anal opening (Fig. 12.1). Anal opening shown as blue spot. External opening, posterior to this line, opens in midline posteriorly (shown as black dots).

- Anterior perianal fistulas have a radial tract (shown as black dots).
- Exception (shown as red dots) (Fig. 12.1).
- Anterior external opening 3 cm away from the anal verge may take a curvilinear tract and open in the midline posteriorly.
- Very low short straight posterior fistulas may have radial tract.
- Anterior horse-shoe fistulae in ano is a well-known condition which obviates this rule (Fig. 12.2).
- Goodsall's rule has more-exceptions-than-rule statements.

12.3.2 Park's Classification Based on Study of 400 Cases [2]

Primary internal opening is always at dentate line corresponding to effected anal gland.

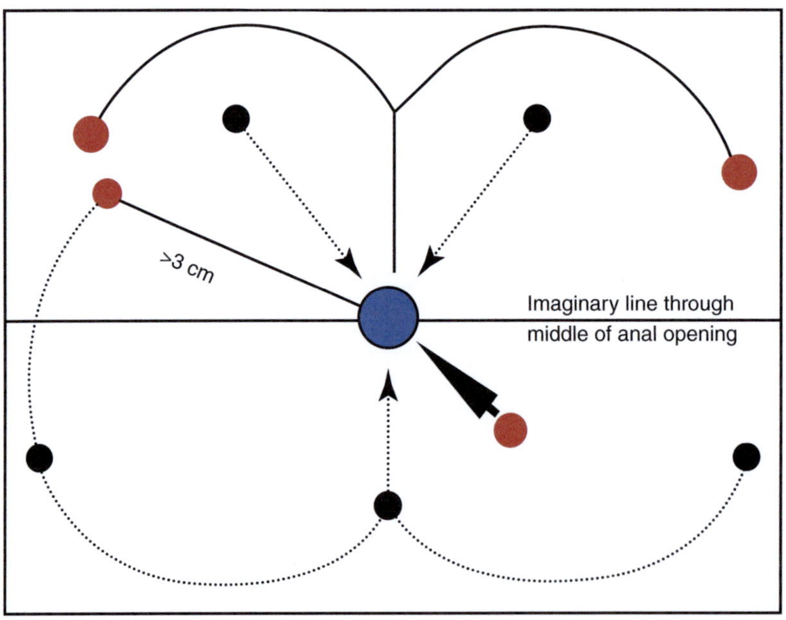

Fig. 12.1 Depicting DH Goodsall's observations eponymously known as Goodsall's rule and its exceptions (as patient in lithotomy position)

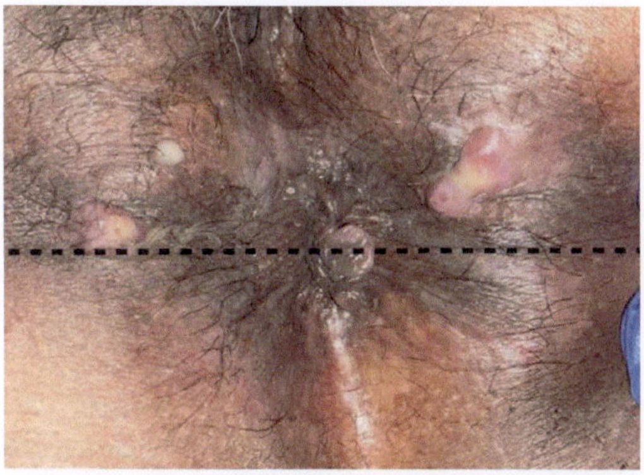

Fig. 12.2 Patient in lithotomy position, imaginary line across anal opening divides perianal space in to anterior and posterior halves. Right and left external openings take curvilinear path and join in the anterior midline before opening in to anal canal

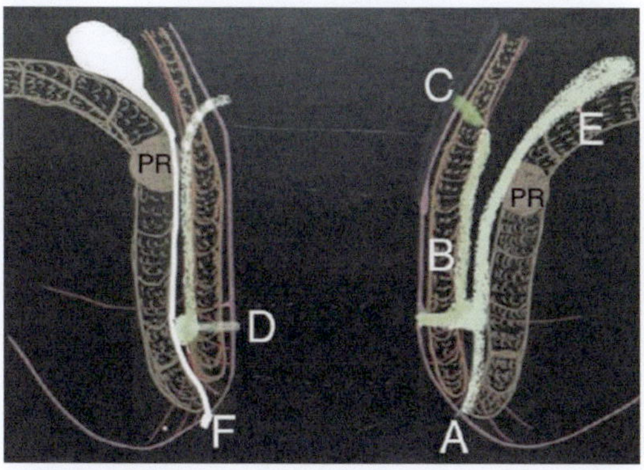

Fig. 12.3 Different variants of intersphincteric fistulae as Park's classification, type "F" shown in white colour is not from cryptoglandular origin, instead manifestation of pelvic disease. (PR) puborectalis

Fistula are classified according to the route taken by the tract before it opens on the skin or ends as blind sinus short of it.

Type 1 inter sphincteric fistula 183 (45%) cases (Fig. 12.3). Tract breaches internal sphincter only and travels in between the internal and external sphincter. It may have many variants (Fig. 12.3):

A. Simple (137).
B. High blind tract (15).
C. High tract opening in to lower rectum (9).

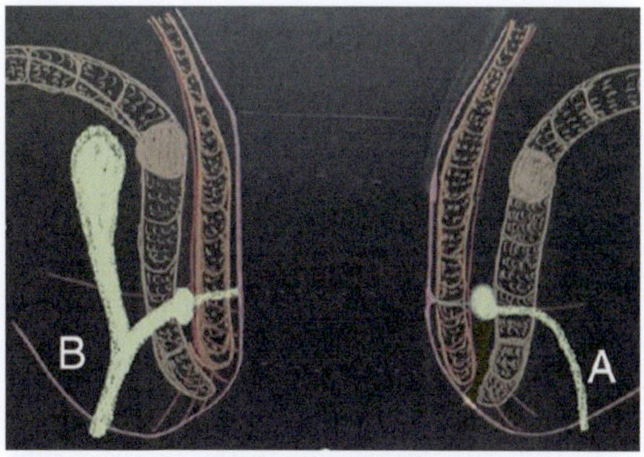

Fig. 12.4 Two variants of trans-sphincteric fistula

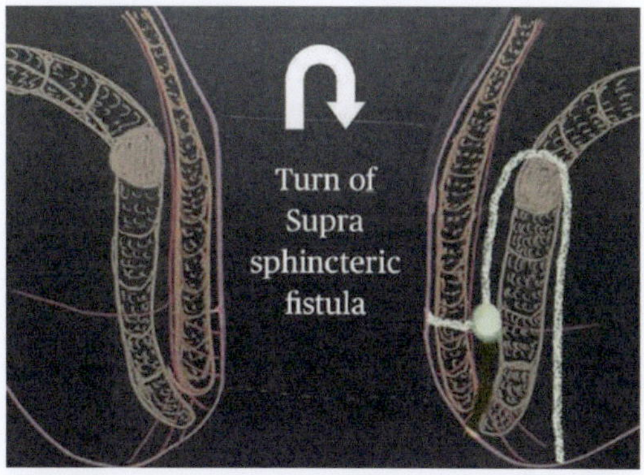

Fig. 12.5 Suprasphincteric fistula taking U turn over the puborectalis

D. High intersphincteric without perineal opening (5).
E. High intersphincteric with pelvic extension (15).
F. Intersphincteric fistula from pelvic disease (2).

Type 2 Transphincteric fistula 116(30%) (Fig. 12.4).

If tract breaches external sphincter.

A. Uncomplicated (83)
B. With a high blind tract (34).

Type 3 Suprasphincteric fistula 78(20%) (Fig. 12.5).

- If tract ascends in intersphincteric space over to puborectalis and then takes a U turn to breach iliococcygeous muscle, to enter in ischiorectal fossa.

Type 4 Extra sphincteric fistula 20 (5%) (Fig. 12.6).

- Tract from skin goes outside the sphincter complex and breach levator-ani and enters rectum high. Usually post traumatic or iatrogenic.
- It has following variants.
  A. Secondary to trans-sphincteric fistula (10).
  B. Due to trauma (2).
  C. Due to specific anorectal diseases like Crohn's, ulcerative colitis and carcinoma. Excluded from study by Park as these fistulae have bizarre pattern [2].
  D. D. Due to pelvic inflammatory disease (8).

Submucous fistula recently added in the Parks classification by American Association of Colon and Rectal Surgeons [3]. (Fig. 12.7).

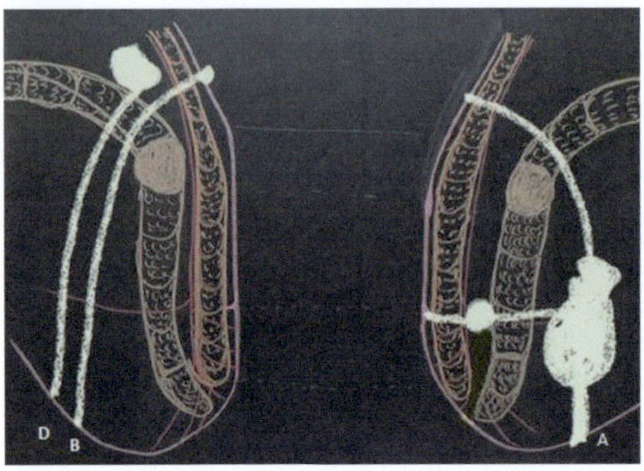

Fig. 12.6 Variants of extra sphincteric fistula, type A on Rt. side and type B and D on the Lt. Side of the sketch

When submucous abscess ruptures but the retained epithelium of gland persists as non-healing sinus.

Analysis of the Parks classification.

- Strong points.
  - First comprehensive anatomical classification of fistula in ano to be used widely.
  - Based on clinical data of 400 patients.
  - Excellent classification proposed by surgeons, when MRI/transrectal ultrasound (TRUS) were not available.
- Weak points.

Complexity of fistulae treatment has been explained clearly in the paper by Parks, though not graded in classification [2].

Usually in day-to-day practice, we use.

The Parks working classification of fistula in ano (Fig. 12.8), which broadly categorises fistula in ano into following types:

- Inter-sphincteric.
- Trans-sphincteric.
- Suprasphincteric.
- Extra sphincteric.

12.3.3 Classification of Fistula in Ano Based on MRI (4)

MRI plays a significant role in defining the routes taken by fistula and associated abscess.

Fig. 12.7 Submucous fistula in ano

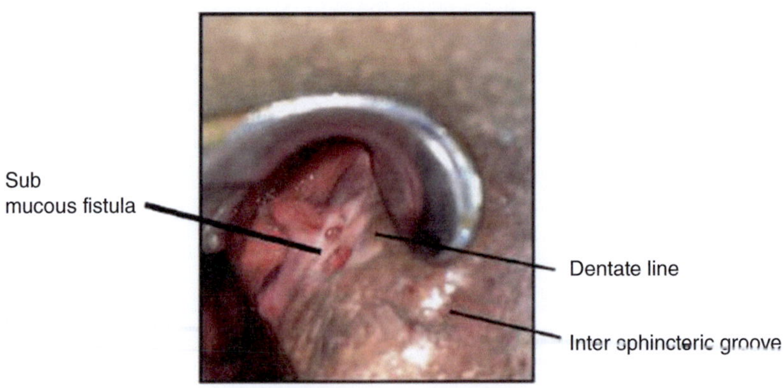

12.3.4 St. James University Hospital Classification [4] (Fig. 12.9)

- Grade 1: Simple linear intersphincteric fistula.
- Grade 2: Intersphincteric fistula with abscess or secondary tract.
- Grade 3: Trans-sphincteric fistula.
- Grade 4: Trans-sphincteric with abscess or secondary tract within the ischiorectal fossa. Suprasphincteric is also clubbed in it.
- Grade 5: Supralevator and trans-levator extension.

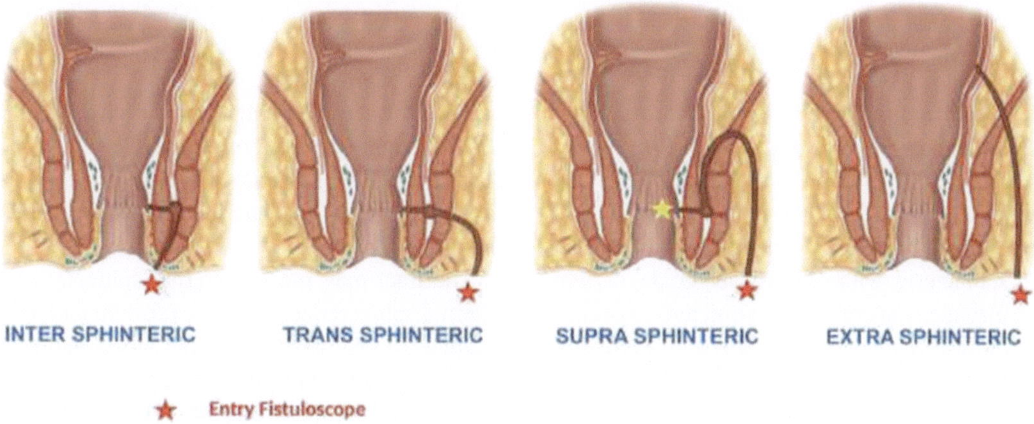

Fig. 12.8 Parks working-classification for fistula in ano. Red star shows entry point for fistuloscope in case of endoscopic management of fistula

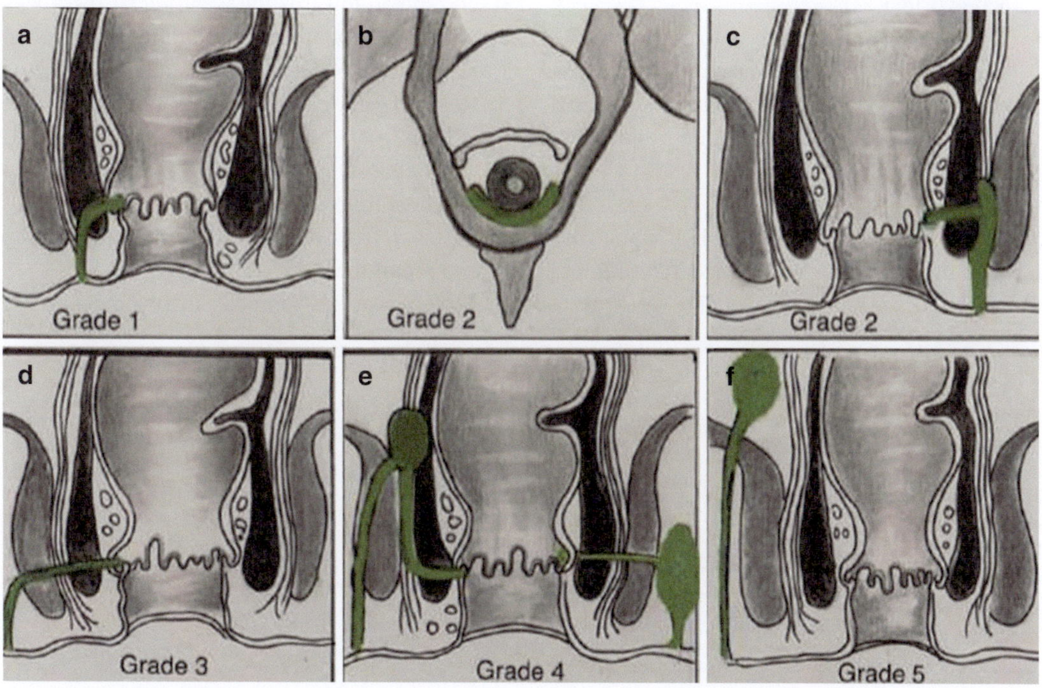

Fig. 12.9 St. James University Hospital classification of fistula in ano. (**a**) Grade 1: Intersphincteric fistula. (**b**) Grade 2: Intersphincteric fistula with horse-shoe extension. (**c**) Grade 2: Intersphincteric fistula with intersphincteric abscess. (**d**) Grade 3: Trans-sphincteric fistula. (**e**) Grade 4: Trans-sphincteric fistula with ischioanal abscess, suprasphincteric fistula clubbed in grade 4. (**f**) Grade 5: Supralevator extension

Analysis of the St. James University Hospital classification of fistula in ano:

Strong points in favour of the St. James University Hospital classification are as following:

- MRI-based widely used classification.
- Supralevator, translevator and extrasphincteric fistulae are grouped together as grade 5, as these fistulae need special attention.

Weak points against the St. James Hospital classification are following:

- Grading not correlated with severity.
- Suprasphincteric clubbed with trans-sphincteric with abscess as grade 4, while management of suprasphincteric fistula is more difficult as compared to trans-sphincteric fistula.
- All supralevator grouped in category 5 but management of supralevator abscess (SLA) from pure intersphincteric extension is different from SLA from trans-levator extension or pelvic origin.
- Very important information for surgeons, i.e., the vertical level of external sphincter involvement/height of breach in external sphincteric is not defined, that's why not reported by radiologists.

Considering importance of MRI in the treatment of fistula in ano, we propose the following check-list before reporting a MRI.

12.3.4.1 Reporting Checklist MRI for Fistula in Ano

Start reporting from inside out, that is, as disease starts and spreads.

Like collection or tract in intersphincteric space, breach in internal sphincter and internal opening if traceable.

Then any intersphincteric spread either circumferential or vertical (along wall of rectum in between the circular and longitudinal muscles of rectum or supralevator).

Level of vertical breach in external sphincter (LOVE) and circumferential breach at one place in midline posteriorly or at two places as shown in a case of posterior horse-shoe fistula (Fig. 12.10).

The tract may breach internal sphincter and external sphincter at 6′ o clock position and then bifurcates into two in post-anal space or intersphincteric collection and may breach external sphincter at two places and two tracts open separately in each ischiorectal fossa (Fig. 12.10).

For spread lateral to external sphincter, check any spread between the external sphincter and its fascia, spread towards the ischiorectal fossa, circumferential or vertical spread in the ischiorectal fossa. External opening on the skin.

Reporting checklist of MRI should include.

- Origin and internal opening—when traceable or where tract comes closest to anal mucosa.
- Distance from anal-verge of internal opening and top of the tract.
- Type of fistula—sphincter involvement.

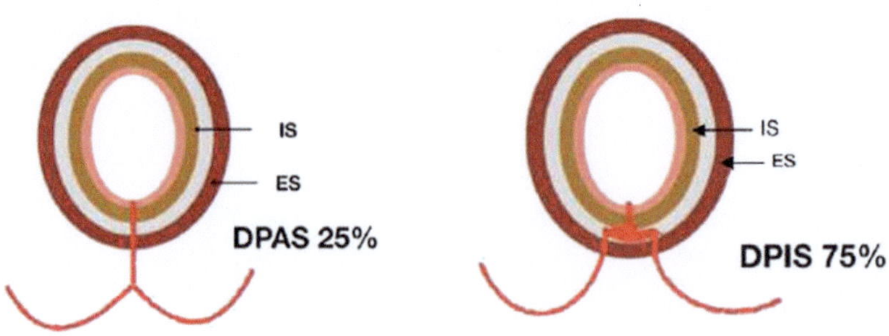

Fig. 12.10 Two deep posterior perianal spaces and routes taken by posterior horse shoe-shaped fistulae. DPAS, Deep post anal space DPIS, Deep posterior intersphincteric space [5]

- Extent of (height) external sphincter involvement is fairly accurate in MRI, but not reported as it is not included in the St. James classification.
- Associated abscess and its spread—vertical or circumferential.
- Involvement/odema of muscle or adjacent organ.
- Supralevator component and its origin—from pure intersphincteric extension, associated with suprasphincteric fistula, translevator extension or from pelvic origin.

If taken care, MRI and reports will be more useful to surgeons in patient care and research.

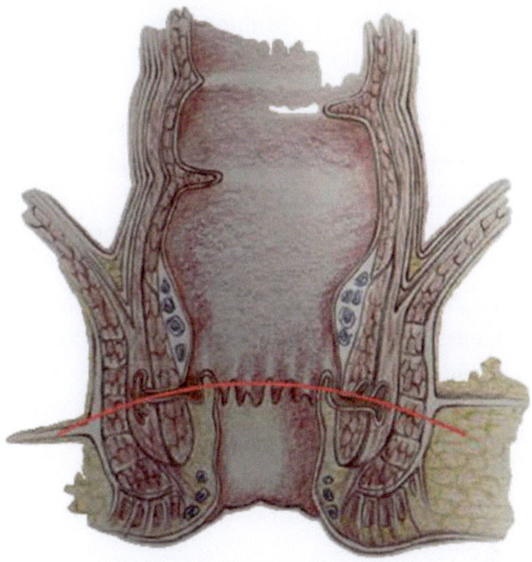

Fig. 12.11 Simple and complex fistulae based on sphincter complex involvement, simple below the red line and complex above the red line

12.3.5 Standards Practice Task Force Simplification [6]

Standards Practice Task Force of the American Society of Colon and Rectal Surgeons published a classification in 2011 to simplify the management of fistula in ano, keeping general surgeon in mind who does not have specialist colorectal training.

Classification proposed by standard practice task-force is as follows (Fig. 12.11):

- Simple fistula:

Involving less than one-third of sphincter complex (fistulotomy is possible without risk of incontinence).

- Complex fistula:

Involving more than one third of sphincter complex (fistulotomy has high risk of incontinence).

High fistula, supralevator fistula, fistula with multiple tracts, horse-shoe tracts, anterior fistula in a female and fistula with associated abscess, Crohn's disease, malignancy or existing continence disturbance.

Strong point of standard-practice task-force classification is its feasibility to be applied by general surgeon with no specialised training in ano-proctology.

Weak point of standard practice task force classification is in its over-simplification, leading to grading of many inter sphincteric fistulae as complex ones, contrary to real scenario.

12.3.6 Garg Classification of Fistula in Ano [7, 8]

Dr. Pankaj Garg classified fistula in ano on the basis of involvement of vertical extent of external sphincter. Feasibility of fistulotomy has been kept as a bench mark while defining management.

Grade I: LOW (less than 1/3 of external sphincter involvement)—single tract (intersphincteric or trans-sphincteric).

Grade II: LOW—Multiple tracts or associated abscess or horse-shoe tract (intersphincteric or trans-sphincteric). Grade III: HIGH (more than 1/3 of external sphincter involvement)—single tract (intersphincteric or trans-sphincteric) or associated comorbidities (anterior fistula in a female or already damaged/weakened sphincter, post-radiotherapy, Crohn's disease.

Grade IV: HIGH—Multiple tracts or associated abscess or horseshoe tract (intersphincteric or trans-sphincteric).

Grade V: Suprasphincteric or supralevator or extrasphincteric and roof of ischiorectal fossa in levator ani (RIFIL) [8].

Strong points of the Garg Classification:

- Grading corresponds to severity of fistula.
- Considers pre-operative weak external sphincter.
- MRI-based large data of 440 operated cases.
- Guides management as proposed by a surgeon.
- Includes new fistula variant called as RIFIL.

Limitations of the Garg classification:

All supralevator fistulae are grouped in Grade 5 while management of supralevator fistula developed from intersphincteric extension is different and easy, as compared to other varieties of supralevator fistula or abscess.

12.4 How Relevant Are Classifications of Fistula in Ano?

- Anatomical road-map of common routes taken by fistula in ano as described in the Parks Classification is relevant to surgeons in the management of this complex disease.
- So-called Goodsall's rule has limited relevance as it has more exceptions to learn as compared to rule statements. There is a saying (exceptions prove the rule) but Goodsall's rule has more exceptions to learn as compared to rule. Moreover, it suggests about horizontal spread only.
- Task-force classification got too simple and it loses its relevance.
- Check-list for MRI reporting tells us that the St. James University Hospital classification is relevant but should be modified to make more relevant to surgeons.
- Grading of anatomical classification of Parks and comparison on MRI and operative findings makes the GARG classification relevant.

12.5 One of the Authors (SKS) Suggests

After clinical examination and support by MRI, one should make a 3D picture of diseased anal canal before operating. For every fistula, management has to be customised.

Look for three components in the anatomy of a fistula (Fig. 12.12):

1. Inner component (inner to skeletal muscle).
2. Middle component (skeletal muscle itself).
3. Outer component (outer to skeletal muscle)
   - Inner component—internal opening, internal sphincter and intersphincteric component and spread in this area of embryonic fusion:
     - Vertical extension—including Deep intersphincteric or supralevator along the wall of rectum or re-entry in to rectum.
     - Circumferential extension–horse-shoe in mid-anal canal in intersphincteric space or in supralevator space.
   - Middle component—the tract through the skeletal muscle. One should know
     - Vertical trans-sphincteric level and suprasphincteric level of breach in external sphincter (level of vertical breach in external sphincter (LOVE)).

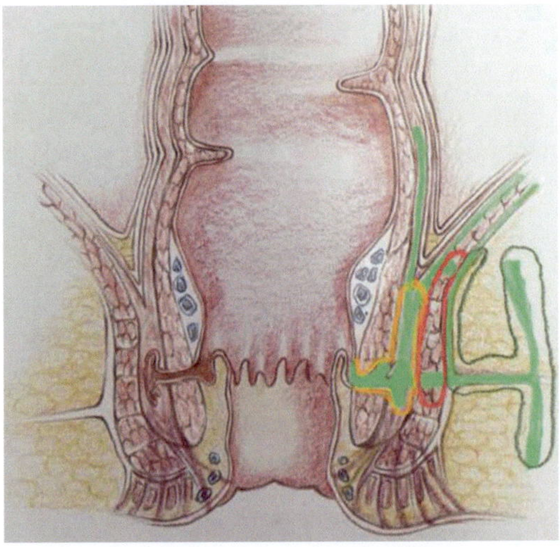

Fig. 12.12 Three components of fistula Inner component internal to skeletal muscle encircled in orange colour Middle component with in the skeletal muscle encircled in red colour outer component outer to skeletal muscle encircled in green colour

- Circumferential breach at one place or two places (as in horse-shoe posterior)
- Outer component spread of fistula.
  - Vertical spread—remaining below the levator or breach in levator, remaining in para-rectal or breach in rectum.
  - Circumferential—horse shoe in extra-sphincteric space.
  - Tract outer to external sphincter and levator ani but within fascia supporting external sphincter and levator ani infer-olaterally and associated collection ascends along the fascia lining the levator called as the tract in roof of ischio-rectal fossa in levator ani (RIFIL) [9].
  - Check pre-operative sphincter status.
  - In pure intersphincteric fistula, there is no middle and external component.
- Once all anatomical components of the fistula under treatment are clear to the surgeon, any complex fistula can be managed by dealing with all the components separately without jeopardising the continence mechanism. Details of this treatment method are described in Chap. 18: New concepts in minimally invasive methods to treat fistula in ano.

Video showing tracts of fistula as per the Parks classification (Fig. 12.13).

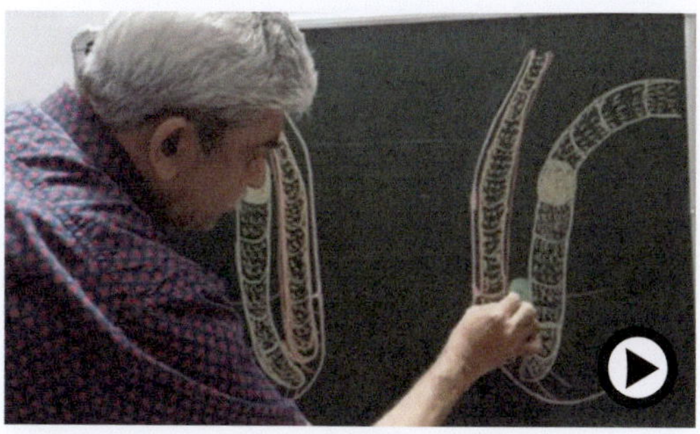

Fig. 12.13 Predictable anatomical routes taken by fistula in ano as proposed by Parks. Park's anatomical routes in detail Strong points First comprehensive anatomical classification of fistula in ano to be used widely Based on clinical data of 400 patients. Excellent classification proposed by surgeons when MRI/TRUS were not available. Video 12.1 Predictable anatomical routes taken by fistula in ano as proposed by Parks (▶ https://doi.org/10.1007/000-hq2)

References

1. Cuiñas K, Williams J. PTU-196 Goodsall's rule – past its sell-by date? Gut. 2015;64:A149.
2. Parks AG, Gordon PH, Hardcastle JD. A classification of fistula-in-ano. Br J Surg. 1976;63(1):1–12.
3. Gaertner WB, Burgess PL, Davids JS, Lightner AL, Shogan BD, Sun MY, Steele SR, Paquette IM, Feingold DL, Clinical Practice Guidelines Committee of the American Society of Colon and Rectal Surgeons. The American Society of Colon and Rectal Surgeons Clinical Practice Guidelines for the Management of Anorectal Abscess, Fistula-in-Ano, and Rectovaginal Fistula. Dis Colon Rectum. 2022;65(8):964–85. https://doi.org/10.1097/DCR.0000000000002473. Epub 2022 Jul 5. PMID: 35732009
4. Morris J, et al. MR imaging classification of perianal fistulas. Radiographics. 2000;20:623–35.
5. Zhang H, Zhou ZY, Hu B, Liu DC, Peng H, Xie SK, Su D, Ren DL. Clinical significance of 2 deep posterior perianal spaces to complex cryptoglandular fistulas. Dis Colon Rectum. 2016;59(8):766–74. https://doi.org/10.1097/DCR.0000000000000628. PMID: 27384095
6. Steele SR, Kumar R, Feingold DL, Raferty JL, Buie WD, Standards Practice Task Force of the American Society of Colon and Rectal Surgeons. Practice parameters for the management of perianal abscess and fistula-in-ano. Dis Colon Rectum. 2011;54(12):1465–74. [PubMed]. [Google scholar]
7. Garg P. garg classification for anal fistulas: is it better than existing classifications?—a review. Indian J Surg. 2018;80:606–8. https://doi.org/10.1007/s12262-018-1788-2.
8. Garg P, Dawka S, Yagnik VD, Kaur B, Menon GR. Anal fistula at roof of ischiorectal fossa inside levator-ani muscle (RIFIL): a new highly complex anal fistula diagnosed on MRI. Abdom Radiol (NY). 2021;46(12):5550–63. https://doi.org/10.1007/s00261-021-03261-y. Epub 2021 Aug 29. PMID: 34455464
9. Garg P, Bhattacharya K, Yagnik VD, Mahak G. Recent advances in the diagnosis and treatment of complex anal fistula. Ann Coloproctol. 2024;40(4):321–35. https://doi.org/10.3393/ac.2024.00325.0046. Epub 2024 Aug 30. PMID: 39228196

13 Fistula in Ano: Sphincter Preserving Procedures Ligation of Inter-Sphincteric Fistula Tract (LIFT)

Abstract

- Ligation of inter-sphincteric fistula tract (LIFT) procedure is based on the secure closure of the internal opening and removal of infected crypto-glandular tissue through the inter-sphincteric approach.
- Essential steps of the procedure, including incision at the inter-sphincteric groove, identification of the inter-sphincteric tract, secure ligation close to internal sphincter, removal of the inter-sphincteric tract to remove the crypto-glandular infection, scraping out all granulation tissue in the rest of the fistulous tract and suturing of the defect at the external sphincter muscle are described by operative photographs and video. Attention to detail is the key for a favourable outcome.
- Reasons of failure and reoccurrence have been mentioned.
- Some modifications to decrease the reoccurrence due to operative factors have been enumerated.

Supplementary Information The online version contains supplementary material available at https://doi.org/10.1007/978-981-96-6190-9_13. The videos can be accessed individually by clicking the DOI link in the accompanying figure caption or by scanning this link with the SN More Media App.

13.1 What One Should Know Before the Procedure

- New concept given and practised by Dr. Arun Rojanasakul in 2007, to intercept fistula in ano-tract in between internal and external sphincter by secure ligation called as ligation of inter-sphincteric fistula tract (LIFT) [1] (Fig. 13.1).
- Central disease that is infected gland area is excised by removing a segment of inter-sphincteric tract.
- As is evident from its name, it is good for trans-sphincteric component of the fistula.

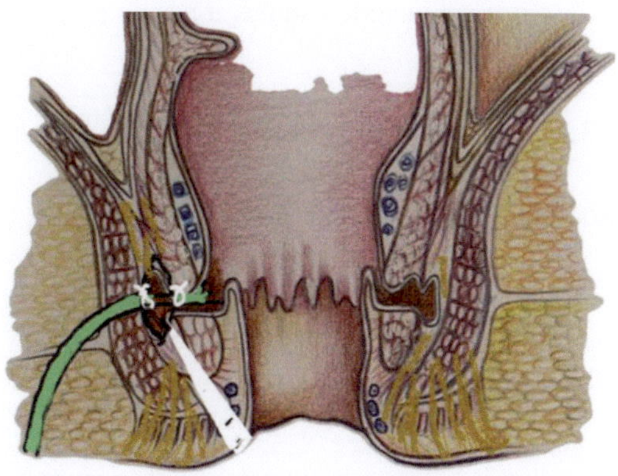

Fig. 13.1 Schematic to show route of entry in inter-sphincteric space (shown as white wedge) and ligation of inter-sphincteric fistula tract/LIFT (shown as green tract)

S. K. Singla, K. Mital, *Operative Manual of Minimally Invasive and LASER Ano-proctology*, https://doi.org/10.1007/978-981-96-6190-9_13

- Inter-sphincteric spread circumferential or vertical is to be dealt with intra-anal fistulotomy or excision of internal component.
- LIFT surgery for fistula became widely popular as it was a sphincter-saving surgery, easy to do and reproducible. Surgeons across the world adapted to it.
- Initial results could not be replicated worldwide.
- Modifications to improve the outcome were suggested by the inventor and other operators.

13.2 Indications

Better reserved for low and mid trans-sphincteric fistulae.

13.3 Contra-Indications

- Pure inter-sphincteric fistuale and/or their supra-levator extensions are dealt by intra-anal fistulotomy or excision of internal component.
- In high trans-sphincteric and supra-sphincteric fistulae, procedure becomes technically highly demanding and not done in routine.
- In extra-sphincteric fistulae, it has no role.

13.4 Equipment

Routine trolley for fistula surgery.

Additional.

Rojanasakul anal speculum (Fig. 13.2(4)).

Tip or proximal side of this speculum is heavy which makes it self-retaining.

- Parks speculum.
- Vaginal speculums various size, lighted.
- Curettes or Volkman's scoupe.
- Electro cautery and monopolar pencil and bipolar coagulator.
- Lahey's forceps/mixter forceps.
- Aneurysm needle.

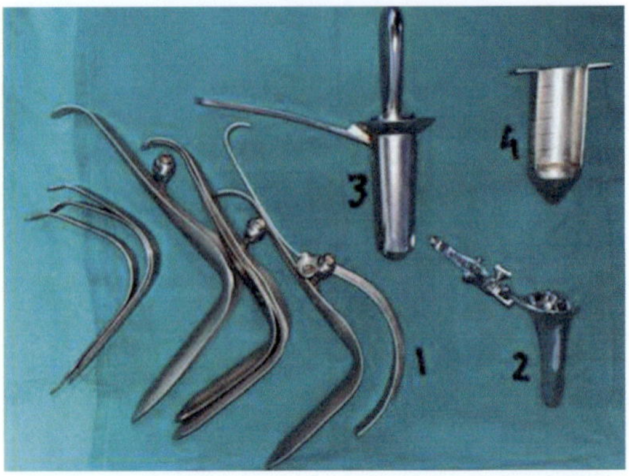

Fig. 13.2 (1) Vaginal speculums. (2) Parks speculum. (3) Proctoscope. (4) Rojanasakul anal speculum for LIFT

- Polyglactin sutures 2.0/3.0 on round body needle.

13.5 Procedure [2]

- Clinical examination under anaesthesia. Look for external opening, induration, swelling, previous scar for any gutter effect of previous surgery (Fig. 13.3a).
- Identify the internal opening.
  - Put Rojanasakul anal speculum in side anal canal or one can use Parks speculum or half speculum.
  - Put diluted dye through the external opening and notice its egress through the internal opening at dentate line.
  - Gently pass a probe through the tract. Passage of a probe if possible facilitates the procedure (Fig. 13.3b).
- Incision at inter-sphincteric groove.
  - Give saline adrenaline solution in inter-sphincteric groove for haemostasis during dissection (Fig. 13.4).
  - Identify inter-sphincteric groove and give curvilinear 2 cm incision over the tract and dissect with electro dissection pencil (Figs. 13.5 and 13.6).
- Dissection through inter-sphincteric plane to find inter-sphincteric fistula tract (Figs. 13.7 and 13.8):

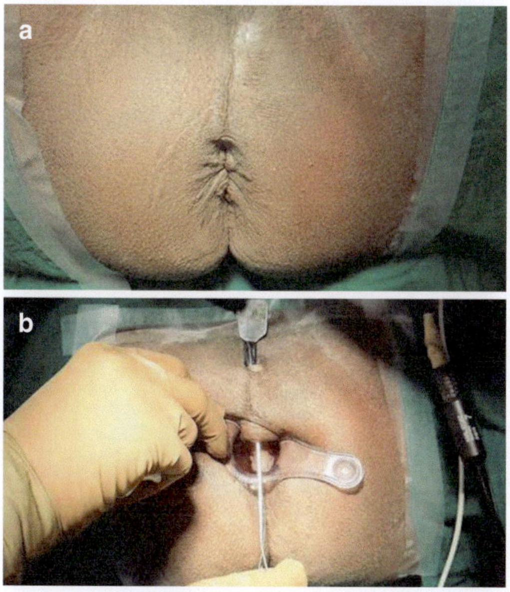

Fig. 13.3 (**a**) Patient in lithotomy, clinical examination on table External opening (EO) left anterior just lateral to perineal raphe, Digital rectal examination (DRE) induration anterior midline at dentate line. (**b**) Probe in the tract

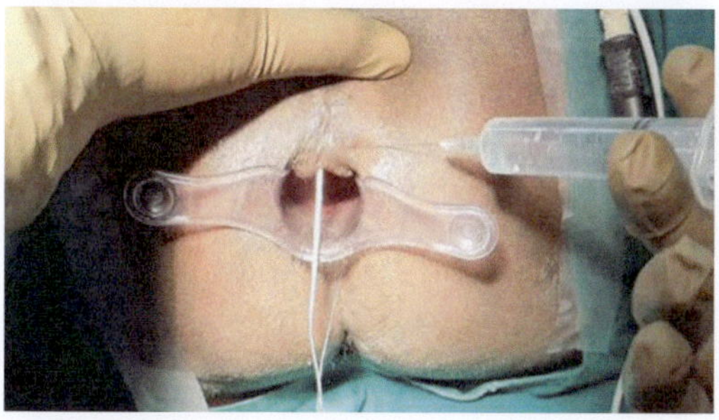

Fig. 13.4 Xylocaine adrenaline Sol. in saline 1:200000, 5–10 ml injected in inter-sphincteric groove

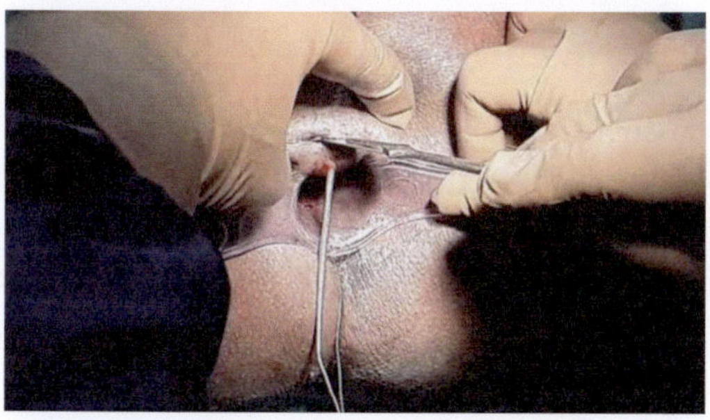

Fig. 13.5 Incision over inter-sphincteric grove

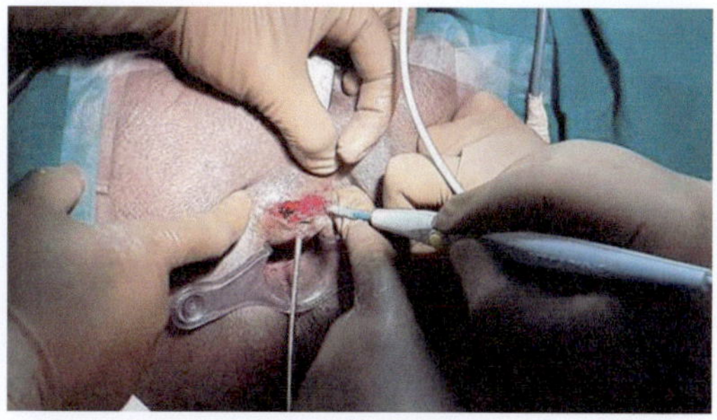

Fig. 13.6 Electro dissection in inter-sphincteric groove

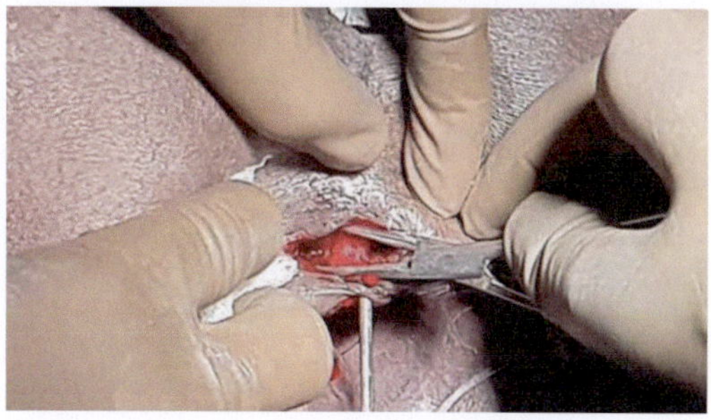

Fig. 13.7 Dissection in the inter-sphincteric space

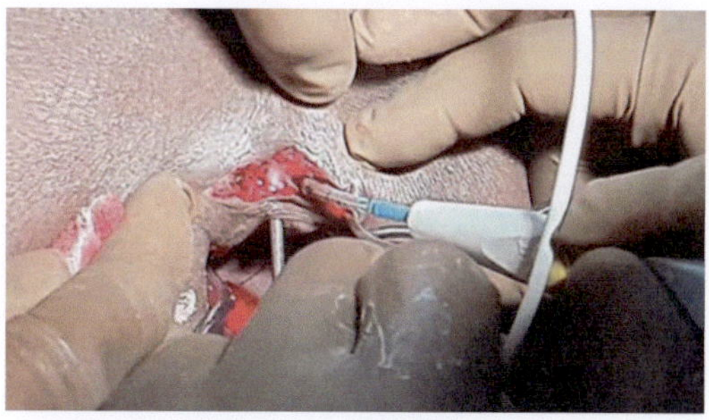

Fig. 13.8 Fistula tract isolated in inter-sphincteric space

- Keep dissection close to external sphincter to avoid damage to internal sphincter, anoderm and mucosa.
- If earlier probe is not put in the tract, put ureteric catheter or malleable probe from external opening in the tract to confirm the position of fistula tract.
- Dissect gently around the fistula tract and then use curved Lahey's forceps to go around the tract.

- Secure suture ligation of inter-sphincteric fistula tract close to internal opening (Fig. 13.9).
  - Pass polyglactin 2.0 suture around the tract with the help of Lahey's forceps and ligate close to internal opening.
- Remove the fistula tract in the inter-sphincteric area and tissue is sent for histopathology (Fig. 13.10).
- Curette fistula tract from external opening (Fig. 13.11).
- Close the external sphincter muscle defect from inter-sphincteric side with 2.0 polyglactin suture (Fig. 13.12).
- Dissect external opening to widen it to avoid premature closure (Fig. 13.13).
- Closure of inter-sphincteric wound.
  - Close the incision given in the beginning by 3 loose sutures of polyglactin (Fig. 13.14).

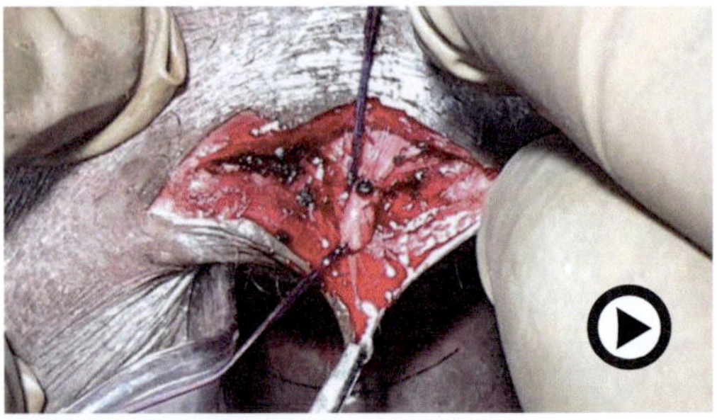

Fig. 13.9 Ligations of the tract with polyglactin 2.0 suture. Video 13.1 LIFT in a case of anterior trans-sphincteric fistula (▶ https://doi.org/10.1007/000-hq3)

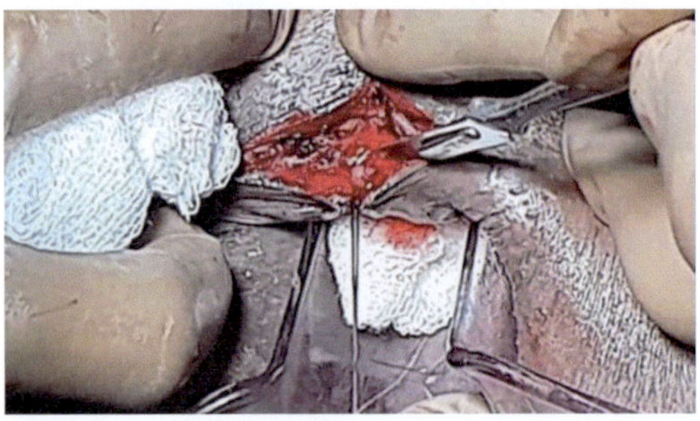

Fig. 13.10 Tract transfixed and portion in the inter-sphincteric area is excised

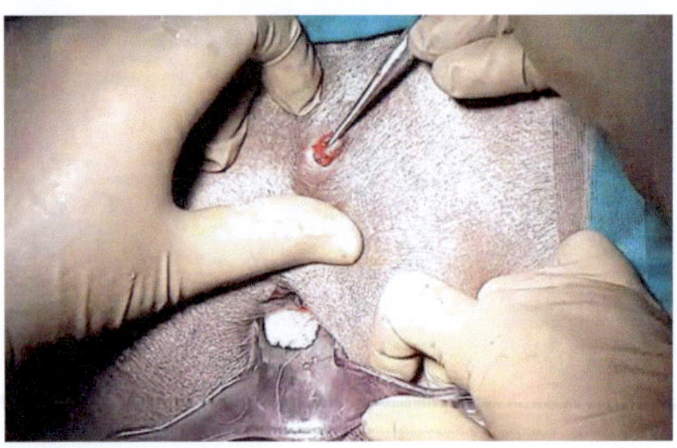

Fig. 13.11 Curette the distal tract

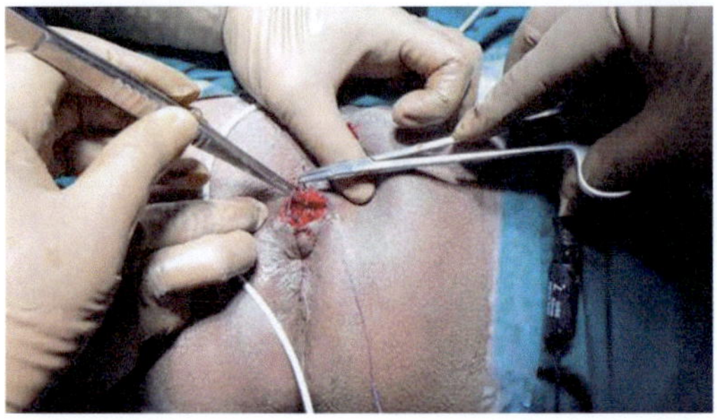

Fig. 13.12 Closure of the external muscle defect from inter-sphincteric side

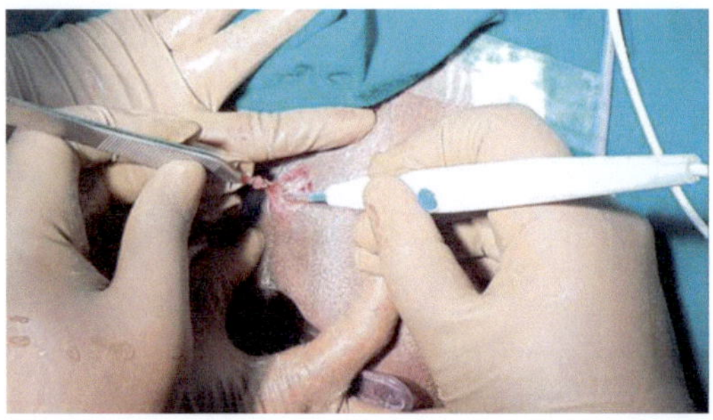

Fig. 13.13 Dissect external opening (EO) to widen it

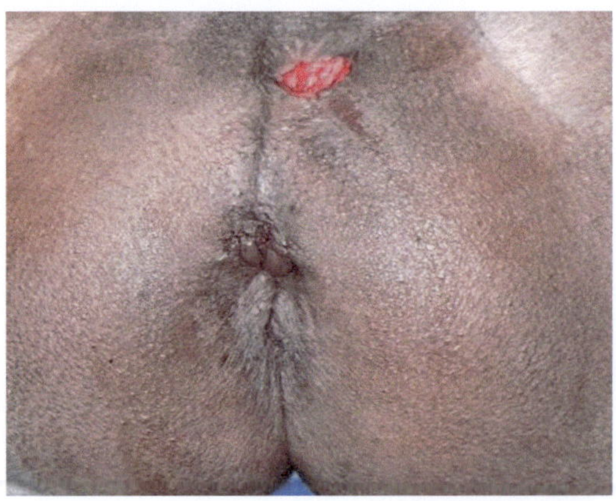

Fig. 13.14 Closure of inter-sphincteric wound and final outcome

13.6 Post-operative Care

- For pain relief oral nonsteroidal anti-inflammatory drugs (NSAIDs) usually suffice.
- Local wound cleansing with water is sufficient.
- Oral antibiotics three dosages, one peri-operative and two shots at 12-hour interval are sufficient to cover the procedure.
- Observation to look for wound dehiscence and healing.

13.7 Complications (Table 13.1)

13.7.1 Causes of Recurrence After LIFT Are Studied as Follows

- Due to disease left in the internal sphincter, internal opening and inter-sphincteric space. It presents as inter-sphincteric fistula during recurrence.
- Disease left within the external sphincter.
- Tracts rejoin.

Table 13.1 Complications of LIFT

Complications	Prevention	Management
Wound dehiscence discharge at the inter-sphincteric wound		Application of silver nitrate Fistulotomy of Inter-sphincteric part
Failure to heal	Follow meticulous detail of the procedure	Refer to causes of recurrence
Recurrence	Follow meticulous detail of the procedure	Refer to causes of recurrence
Incontinence	Avoid damage to any sphincter and over stretching the sphincters	Incidence very low 0 to 20% (18%). Gas and mucous only [3] Kegel's exercise

13.7.2 Different Investigators Found Following Risk Factors for Failure of LIFT

- Horseshoe fistulas, fistulas associated with Crohn's disease, and those with a history of previous fistula surgery has high incidence of reoccurrence [4].
- Collection, fistula tract size more than 5 mm, and the failure of ligating the tract in one attempt [5].
- High trans-sphincteric fistula, previous fistula surgery, diabetes [6].

13.8 Variations Suggested to Improve Outcomes

13.8.1 Laying Open Internal Tract

Amounting to distal internal sphincterotomy has been suggested as a method to improve the results [7].

13.8.2 Bio LIFT

Ligation of inter-sphincteric fistula tract procedure with bio-prosthetic reinforcement [8].

13.8.3 LIFT Plug

Ligation of the inter-sphincteric fistula tract plus a bioprosthetic anal fistula plug [9].

13.8.4 LIFT Plus

Ligation of the inter-sphincteric fistula tract plus a partial core out fistulectomy [10].

13.8.5 Suggestion by Arun Rojanasakul

Bend the tract over itself and then ligate.

13.8.6 Our Views to Prevent Recurrence After LIFT

- Handle spread within intersphincteric space by intra-anal fistulotomy.

In posterior horseshoe fistulae high recurrence after LIFT may be due to pathological anatomy of these fistulae. In 75% of posterior horseshoe fistula, there is spread in posterior inter-sphincteric space and then breach of external sphincter at two places. Probably, it is not managed by single ligation. Appreciation of this arrangement in 75% of posterior horse shoe fistulae is essential to eradicate chronic sepsis.

13.9 Submucosal Ligation of Fistula Tract (SLOFT)

Dr. DU Pathak from Jabalpur, India, invented a procedure where he suggested to intercept the transphincteric fistula tract at the level of sub mucosa and ligate the proximal part. Distal tract is curettaged and LASER ablated [11].

Algorithm for LIFT

History and clinical examination
Spinal anaesthesia
Position lithotomy
Identify the internal opening
Incision over intersphincteric groove
Dissection in the intersphincteric space for identification of the fistula tract
Ligation close to internal sphincter and towards external sphincter
Removal of the part of intersphincteric tract to remove the crypto-glandular infection
Scrap out all granulation tissue in the rest of the fistulous tract
Enlarge external opening
Close the incision made in intersphincteric groove

References

1. Rojanasakul A, Pattanaarun J, Sahakitrungruang C, Tantiphlachiva K. Total anal sphincter saving technique for fistula-in-ano; the ligation of intersphincteric fistula tract. J Med Assoc Thai. 2007;90(3):581–6. PMID: 17427539
2. Rojanasakul A. LIFT procedure: a simplified technique for fistula-in-ano. Tech Coloproctol. 2009;13(3):237–40. https://doi.org/10.1007/s10151-009-0522-2. Epub 2009 Jul 28. PMID: 19636496
3. van Oostendorp JY, Verkade C, Han-Geurts IJM, van der Mijnsbrugge GJH, Wasowicz-Kemps DK, Zimmerman DDE. Ligation of intersphincteric fistula tract (LIFT) for trans-sphincteric cryptoglandular anal fistula: long-term impact on faecal continence. BJS Open. 2024;8(3) https://doi.org/10.1093/bjsopen/zrae055.
4. Emile SH, Khan SM, Adejumo A, Koroye O. Ligation of intersphincteric fistula tract (LIFT) in treatment of anal fistula: An updated systematic review, meta-analysis, and meta-regression of the predictors of failure. Surgery. 2020;167(2):484–92. https://doi.org/10.1016/j.surg.2019.09.012. Epub 2019 Oct 21. PMID: 31648932
5. Sirikurnpiboon S. The risk factors for failure and recurrence of LIFT procedure for fistula in ano rectal surgery. Turk J Surg. 2023;39(1):27–33.
6. Salgado-Nesme N, Alvarez-Bautista FE, Mongardini FM, Docimo L, Hoyos-Torres A, Ruiz-Muñoz EA, Vergara-Fernàndez O, Suastegui HOG, Illanes MFR, Reyes NDM. LIFT procedure: postoperative outcomes, risk factors for fistula recurrence and continence impairment. Updates Surg. 2024;76(3):989–97. https://doi.org/10.1007/s13304-024-01818-2.
7. Bastawrous A, Hawkins M, Kratz R, Menon R, Pollock D, Charbel J, Long K. Results from a novel modification to the ligation intersphincteric fistula tract. Am J Surg. 2015;209(5):793–8. discussion 798. https://doi.org/10.1016/j.amjsurg.2015.01.002. Epub 2015 Feb 16. PMID: 25754846
8. Lau YC, Brown KGM, Cheong J, Byrne C, Lee PJ. LIFT and BioLIFT: a 10-year single-centre experience of treating complex fistula-in-ano with ligation of intersphincteric fistula tract procedure with or without Bio-prosthetic Reinforcement (BioLIFT). J Gastrointest Surg. 2020;24(3):671–6. https://doi.org/10.1007/s11605-019-04305-x. Epub 2019 Jun 25. PMID: 31240556
9. Han JG, Yi BQ, Wang ZJ, Zheng Y, Cui JJ, Yu XQ, Zhao BC, Yang XQ. Ligation of the intersphincteric fistula tract plus a bioprosthetic anal fistula plug (LIFT-Plug): a new technique for fistula-in-ano. Colorectal Dis. 2013;15(5):582–6. https://doi.org/10.1111/codi.12062. PMID: 23067044

10. Sirikurnpiboon S, Awapittaya B, Jivapaisarnpong P. Ligation of intersphincteric fistula tract and its modification: Results from treatment of complex fistula. World J Gastrointest Surg. 2013;5(4):123–8. https://doi.org/10.4240/wjgs.v5.i4.123. PMID: 23671739; PMCID: PMC3646132
11. Raja Ram NK, Chan KK, Md Nor SF, Sagap I. A prospective evaluation of the outcome of submucosal ligation of fistula tract. Colorectal Dis. 2020;22(12):2199–203. https://doi.org/10.1111/codi.15305. Epub 2020 Oct 6. PMID: 32780561

Suggested Reading

Matos D, Lunniss PJ, Phillips RK. Total sphincter conservation in high fistula in ano: results of a new approach. Br J Surg. 1993;80(6):802–4. https://doi.org/10.1002/bjs.1800800651. PMID: 8330181

Parthasarathi R, Gomes RM, Rajapandian S, Sathiamurthy R, Praveenraj P, Senthilnathan P, Palanivelu C. Ligation of the intersphincteric fistula tract for the treatment of fistula-in-ano: experience of a tertiary care centre in South India. Colorectal Dis. 2016;18(5):496–502. https://doi.org/10.1111/codi.13162. PMID: 26476011

Sirany AM, Nygaard RM, Morken JJ. The ligation of the intersphincteric fistula tract procedure for anal fistula: a mixed bag of results. Dis Colon Rectum. 2015;58(6):604–12. https://doi.org/10.1097/DCR.0000000000000374. PMID: 25944433

Tan KK, Tan IJ, Lim FS, Koh DC, Tsang CB. The anatomy of failures following the ligation of intersphincteric tract technique for anal fistula: a review of 93 patients over 4 years. Dis Colon Rectum. 2011;54(11):1368–72. https://doi.org/10.1097/DCR.0b013e31822bb55e. PMID: 21979180

Suggested Video

Video SV 13.1 by inventor https://youtu.be/zHSYutaulK4?si=6txR7bnSJJ0aMo9Y

Fistula in Ano: Sphincter-Saving Procedures Eisenhammer and A.G. Parks Revisited, This Time with Technology (E PARK Tech.)

14

Abstract

- Concept of intermuscular (intersphincteric) sepsis as the source of all anal fistulae of cryptoglandular origin as suggested by Eisenhammer and later shown by A. G. Parks is again emphasised. We designate it as central disease.
- Their method of management of anal fistula is revisited, this time with advanced technology of modern times.
- To honour both, we named our approach after their names as E PARK Tech. (Eisenhammer Park with Technology).
- All steps involved in diagnosing, assessing and operating fistula in ano with technology at hand are fully explained with sketches, clinical photographs and videos.
- Complications in using technology during the procedure are grouped in a tabulated form with methods of prevention and management.
- "Tips and Tricks" section has pearls of wisdom by previous and recent operators.
- "References" and "Suggested Readings" sections will be of interest to the modern aware reader.

Supplementary Information The online version contains supplementary material available at https://doi.org/10.1007/978-981-96-6190-9_14. The videos can be accessed individually by clicking the DOI link in the accompanying figure caption or by scanning this link with the SN More Media App.

14.1 What One Should Know Before the Procedure

- When A.G. Parks originally described his technique in 1961 on 38 patients comparing with fistulotomy, he worked on the basis of sound knowledge of anatomy of spread of fistula tracts [1].
- Eisenhammer had already suggested to open the intermuscular space (intersphincteric space) through anal canal by internal sphincterotomy to treat anal abscess and fistulae [1].
- Parks did not have facility of magnetic resonance imaging (MRI) and availability of fistuloscope, light amplification by stimulated emission of radiations (LASERS) and other devices and delayed degradable sutures in his times.

14.2 Mode of Fistula Formation (Fig. 14.1)

- Crypto glandular fistulas start as an infection in anal glands, a component of which lies in intersphincteric space. Suppuration extends in this narrow space circumferentially or vertically and may go up to supralevator space and remains trapped.
- Suppuration may seep out through lower border of intersphincteric space or trans-sphincteric through external sphincter.
- Rarely it loops over the external sphincter and enters ischiorectal fossa.

S. K. Singla, K. Mital, *Operative Manual of Minimally Invasive and LASER Ano-proctology*,
https://doi.org/10.1007/978-981-96-6190-9_14

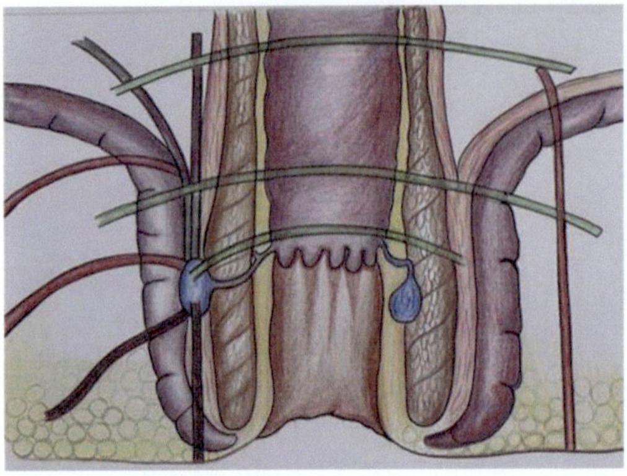

Fig. 14.1 Spread of anal gland infection and latter mode of fistula formation Laying open of red tracts is risky

Review our video in the previous chapter for some predictable anatomical routes taken by fistulae in ano (Video 12.1).

14.3 Pre-operative Requisition

- After history, a detailed local digital examination is must (Fig. 14.2). It is supplemented by properly done magnetic resonance imaging (MRI) of anal and perianal spaces in appropriate cases.

MRI increases yield in the following cases [2].

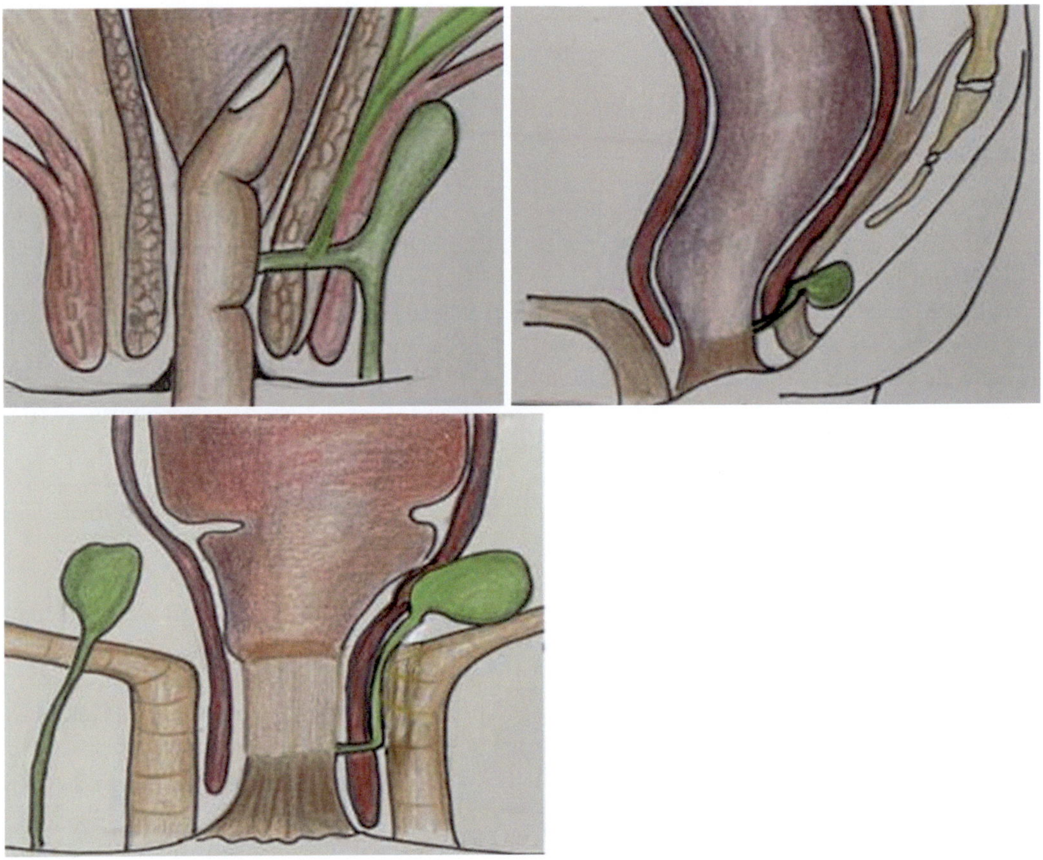

Fig. 14.2 Palpate for any induration, dimple or irregular surface vertically as well circumferentially, at mid-anal canal (the level of dentate line) as well as at the level of anorectal ring

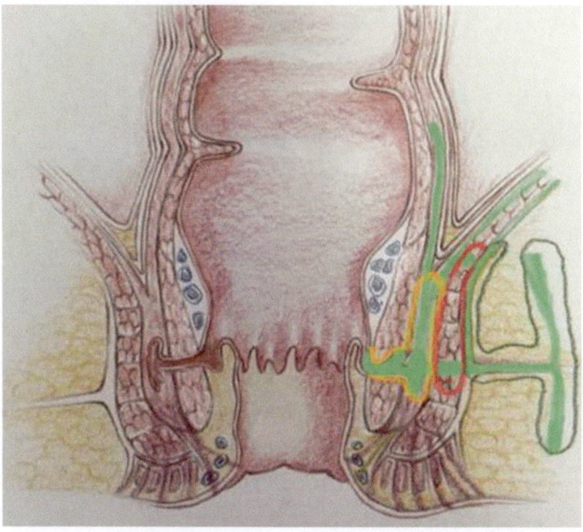

Fig. 14.3 Three components of Fistula. Inner component internal to skeletal muscle encircled in orange colour. Middle component within the skeletal muscle encircled in red colour. Outer component outer to skeletal muscle encircled in green colour

- On examination complex cases—with multiple external openings, on digital rectal examination (DRE) induration extending from internal opening circumferentially or vertically, tight lower anorectum due to fibrosis at mid-rectum or at anorectal ring.
- All posterior horse-shoe-shaped fistulae.
- External opening 2 cm away from anal verge.
- Recurrent cases.

Make a 3D picture of anatomy of fistula considering involvement inner to skeletal muscle, within skeletal muscle and outside the skeletal muscle (Fig. 14.3) in cortex diary.

14.4 Indications

- All sorts of crypto glandular anal fistulae can be effectively managed by E PARK Tech. with very less recurrence and without damaging the external sphincter.

With very low fistulae, it may sound like fistulotomy but sparing part of skin between external opening and anal canal, sparing even few fibres of subcutaneous external sphincter maintains the shape of anal orifice and hastens recovery without increasing any recurrence.

14.5 Contra-Indications

Non-cryptoglandular fistulae.

14.6 Equipment (Fig. 14.4)

- Routine trolley for fistula surgery.
- Parks speculum.
- Vaginal speculums of various sizes, preferably lighted.
- Curettes or Volkman's scoupe.
- Electro cautery with monopolar pencil and bipolar coagulator.
- FiXcision/coring device (Fig. 14.5).
- LASERS 1470 diode with radial LASER fibre.
- Fistuloscope (optional).

We use these gadgets to ensure complete eradication of central disease (cryptoglandular disease component in intersphincteric space) and

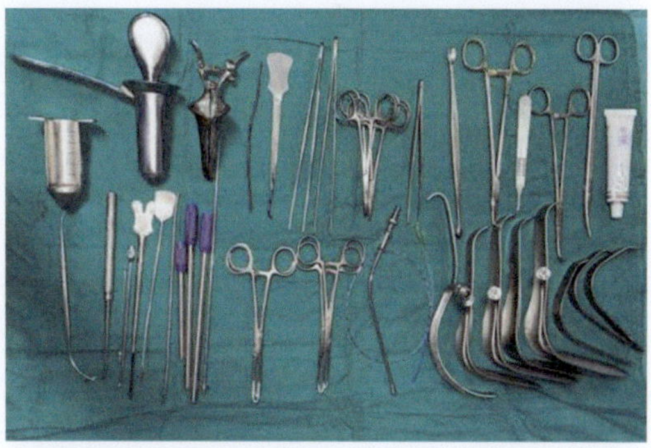

Fig. 14.4 Equipment trolley for E PARK Tech. Procedure

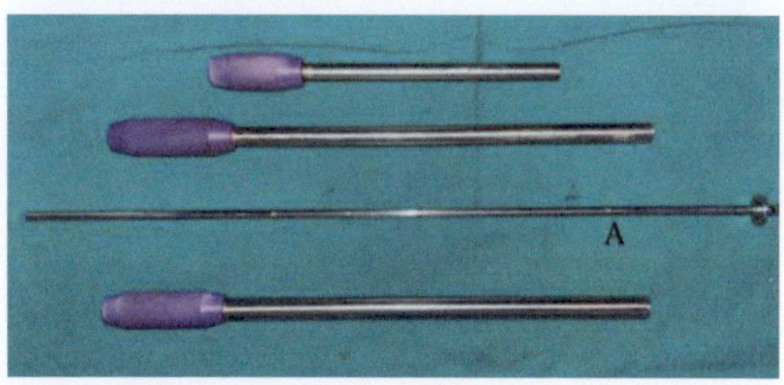

Fig. 14.5 FiXcision/coring devise to core out fistula tract. (A) Central rod with detachable stud/base plate, all other are cutting cylinders of various diameter with sharp edge at the tip

epithelium of the distal tract, under vision, while working by minimal access in narrow space.

- PDS suture 2.0 on round body needle.
- Polyglactin sutures 2.0 on round body needle.

14.7 Procedure (Video 14.1)

14.7.1 Anaesthesia

- Spinal or general anaesthesia, usually done under spinal anaesthesia.

14.7.2 Position of the Patient

- Lithotomy/prone. Prone position may improve the exposure in case of anterior fistula.

14.7.3 Stepwise Approach

14.7.3.1 Identification of Internal Opening as Disease Lies Beneath It

- Reassessing Pre-operative MRI.
  - MRI can detect internal opening or can tell where the tract is closest to the anal canal lumen.
- Clinical examination under anaesthesia (Fig. 14.6).
- Put Parks speculum in the anal canal and then inject very diluted methylene blue from external opening and identify internal opening by its egress in the lumen (Fig. 14.7).
- Mark internal opening by a stroke of electrocautery pencil.
- Gentle probing under anaesthesia can be done without damaging walls of the tract.

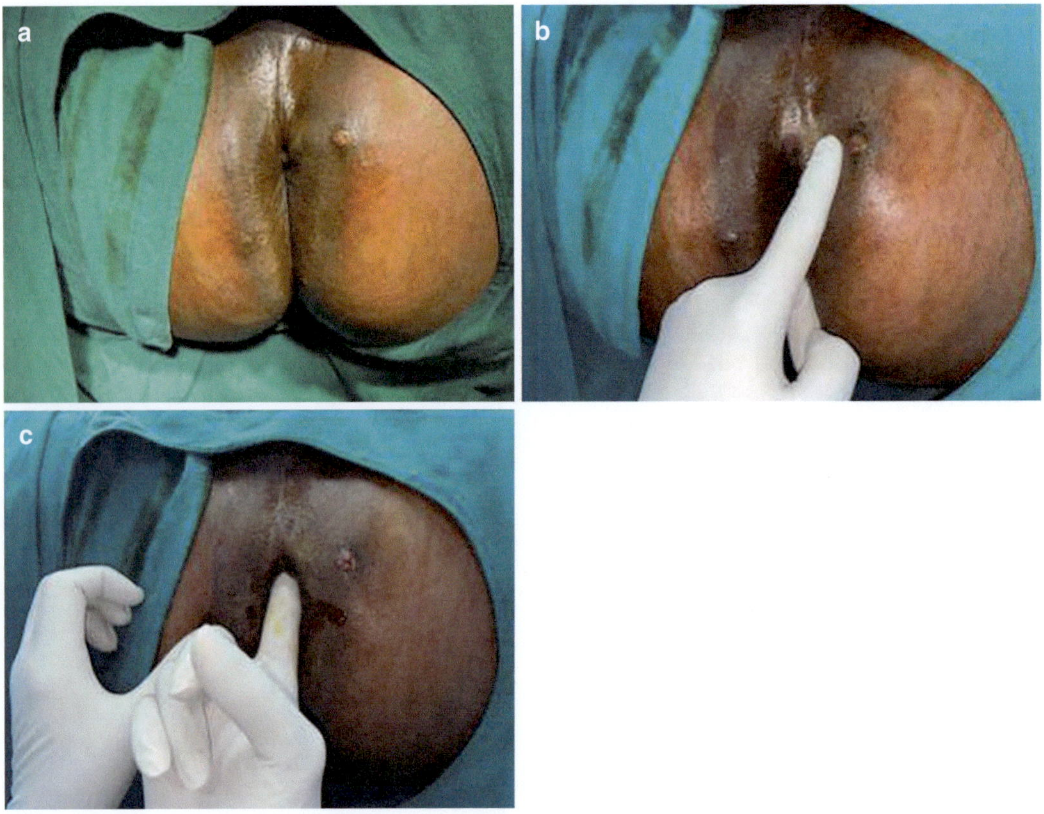

Fig. 14.6 Patient in lithotomy position. (**a**) Inspection. (**b**) Palpation of the induration caused by tract. (**c**) DRE to locate internal opening by induration/dimple in the area of dentate line and any induration around the circumference or vertically up

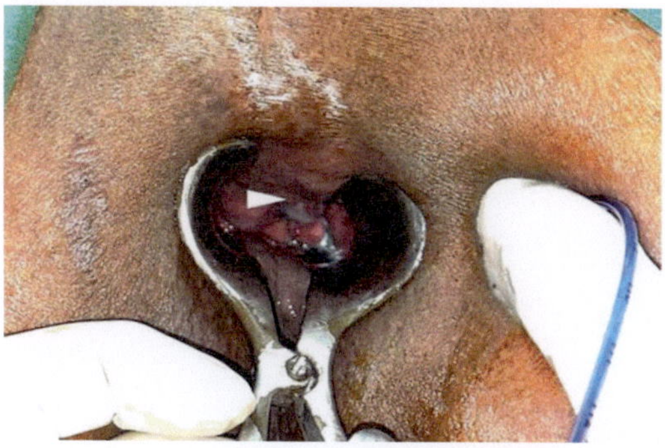

Fig. 14.7 Locate internal opening (shown with white arrow head) by checking egress of the dye instilled from external opening

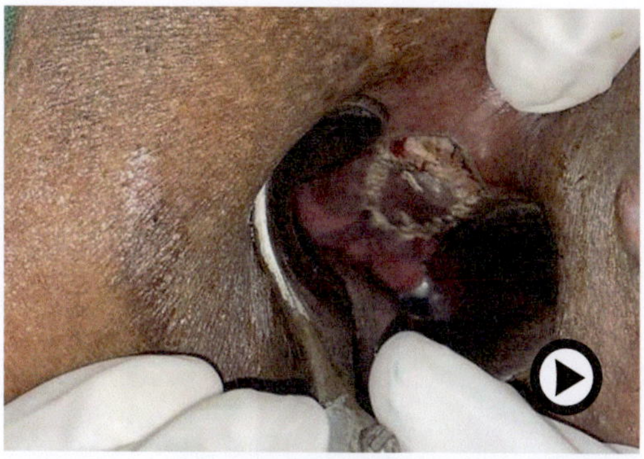

Fig. 14.8 Incision 5 mm around the internal opening (at 1 0′ clock position) and distal limit up to lower border of the internal sphincter. Video 14.1 PARK Tech. Trans sphincteric fistula (▶ https://doi.org/10.1007/000-hq5)

14.7.3.2 Incision Around Internal Opening

- Mark an area of 5 mm around internal opening and extend the mark in an oval manner to touch the anal margin up to the lower border of the internal sphincter (Figs. 14.8 and 14.9).
- Incise the mucosa to expose distal internal sphincter (Fig. 14.9).

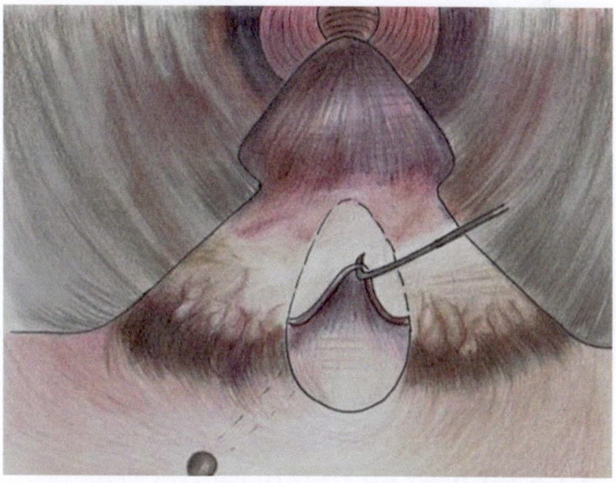

Fig. 14.9 Parks speculum opened to expose internal opening (at 6 0′ clock position). Incise mucosa almost 5 mm all around internal opening to bring the distal internal sphincter in view

14.7.3.3 Dissect the Intersphincteric Space and Remove the Source of Original Abscess k.a. Central Disease

- Inject diluted adrenaline lignocaine 1:200000 solution in submucosal area around the internal opening to have comparatively avascular field of dissection.
- A segment of internal sphincter is excised corresponding to mucosal incision, as it is lifted off the external sphincter and the longitudinal layer, one may encounter a small abscess of origin also called as central disease (Figs. 14.10 and 14.11).
- Any intersphincteric extension circumferential or vertical (either detected by MRI or assessed on clinical examination) can be either excised or laid open by gentle electro-dissection between the mucosa and circular fibres on one side and external sphincter fibres on the other side.

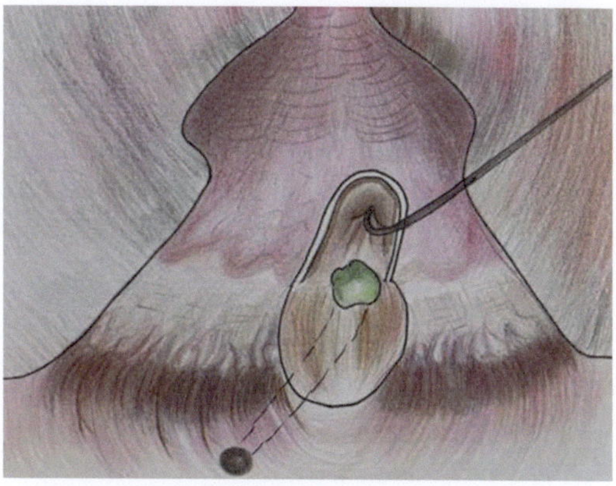

Fig. 14.10 A segment of internal sphincter is incised and lifted off the longitudinal layer of conjoint longitudinal muscle (CLM) to enter intersphincteric space which deroofs the cryptoglandular abscess [1]

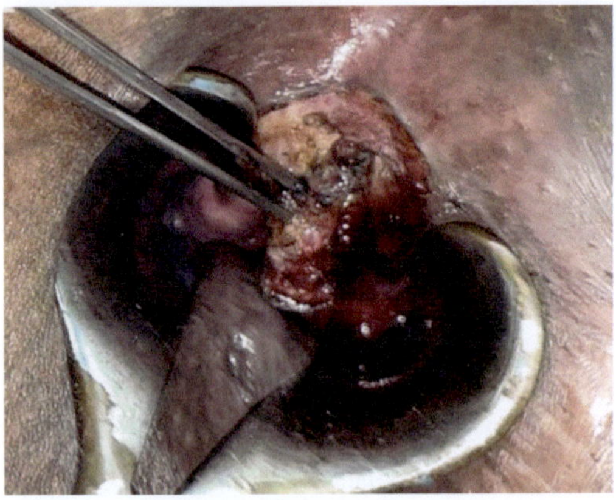

Fig. 14.11 Exposure of abscess of origin of the disease also called as central disease after trans-anal incision of fibres of internal sphincter to enter intersphincteric space

- Attain complete haemostasis by compression with saline-soaked gauge, and/or bipolar coagulation as this area of dissection may have engorged submucosal cushions.
- Reinstill the diluted dye through the external opening and ascertain the site of internal opening, which is now an opening in fibres of external sphincter.

14.7.3.4 Core Out the Distal Tract by FiXcision Device [3]

- Pass probe through the tract followed by a dilator (Fig. 14.12).
- Pass FiXcision probe through the tract.
- Screw the stud/base plate on inner end as a stopper (Fig. 14.13).
- Pass the round cutter over the FiXcision probe.
- Make proper alignment and rotate the circular cutter to core out the whole tract, stopper stud/base plate will avoid injuring the mucosa on opposite side (Fig. 14.14).
- Stop when coring is finished.
- Unscrew the stud/base plate.
- Remove the cutter and retrieve the whole tract which is submitted for histopathology (Figs. 14.15 and 14.16).
  - Coring by this device decreases size of the wound and accelerates healing as compared to coring done manually (Fig. 14.17).
  - Coring by FiXcision device is possible in case of a mature tract.

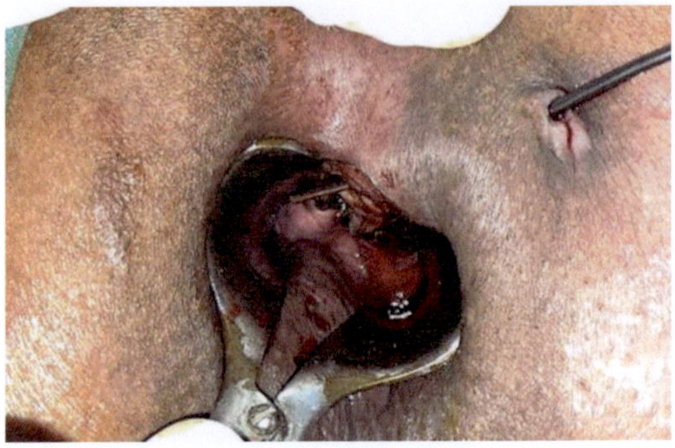

Fig. 14.12 Fistula probe passed through the tract

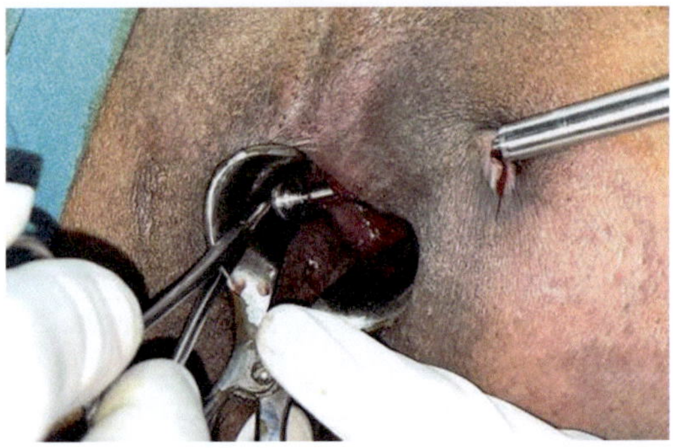

Fig. 14.13 FiXcision probe in the tract with stud/base plate fixation at inner end

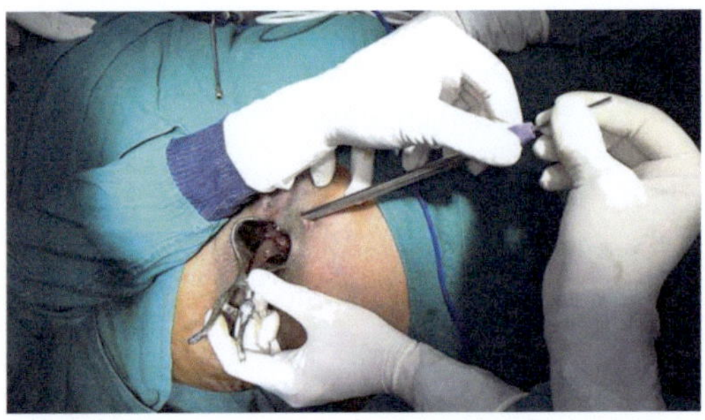

Fig. 14.14 Cutting cylinder over the probe. Coring by rotation and constant push on cylinder, stud/base plate at the inner end prevents over shooting

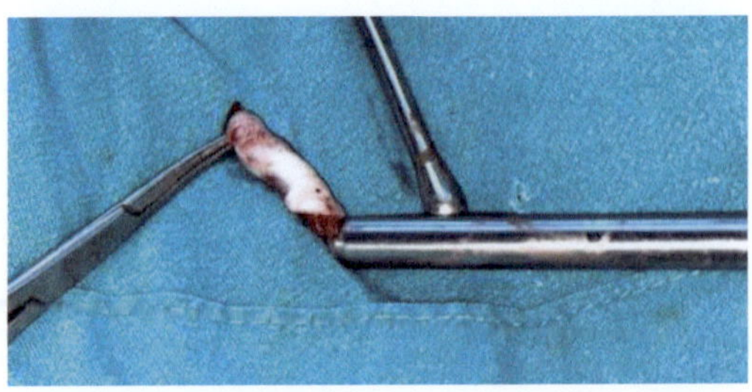

Fig. 14.15 Retrieved distal tract from device

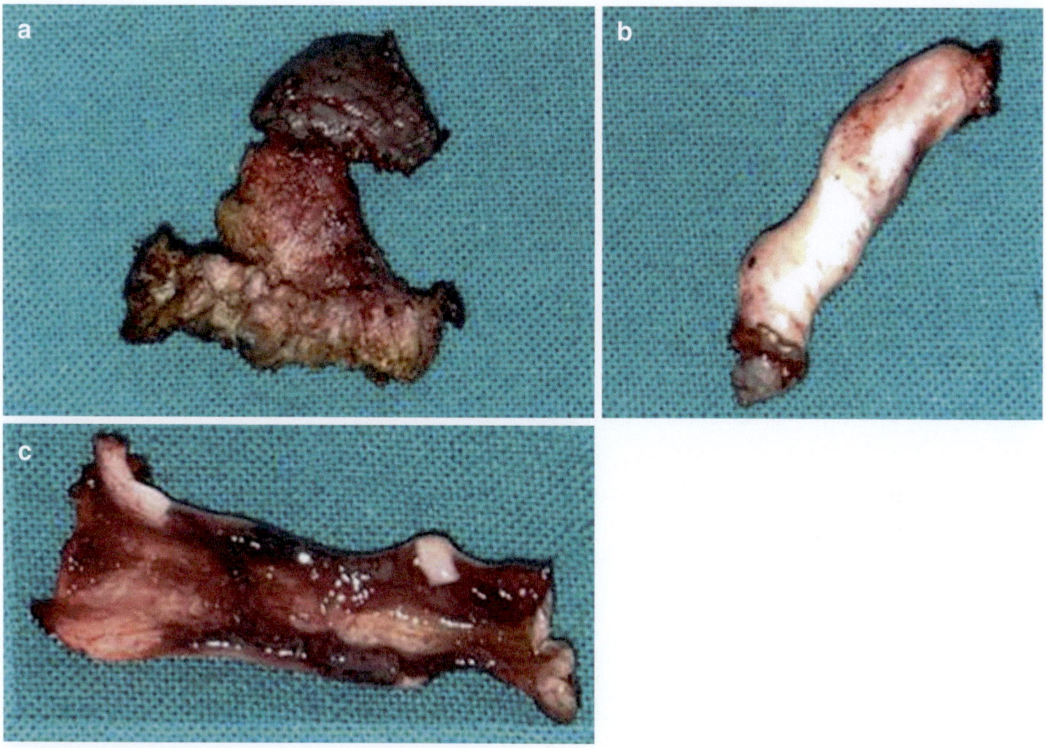

Fig. 14.16 All components of the fistula. (**a**) Inner component, i.e., central disease. (**b**) Part of the tract within external sphincter and outer to the sphincter. (**c**) Tract slit open showing no macroscopic muscle tissue

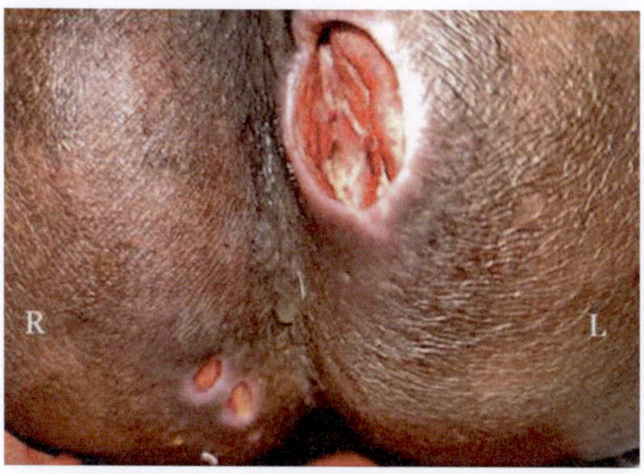

Fig. 14.17 Healing at 2 weeks in a posterior horseshoe fistula, coring done by FiXcision on right side and by manual dissection on left side. Left side there was associated abscess and the tract was immature

- In case of associated abscess and immature tract, better to do manual coring as instrumental coring by FiXcision is not possible and is inadequate.

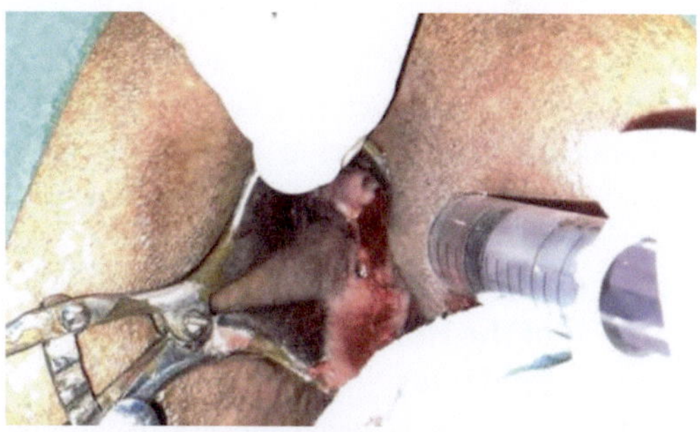

Fig. 14.18 Flush the tract with saline mixed with few drops of H_2O_2 to remove all debris

- Coring removes the fibrous tissue around the tract thereby tract collapses fast and heals early.

- Thoroughly wash the tract with saline and hydrogen peroxide solution (Fig. 14.18).

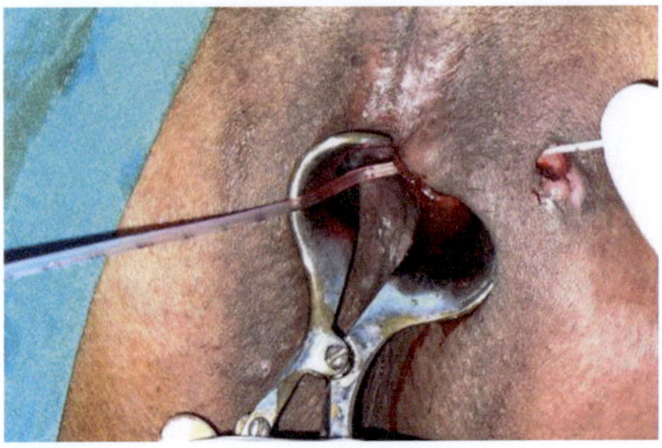

Fig. 14.19 Radial fibre passed through the tract protected in the cover of infant feeding tube

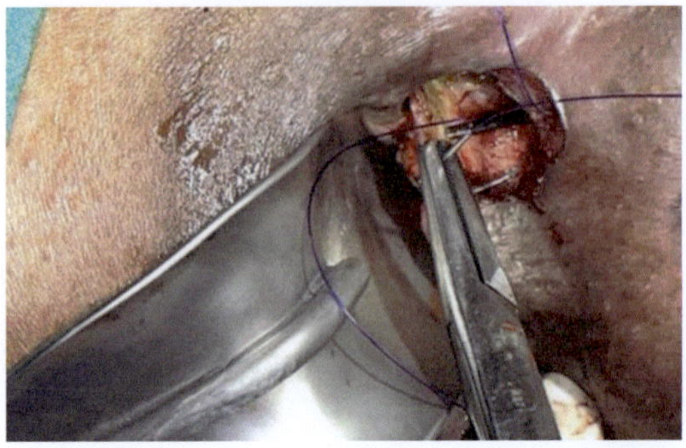

Fig. 14.20 Opening in external sphincter is closed over a probe with PDS 2.0 suture

14.7.3.5 Fulgration of Any Leftover Granulation in the Tract

- During coring at times, part of the tract is breached due to curvilinear tracts.
- Wear LASER-protective glasses.
- Put 1470 nm diode radial LASER fibre through the tract. Keep the tip at the inner end and give LASER energy 10 watts continuous wave and withdraw at a speed of 1 mm per second. LASER energy helps to stop bleeding as well as fulgrates any leftover granulating epithelium (Fig. 14.19).
- In case the tract is very wide, put fistuloscope and ensure that no granulation epithelium is left in the tract which can be fulgrated with LASER energy delivered by LASER fibre through the operative channel of the scope.

14.7.3.6 Trans-anal Suturing of the Hole in External Sphincter

New internal opening created after coring through the external sphincter is closed to avoid early soiling and fast closure of the tract.

- Before suturing, change the Parks speculum with lighted vaginal speculums of appropriate size. It decreases the traction on tissue and facilitates suturing.
- Inner opening in external sphincter which is now the proximal end of distal tract is closed with PDS 2.0 suture over a probe (Fig. 14.20).
- Probe is withdrawn and suture is tied firmly (Fig. 14.21).

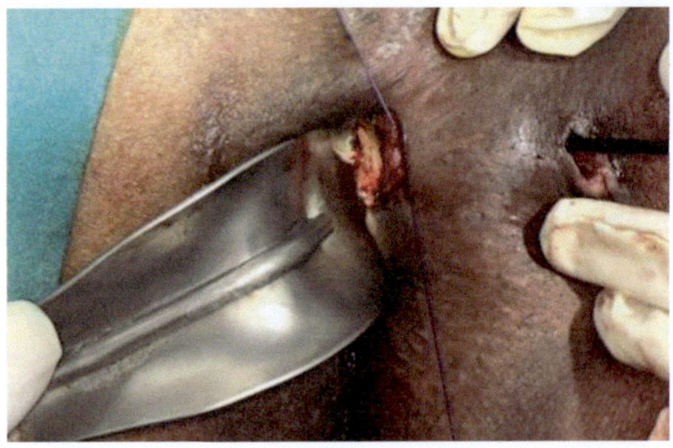

Fig. 14.21 Probe withdrawn—suture tied to approximate the sphincter fibres

- Do not tie the suture too tight otherwise tissue will crush and slough latter.
- After excision of infected area and fibrosis around by FiXcision, tissue is supple enough to come closer by sutures.
- Wash the area and do marsupialisation of the anoderm and mucosal wound with polyglactin 2.0 interrupted sutures.
- Marsupialisation helps prevent bleeding in post-operative course, causes less impairment in squeeze pressure after 3 months and thereby decreases incontinence rate [4, 5].
- Do check proctoscopy on table.

14.7.3.7 Injecting Methylene Blue for Prolonged Analgesia

- We inject 1% methylene blue solution with 0.25% bupivicane in 1:5 ratio in intradermal plain, in any dissection below the dentate line.
- Fine 27 gauge needle is used for the purpose.

- 5–10 cc solution is sufficient for most of the surgeries.
- It keeps the area numb for 3–4 days.
- Caution the patient for violet tinge in urine after methylene blue injection.
- Do not pack the anal canal. Just keep a sterile pad over the wound area.

14.8 E PARK Tech. in a Case of Suprasphincteric Fistula (Fig. 14.22; Video 14.2)

- Higher the fistula, i.e., more the bulk of external sphincter involved, more is the advantage to the patient.

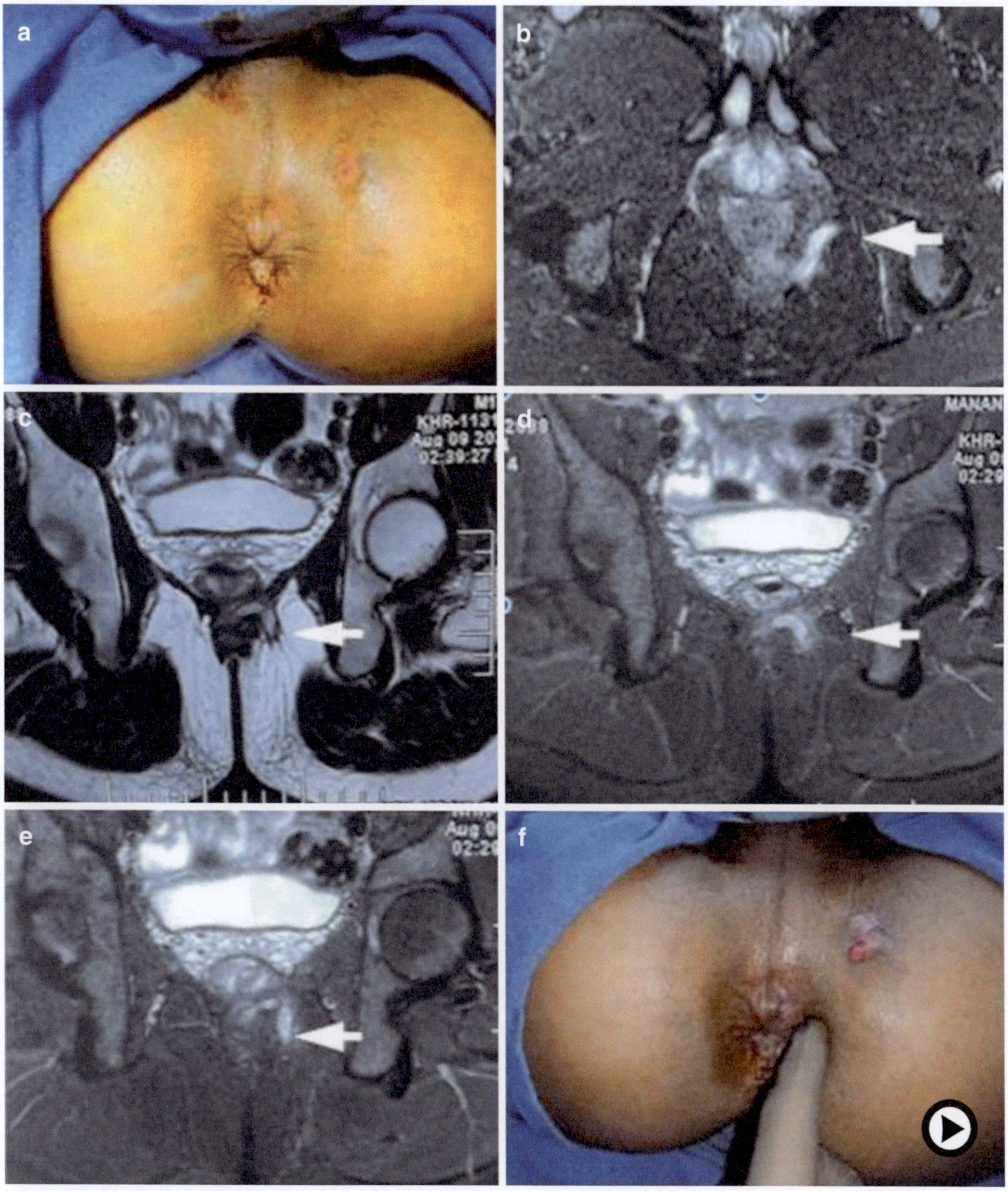

Fig. 14.22 Assessment of fistula anatomy. (**a**) In lithotomy external opening (EO), (**b**) MRI axial plane transphincteric spread from 6 0′ to 2 0′. (**c**–**e**) MRI coronal plane showing inverted U loop of supra sphincteric fistula. (**f**) Pointed finger to EO tract in ischiorectal space. Video 14.2 PARK Tech. Supra sphincteric fistula (▶ https://doi.org/10.1007/000-hq4)

- Coring by device may be incomplete, but it straightens the path for fistuloscope and one can fulgrate the residual granulation tissue under vision.
- One can use LASER fibre to fulgrate the granulation as lateral damage is limited to 2 mm only.

14.8.1 Pre-operative Assessment (Fig. 14.22)

Disease started at 6 0′ post-midline in intersphincteric space with internal opening (IO) at same site.

Spreads from 6 0′ to 4 0′ in intersphincteric space circumferentially, thereafter the tract ascends in the intersphincteric space crosses above puborectalis and takes a U turn through levator ani at 4 0′ to enter ischiorectal space. Tract then travels from 4 0′ to 2 0′ inferolaterally to open on the skin as external opening (EO).

14.8.2 Steps of Operation

- Suprasphincteric fistula—assessment of anatomy of the tract (Fig. 14.22).
- Suprasphincteric fistula—confirmation of anatomy and excision of central disease (Fig. 14.23).
- Suprasphincteric fistula-coring out the distal tract with FiXcision device and fulgration of residual granulation with LASER (Fig. 14.24).
- Suprasphincteric fistula PARK Tech.—closing the new IO and marsupialisation of the anal canal wound after central disease excision (Fig. 14.25).

14.8.3 Post-operative Care

- Wash the wound and apply ointment metronidazole and povidine combination and sterile pad.
- Just keep a clean self-sticking sanitary napkin in rear side of undergarment as a pad.
- Laxatives for a three weeks.
- Avoid squatting for initial post-operative period.
- Post-operative anti-bacterials like ofiaxacin and metronidazole for 5 days or till any cellulitis exists.
- Usual healing time is two to three weeks for external wound and epithelisation of internal wound takes a little longer.

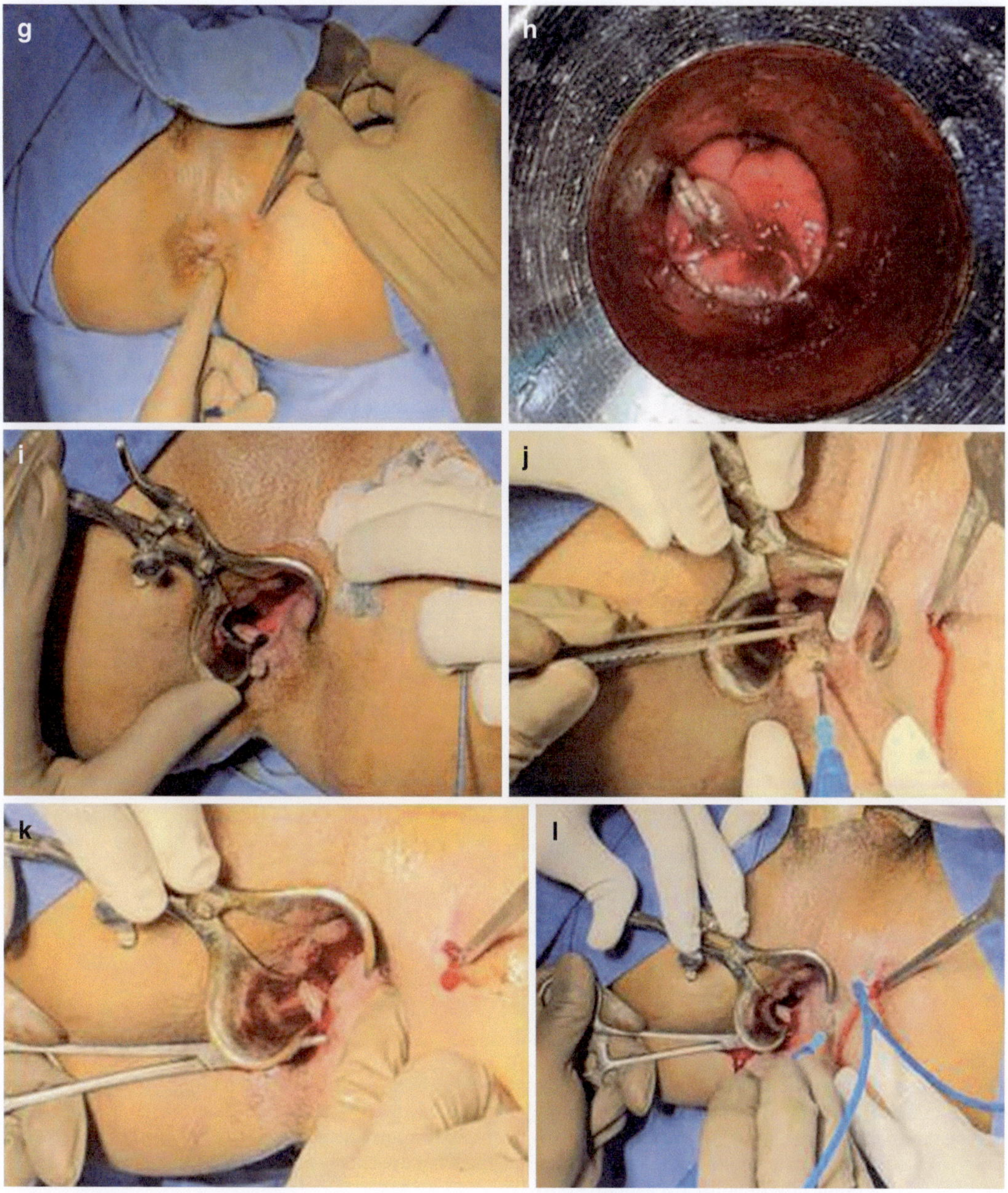

Fig. 14.23 (**g**) Gental probing possible for part of tract in ischiorectal fossa. (**h**) IO seen through proctoscope. (**i**) Instill dye from EO to appear at IO at 6 0′. (**j**) Central disease excision at 6 O′. (**k**) Probing fistula from both sides gently, using Lahey's forceps from inside to loop over the sphincters. (**l**) Tip of Lahey's felt lateral to external sphincter at 4 O′ and skin incised over the tip. This step done to divide tortuous tract in two relatively straight tracts

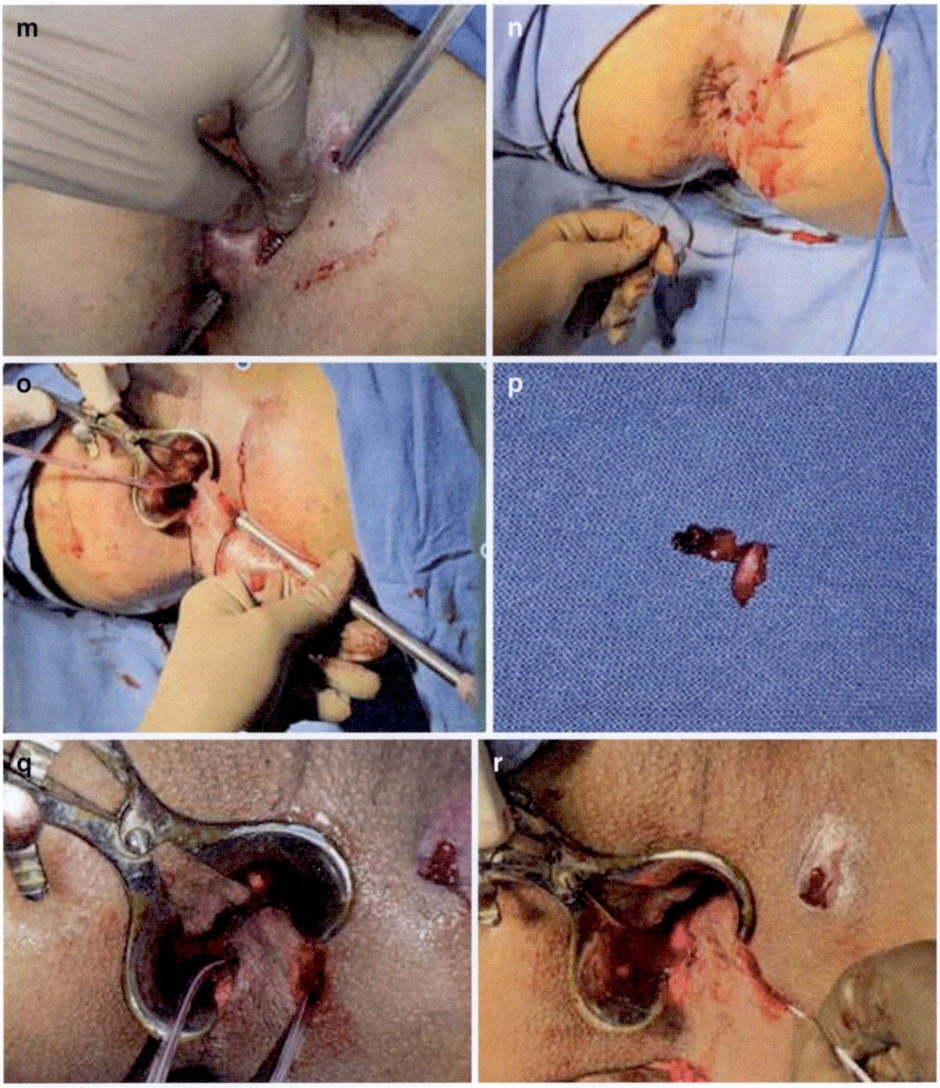

Fig. 14.24 (**m**) Lahey's forceps tip in the new opening created in the skin. (**n**) Suprasphincteric tract secured by passing thread through the inverted U loop. (**o**) FiXicison device in the tract and coring done. (**p**) Cored out specimen. (**q**) Infant feeding tube (number 10) with tip excised passed in inverted U loop of the tract. Note the bulk of tissue involved (R)1470 nm diode radial LASER fibre passed through the tube and tract fulgrated—10 watts continuous wave energy and with drawl@ 1 mm/second

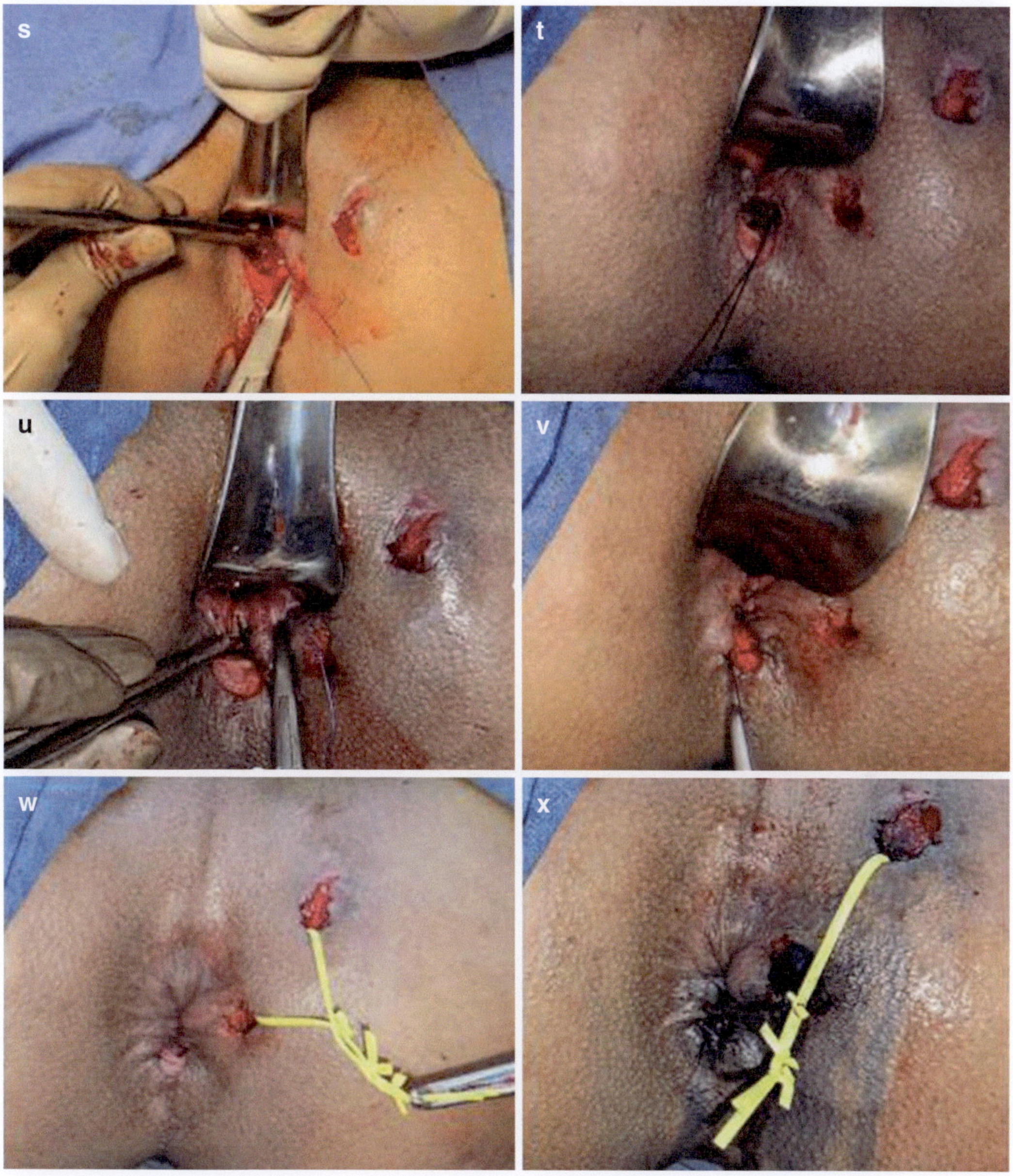

Fig. 14.25 (**s**, **t**) Trans-anal closure of opening in levator ani by 2.0 PDS. (**u**, **v**) Marsupialisation of internal wound also helped to cover the muscle stitch with a mucosal flap. (**w**) Vascular loop as draining set on for distal tract outside the external sphincter. (**x**) Tattooing with diluted methylene blue for all wounds distal to dentate line

14.9 Complications of E PARK Tech. (Table 14.1)

Table 14.1 Complications, prevention and management

Complications	Prevention	Management
Bleeding near submucosal cushions	Apply adrenaline solution in the area 1.200000	Press with saline soaked gauge Coagulate bleeding point with bipolar forceps or suture
Difficulty putting fiXicision rod in curvilinear tract	Dilate tract little bit with Haeger dilator and then align the axis and negotiate	Rail road on a 10f infant feeding tube which is passed on a narrow fistula probe
Breach in cored out tract	Align axis of fiXicison device cutter with original axis of fistula tract	Fulgrate the residual epithelial granulation in the residual tract with LASER fibre in the scope
Not able to excise the deep intersphincteric tract extensions	Clean the area and use lighted retractors to improve the illumination	If excision of extensions is difficult, lay them open over a probe or tip of curved haemostat. One can scope from inside to ensure right tract and fulgration with LASER energy

14.10 Tips and Tricks

- While dissecting around IO, be very slow with electrodissection and attain complete haemostasis by compression with saline-soaked gauge and/or bipolar coagulation, as this area of dissection may have engorged submucosal cushions.
- Field should be clean to differentiate between whitish internal sphincter fibres and reddish brown external sphincter fibres.
- Ensure complete removal of intersphincteric chronic suppurated tissue. Fibrosis around deep tracts helps to locate them.
- Remove all residual epithelial granulation tissue after FiXcison, with curettage and under vision fulgration with LASER.
- Before suturing the new internal opening, change the Parks speculum with lighted vaginal speculum of appropriate size. It decreases sideways traction and helps in suturing.
- Enlarge external opening adequately for drainage or put a drain for 5–7 days. Transfix the drain flushed with skin.
- Whenever LASER energy is delivered in continuous mode, due to a rise in temperature, carbonization occurs at the tip of LASER fibre. It increases resistance to further transmission of energy. This carbon deposition should be wiped off by a swab soaked in diluted H2O2 by moving the swab from tip to body of the fibre. Wiping in the reverse direction, i.e., from body to tip, may loosen the tip, which may get dislodged from the body of the fibre.

Algorithm for E PARK Tech

Clinical history and examination with DRE
MRI for fistula in ano
Make 3d picture of anatomy in cortex diary
Spinal anaesthesia/lithotomy position
Reassess the anatomy
Locate internal opening
5 mm incision in anal mucosa all around the internal opening and distal limit up to anal verge
Incise mucosa and few fibres of internal sphincter(IS) to lift IS from longitudinal fibres of conjoint longitudinal muscle
This opens intersphincteric space
Locate central disease excise it from external sphincter
LASER ablate external tract
Do fixcision or core out distal tract
In high tracts, one can use fistuloscope
Residual granulation can be ablated with LASER under vision
Curette the distal tract thoroughly
Wash with saline H_2O_2 solution
Put a probe through the tract
Close opening in external sphincter from anal side by horizontal interrupted sutures of 2.0 PDS over the probe to ensure closure
Marsupialise the mucosal wound with 2.0 polyglactin sutures
Keep the external wound wide open for drainage

References

1. Parks AG. Pathogenesis and treatment of fistula-in-ano. Br Med J. 1961;1(5224):463–9. https://doi.org/10.1136/bmj.1.5224.463. PMID: 13732880; PMCID: PMC1953161
2. Konan A, Onur MR, Özmen MN. The contribution of preop-erative MRI to the surgical management of anal fistulas. Diagn Interv Radiol. 2018;24(6):32137. https://doi.org/10.5152/dir.2018.18340.
3. Kasiri MM, Riss S, Stift A, Binder AD, Kogovaek U, Huth M, Kronberger IE. Optimized fistulectomy using the novel FiXcision® device: a technical feasibility study and evaluation of short term healing rates. Tech Coloproctol. 2019;23(6):579–82. https://doi.org/10.1007/s10151-019-02025-7. Epub 2019 Jul 3. PMID: 31270652; PMCID: PMC6677700
4. Ho YH, Tan M, Leong AF, Seow-Choen F. Marsupialization of fistulotomy wounds improves healing: a randomized controlled trial. Br J Surg. 1998;85(1):105–7. https://doi.org/10.1046/j.1365--2168.1998.00529.x. PMID: 9462396
5. Pescatori M, Ayabaca SM, Cafaro D, Iannello A, Magrini S. Marsupialization of fistulotomy and fistulectomy wounds improves healing and decreases bleeding: a randomized controlled trial. Color Dis. 2006;8(1):11–4. https://doi.org/10.1111/j.1463--1318.2005.00835.x. PMID: 16519632

Suggested Reading

Cedric B. Fistula-in-ano and Stephen Eisenhammer (1906–1995): Putting the record straight. S Afr J Surg [Internet]. 2016 [cited 2024 Sep 08]; 54(1): 2–3. Available from: http://www.scielo.org.za/scielo.php?script=sci_arttext&pid=S0038-23612016000100001&lng=en

https://www.ncbi.nlm.nih.gov/pmc/articles/PMC1953161/ pdf/brmedj02881-0047.pdf

Zhang H, Zhou Z-y, Hu B, Liu D-c, Peng H, Xie S-k, Su D, Ren D-l. Clinical significance of 2 deep posterior perianal spaces to complex cryptoglandular fistulas. Diseases Colon Rectum. 2016;59(8):766–74. https://doi.org/10.1097/DCR.0000000000000628.

15 Fistula in Ano: Sphincter-Saving Procedures VAAFT/Video-Assisted Anal Fistula Treatment

Abstract

- Video-assisted anal fistula treatment (VAAFT) is video-assisted minimally invasive sphincter-preserving treatment for complex fistula in ano developed by Prof. Piercarlo Meinero.
- Indication and contraindications have been defined, along with very specific indication in inter-sphincteric fistula going supralevator.
- Great deal on how to use and maintain the Meinero's scope has been described with emphasis on ways to avoid damage of delicate instrument accessories of the scope.
- Procedure details in trans-sphincteric and deep inter-sphincteric fistula are explained well with operative photographs and video.
- Different ways to close the internal opening have been mentioned along with our preference with its rationale.
- Complications and difficulties while performing the procedure, their prevention and management are presented in tabulated form for easy understanding and ready reference.
- "Tips and Tricks" section deals with troubleshooting and our ways to achieve better results.
- One can go through multimedia presentation in suggested viewing section.
- For more details by the inventor of the procedure, reader can refer to suggested reading section.

15.1 What One Should Know Before the Procedure

15.1.1 VAAFT

- It is minimally invasive sphincter preserving, video-assisted anal fistula treatment (VAAFT), developed by professor Piercarlo Meinero in an attempt to save the integrity of muscle of anal continence [1].
- Special scope designed by Meinero and manufactured by KarlStorz is used as fistuloscope (Fig. 15.1).
- Everything is done under vision from within fistula tracts without jeopardising the integrity of muscles of continence.
- Procedure is done in two parts.

Supplementary Information The online version contains supplementary material available at https://doi.org/10.1007/978-981-96-6190-9_15. The videos can be accessed individually by clicking the DOI link in the accompanying figure caption or by scanning this link with the SN More Media App.

S. K. Singla, K. Mital, *Operative Manual of Minimally Invasive and LASER Ano-proctology*,
https://doi.org/10.1007/978-981-96-6190-9_15

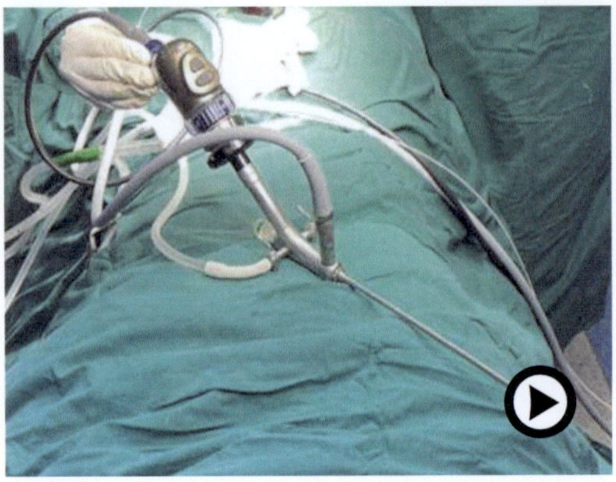

Fig. 15.1 Meinero's scope attached with endo camera, fibre optic light source and fluid channel. Video 15.1 Meinero's fistuloscope manufactured by Karl Storz Germany (▶ https://doi.org/10.1007/000-hq8)

15.2 Diagnostic Part

- Identification of tract, secondary tracts, associated abscess and internal opening.

15.3 Operative Part

- Fulgration of the distal tract and debridement.
- Closure of internal opening.

15.4 Indications

- Primary perianal and anal abscesses of cryptoglandular origin—fulgration and debridement can be done under vision without giving big skin incision (Fig. 15.2; Video 15.2).
- Complex fistula in ano including tuberculosis and Crohn's. Of course, medical management of tuberculosis and Crohn's is very essential.
- Horse-shoe-shaped fistula.
- Suprasphincteric and extra-sphincteric fistulas.
- Inter-sphincteric fistulas with supralevator extension especially going up to precoccygeal space is a special indication (Fig. 15.3).
- Longer the fistula, more is the advantage of the scope like fistula opening in the thigh, legs and on abdominal wall.

15.4.1 Prerequisites Are

- Better to have mature tract.
- Magnetic resonance imaging (MRI) for preoperative assessment of secondary tracts.

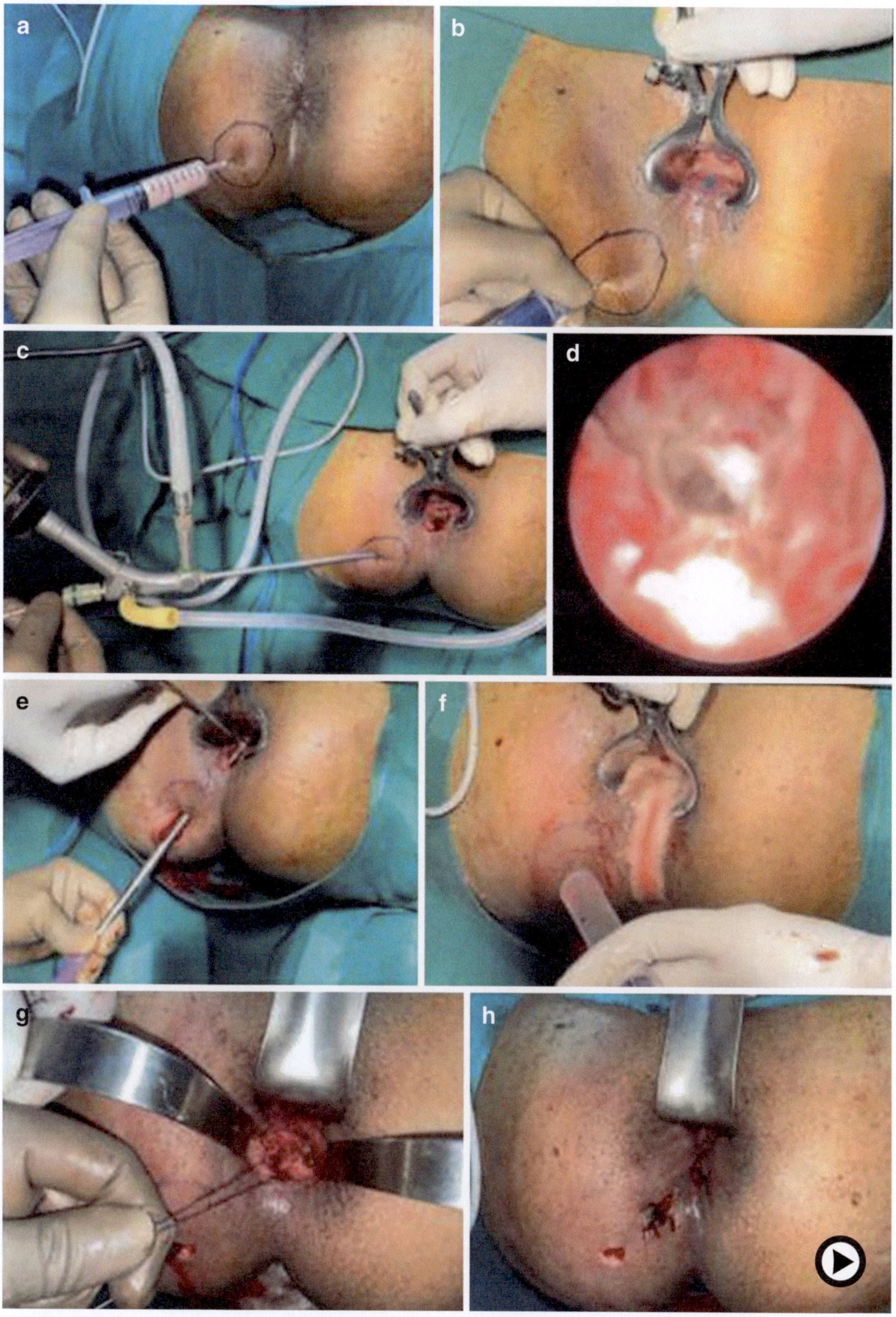

Fig. 15.2 (**a**) Needle aspiration of pus. (**b**) Internal communication at dentate line. (**c**) Centeral disease excision and fistuloscope insertion with LASER fibre. (**d**) Internal view of abscess cavity -fulgration by LASER. (**e**) Fixicision (**f**) Lavage with H_2O_2 and saline. (**g**) Closure of internal opening in external sphincter by PDS 2.0. (**h**) Drain in abscess cavity. Video 15.2 Transphincteric abscess with fistula (▶ https://doi.org/10.1007/000-hq7)

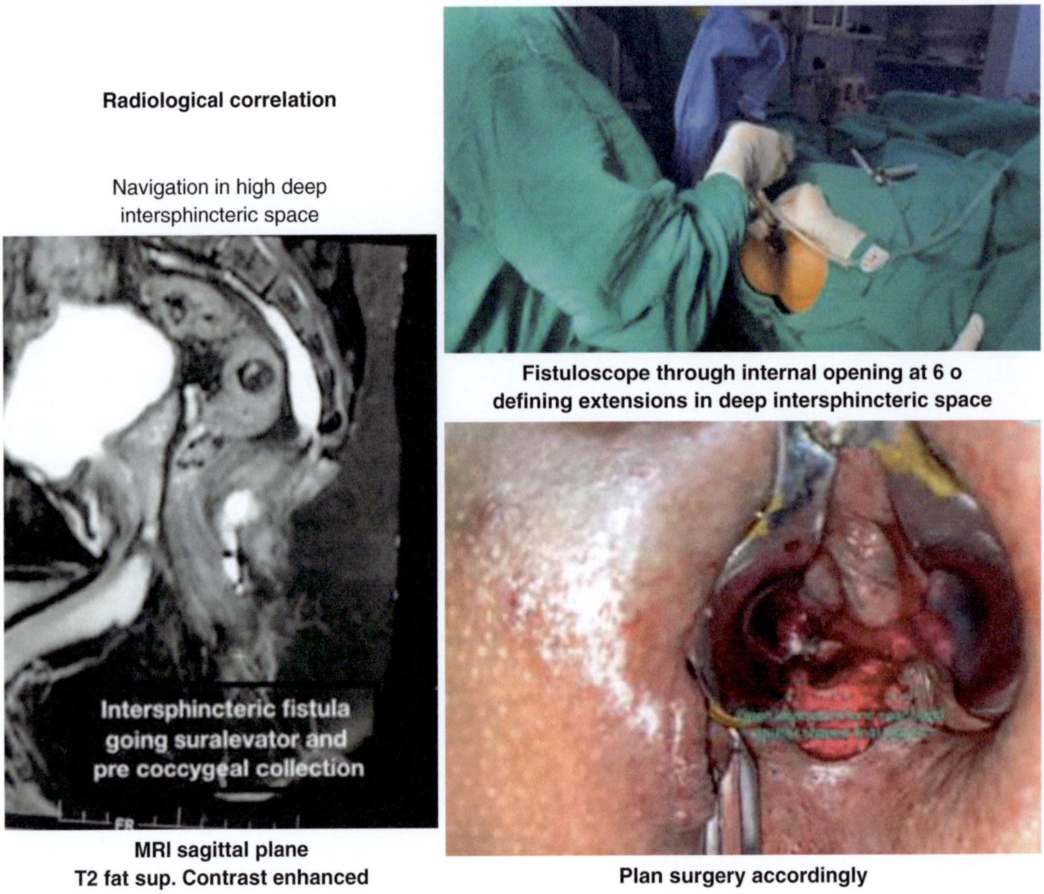

Fig. 15.3 Inter-sphincteric fistula with supralevator pre-coccygeal collection Fistuloscope comes very handy to enter and fulgrate this deep gorge. Lower end of the wound kept open and wide by incising internal sphincter below the dentate line and making saucer shape wound at anal verge for easy dressing and wash

15.5 Contra-Indications

- Simple fistulas—straight low inter-sphincteric or low straight trans-sphincteric fistulas are better treated by fistulotomy and marsupialisation with less recurrence and minimal change in continence to flatus.
- Fibrosed tracts or very thin tracts where even after dilatation of external opening, scope cannot be negotiated.
- Suspected malignancy and irradiated area.

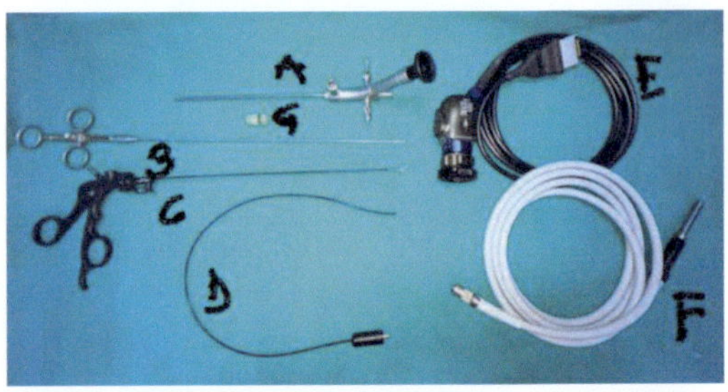

Fig. 15.4 Fistuloscope (**a**) (Meinero's type Storz) and associated accessories, brush (**b**), forceps (**c**), bug bee monopolar electrode (**d**), camera (**e**), fibroptic cable (**f**), water tight washer (**g**)

15.6 Equipment (Fig. 15.4)

- Meinero's fistuloscope manufactured by Karl Storz Germany (Fig. 15.1; Video 15.1).
- It has 8° angled eyepiece and is equipped with an optical, working and irrigation channel.
- Its antero-posterior diameter is 10F–14F from tip to handle.

- Its operative length is 18 cm which decreases to 14 cm when handle is attached but handle allows easier manoeuvring and provides stability (Fig. 15.5).
- In new model, removable handle can be rotated by 180 degrees so that manoeuvring is not limited by buttocks in different positions of fistula in ano.
- The fistuloscope has two taps—one of which is connected to irrigants which comprises of
  - 3-litre bag of 1.5% w/v glycine, mannitol 20% w/v 100 ml solution. Mannitol decreases absorption and increases excretion of glycin.
  - Normal saline 1 litre pack for diagnostic part.
- Transuretheral Resection of prostate (TURP) set is used as connector.
- Accessories with fistuloscope:
- An obturator, endo-forceps, unipolar bug bee electrode, an endo-brush and a water seal or washer (Figs. 15.4, 15.5, 15.6, and 15.7).
- Volkman's scoupe.
- Anal scopes, Parks speculum, self-lighted vaginal speculum of various size.
- Equipment for closure of internal opening depends on the way one closes internal opening.
- Stapler.
- Sutures, scissors and monopolar pencil for advancement flap or closure of opening in external sphincter after excision of central disease. (Central disease means internal opening with internal sphincter and inter sphincteric area.)
- Endoscopy tower/trolley.

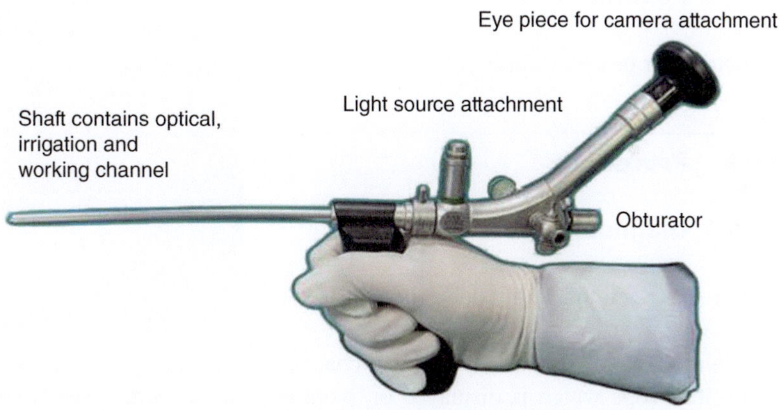

Fig. 15.5 Fibre optic rigid scope Meinero's type 18 cm long

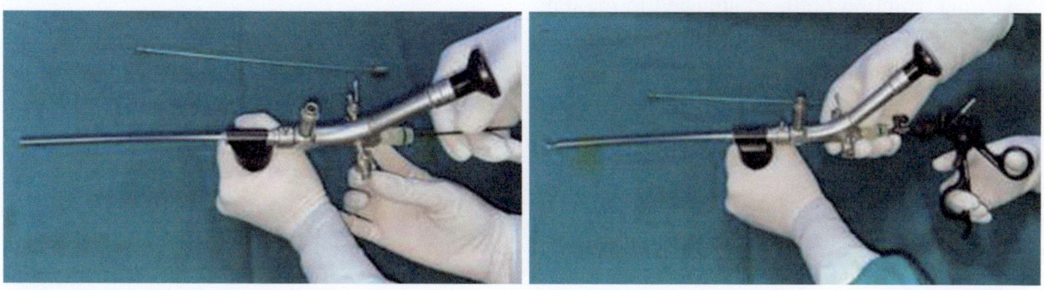

Fig. 15.6 Obturator is replaced with long delicate endo forceps which is threaded through attached water seal by assistant with two hands and scope is supported by surgeon

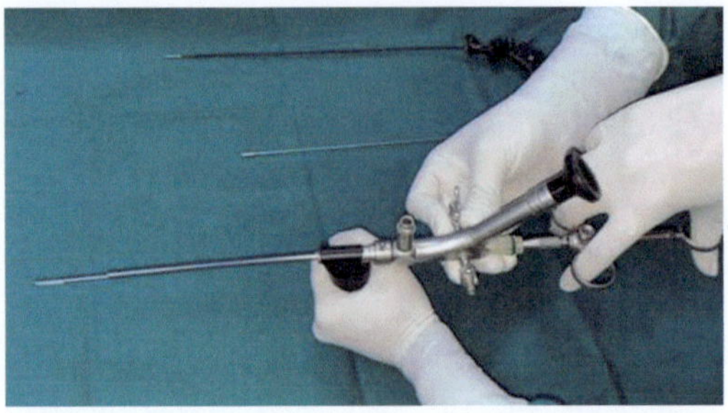

Fig. 15.7 Endobrush is pushed out of its sleeve after entering the fistula cavity and scope is supported by the assistant

15.7 Anaesthesia

Spinal anaesthesia or general anaesthesia as per patient requirment.

15.8 Position

Lithotomy or prone position.

15.9 Procedure

15.9.1 Diagnostic phase

- Camera head and light source is attached to the scope.
- White balancing is done and setting is changed to fibroscope which is displayed on monitor screen.
- Glycine solution bottle is attached to one tap with TURP set and device to increase the pressure of irrigation bottle is attached.
- We insert the fistuloscope through the external opening after dilating the opening as per requirement (Fig. 15.8).
- At times if the external opening is surrounded by tough scar tissue, it needs excision to allow easy entry of the scope.
- Moon crescent of the obturator is visible at the lower edge of the screen and ensures the correct orientation of the fistuloscope (Fig. 15.9).
- The fistula tract is identified by loose granulation visible on the screen (Fig. 15.10).
- We keep the tip of fistuloscope against it and wait for the glycine–mannitol solution to open the fistula tract.
- Navigate fistuloscope along the tract using slow movements, sideways and up/down.
- These movements and continuous water jet allow the fistula to get straightened and accommodate the fistuloscope.
- Continuous navigation under vision, keeping lumen in the centre helps one to reach as far as the internal opening or just below the mucosa.
- Look for side tracts and associated abscess.

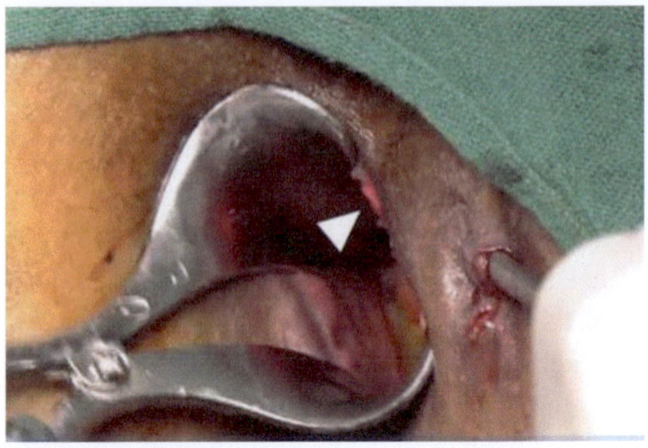

Fig. 15.8 Entry of the fistuloscope through the external opening and transillumination at the site of internal opening (arrow head)

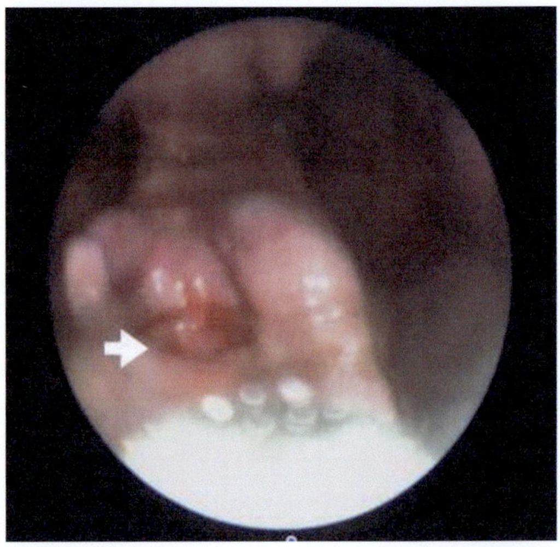

Fig. 15.9 Entry point of scope internal opening at dentate line (white arrow head) moon crescent of the obturator seen at lower edge of the figure

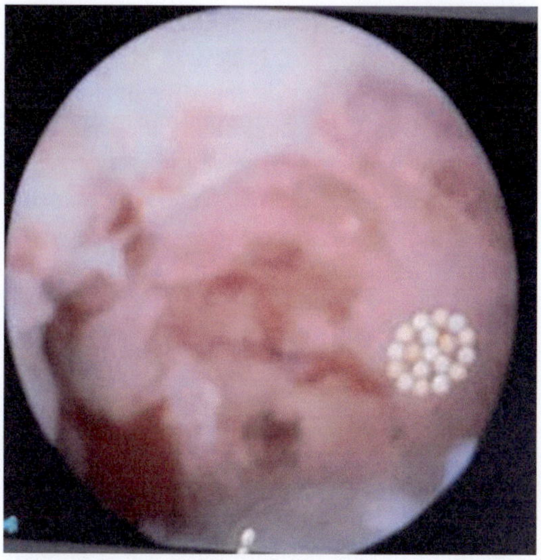

Fig. 15.10 Tract with granulation tissue and debris

- Insert an anal retractor and confirm internal opening either by the egress of water-jet or transillumination of anorectal mucosa in case opening is very narrow or closed.
- Mark the internal opening with a stroke of cautery or marking sutures.

15.9.2 Therapeutic Phase

- Remove the obturator and replace it with a sealing cap or washer over the operating channel.
- 2 mm endo-forceps with jaws closed is threaded by the assistant with both hands into the operative channel and when it is visible out of the shaft, surgeon holding the handle of the scope in the left hand now works with handle of the endo-forceps in the right hand (Fig. 15.6).
- Remove the granulation tissue and debris from the tract and make way forward towards the internal opening.
- After initial debridement forceps is replaced with bug bee electrode. Ball point electrode is connected to the electrosurgical unit and inserted through the sealing cap in the operating channel. It is very important to keep the tip of the electrode at least 1 cm away from lens of the scope to avoid any thermal damage to the lens.
- On way back from inner opening to external opening, one can fulgrate the tract bit by bit with bug bee monopolar electrode and look for secondary tracts.
- Keep electrode tip fixed 1 cm away from tip of the lens and with draw the scope as a whole.
- Debride the tract with endobrush or Volkman's scoupe. While using endobrush, note that the covering sheath remains in the instrument channel and only the brush moves to and fro. Otherwise, if the outer sheath is pushed in the tract, there would be no space for the movement of the brush.
- Irrigate the tract with saline hydrogen peroxide solution and finally lavage with saline.

Now is the time to close the internal opening which can be done by following methods:

- Stapler.
- Advancement flap.
- Suture the opening in external sphincter after central disease excision.
- Xenograft (*Bovine myocardium* biological mesh).
- Autologous fat graft.
- Others combine ligation of intersphincteric fistula tract (LIFT) with VAAFT.
- Success rate varies with the method of closure of internal opening in a given case.
- The high pressure in the anal canal exerted by the sphincter blows away any simple suture.
- Usually, the internal opening is surrounded by scars and tough tissue, especially in recurrent cases.

15.10 Use of a Linear or Semicircular Stapler

- This is one of the first methods for closing the internal opening proposed by the inventor.
- In cases without prior history of surgery and supple mucosa at dentate line area, the mucosa

is lifted by applying traction on two stitches placed on either side of the internal opening. Margins around internal opening are raised like a volcano. Depending on the position of internal opening and level of the raised mucosa, a linear or a semicircular stapler is fired at the base of this elevation to close the internal opening.

- In our experience, this led to early recurrence and we do not use this method any more. Meinero uses this method in about 10% of cases.

15.11 Advancement Flap

- In patients with sclerosed internal opening which is surrounded by tough tissue, mechanical suturing device fails.
- In such cases following removal of the entire scar tissue around internal opening, a full thickness mucosal muscular (fibres of internal sphincter) flap can be advanced to cover the internal opening.
- In our current practice, we sparingly use this closing procedure. Meinero uses this method in about 20–25% of his cases. The postoperative incontinence rate after making such a flap varies from 10% to 20% [2]. In our opinion, an unacceptable risk that is not worth-taking in minimally invasive procedure.

15.12 Trans-anal Suturing the Opening in External Sphincter

- In our practice, we rely on excising the 5-mm tissue around internal opening and opening intersphincteric space by removing a small fragment of internal sphincter as in Park's procedure and close the opening in supple external sphincter with PDS 2.0 by taking sutures in vertical manner.
- Put a probe in tract and take a figure-of-8 or u-shaped suture around the opening and tighten the suture while withdrawing the probe. Recheck for firm closure by gentle advancement of probe, which should not go now in the anal canal lumen.
- This method removes the offending central disease completely and closes the tract from inside to avoid any early soiling.
- Marsupialisation of this wound by suturing mucosa with sphincter muscles, keeps the wound fiat, improves healing and maintains anal squeeze pressure better at 3 months [3].

15.13 Use of a Bioabsorbable Mesh (Xenograft)

- The use of a bioabsorbable mesh (a xenograft made of bovine pericardium), which is interposed between the mucosa and the internal sphincter.
- Indication—excessive scar tissue around the internal opening.
- Sclerotic area is completely removed, a linear horizontal incision is made in mucosa, close to internal opening to raise a flap of mucosa around 2.5 cm^2.
- A patch of biological mesh is trimmed to fit the area of the defect and is fixed tension-free over internal sphincter covering internal opening defects with interrupted PDS stitches.
- Mucosa is repaired over the mesh with polyglactin sutures.

15.14 Autologous Dermis Graft

- An autologous dermis graft of adequate size is harvested from the margin of the external opening.
- Internal opening in internal sphincter is exposed by making an incision in mucosa around internal opening. Dermis graft is secured over the opening in internal sphincter by PDS 3.0 suture.
- The autologous dermis graft, acts as an airtight barrier and scaffold as well for tissue repair [4].
- A thorough hemostasis is achieved before closing the overlying mucosa with polyglactin sutures.
- Combination of ciprofioxacin and metronidazole given for 7 days.

15.15 VAAFT Combined with LIFT Procedure

- It is good idea to ligate intersphincteric fistula tract to close and isolate internal opening from the distal tract. LIFT is done after diagnostic part of VAAFT.
- Especially done when the internal opening is surrounded by scar and tough tissue after recurrence of fistula in ano [5].
- LIFT is easy to perform when tract is not very deep or high.
- Meinero team currently use this method in about 15% of cases.
- One of our colleagues, Dr. Arshad Ahmed from Lucknow, uses this method and his video is shown in procedure video 15.3 (Fig. 15.11).

VAAFT for inter sphincteric fistula going supra levator video 15.4 (Figs. 15.12, 15.13, 15.14, and 15.15).

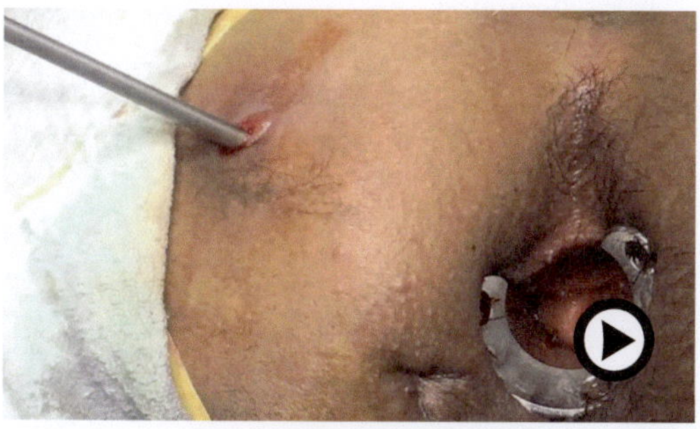

Fig. 15.11 VAAFT combined with LIFT Procedure. Video 15.3 (▶ https://doi.org/10.1007/000-hq6)

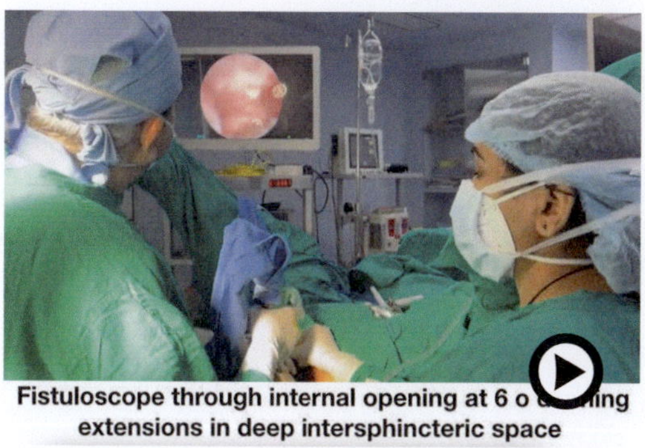

Fig. 15.12 VAAFT for inter sphincteric fistula going supra levator. Video 15.4 (▶ https://doi.org/10.1007/000-hq9)

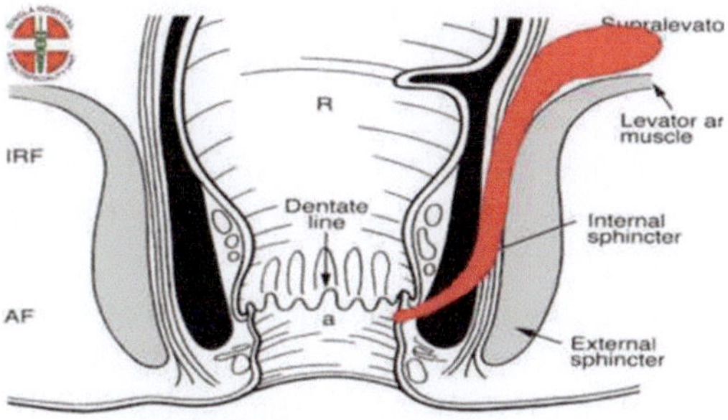

Fig. 15.13 MRI findings in coronal section intersphincteric fistula going supra levator

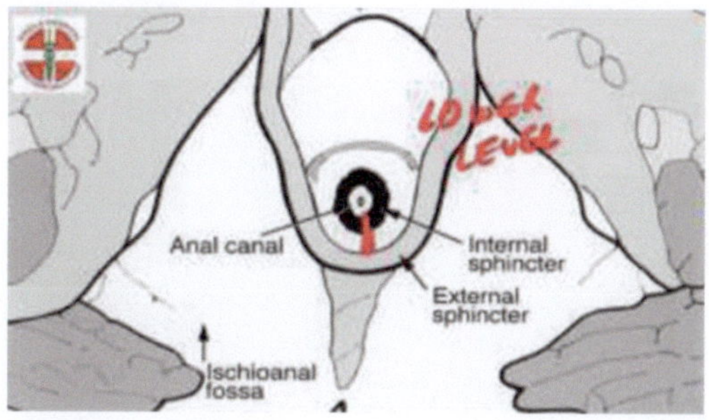

Fig. 15.14 MRI axial section at dentate line

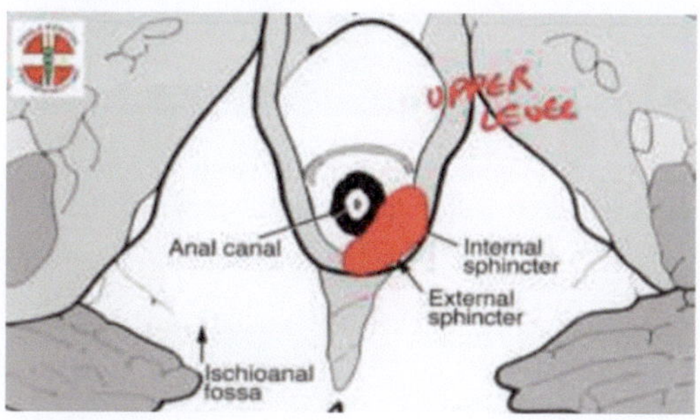

Fig. 15.15 MRI axial section at supra levator level

- Entry point of scope is from inside the anal canal at dentate line (Fig. 15.9). Rest is same as for diagnostic part except that following the tract inside the anal canal keeping the fistuloscope as per MRI guidance and slowly up towards the supralevator or precoccygeal space.
- Remove the debris with endo-forceps to create space.
- One can fulgrate the granulation tissue in sinus cavity wall while coming back either with bug bee or with 1470 nm diode LASER

using radial fibre, delivering 10 watts energy as continuous wave. Withdraw fibre with scope at the rate of (@) of 1 mm per second with flow decreased to minimum so that walls of the sinus cavity collapse over the LASER fibre (Fig. 15.16).
- Curette with endo-brush or Volkman's scoupe.
- To facilitate postoperative flushing till the tract heals from top to bottom, enlarge the lower end of the tract cephalic to dentate line by incising almost 1 cm.
- For the same reason, lower end of the internal sphincter in incised and wound is made saucer-shaped at anal verge (Fig. 15.17).

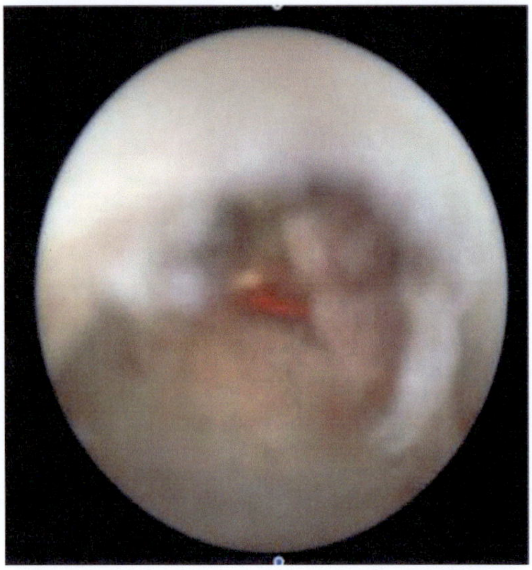

Fig. 15.16 Fulgration of the tract with LASER fibre, water flow decreased so that tract collapses over the fibre to facilitate 360-degree fulgration

15.16 Post-operative Management

- All patients are given written instructions on diet and defecatory habits.
- Keep open the distal opening with help of clean autoclaved ear buds and pressing the tract from medial to lateral every fourth day till two weeks. This method lets the secretions to flow out through the external opening.
- For pure intersphincteric fistula, flush the wound to keep lower end open for drainage.
- Encourage patients to start walking as soon as possible after the effect of anaesthesia is over.
- Avoid squatting in initial phase to save sutures from disruption.

15.17 Complications of VAAFT (Table 15.1)

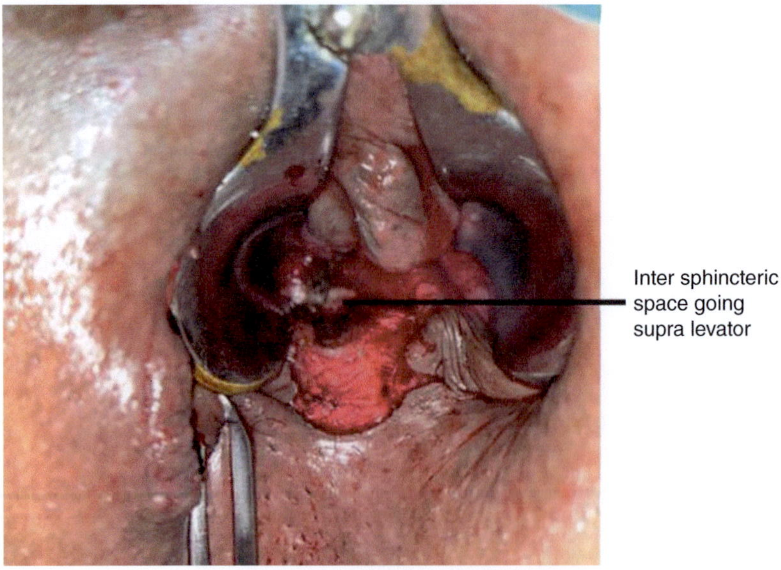

Fig. 15.17 One cm portion of internal sphincter cephalic to dentate line and lower portion of internal sphincter incised to make wound saucer shape for easy flushing with saline

Table 15.1 Complications of VAAFT

Complications	Prevention	Management
Creation of false tract and leakage of irrigation fluid into surrounding tissue.	Keep scope on entry point and wait to let the fluid open up the tract. Don't force scope. Pre-op MRI should guide the direction. While advancing the scope. Keep lumen in the center.	Stop irrigation, especially under pressure. If detected early withdraw scope in normal tract and try to pass terumo guide wire to negotiate around breach area. Thread scope over guide wire. If not possible convert to open procedure or core out the tract.
Unable to reach internal opening due to collapsed or narrow tract	Wait at entry point with irrigation on, let the tract open with fluid pressure.	Pass guide wire or bug bee electrode. Slowly rail road the scope over the wire or bugbee electrode.
Skip areas and wide tract.	Use bugbee electrode under vision.	Decrease pressure in tract, keep electrode ball 1 cm distal to tip of the scope. Stop irrigation and fulgrate while withdrawing scope 1mm per second. Recheck for skip areas.
Damage of instruments especially endo forceps. Jaws and shaft are very vulnerable.	2 mm instruments are very delicate and long, it needs two hands of the assistant to thread them in to the instrument channel of the scope. Entry without the closed jaws will break the grasper tip. While using endo forceps try to keep handle in alignment with shaft otherwise shaft bends at shat handle junction. On taking out unhealthy tissue, take out the whole assembly, as more often the grasper is taken out which increases the chances of damage. Additionally, the tissue doesn't come out, as it gets stuck in washer(seal cap) at the instrument channel entry. While holding the tissue, either pull it or rotate it with the rotation wheel on the handle. Keep VAAFT instruments on separate trolley.	Better prevention than cure. These instruments cannot be repaired, only need replacement.
Thermal damage to optical tip causing optical fibre loss.	Keep bug bee electrode tip/radial LASER fibre tip at least 1 to 1.5 cm away from tip of the scope	Repair of damaged optical fibres is not possible, one has to replace the scope.

15.18 Tips and Tricks

How to locate the internal opening IO.

- Read MRI again and display in OT.
- Entry of scope from EO towards IO, bright light can be seen at the internal opening (Fig. 15.18).
- The fistuloscope can be inserted in the anal canal to visualize the IO.
- Use Terumo guide wire or the bug-bee tip as a guide and advance the scope over it.

Secondary track must be found in accordance with pre-op. MRI.

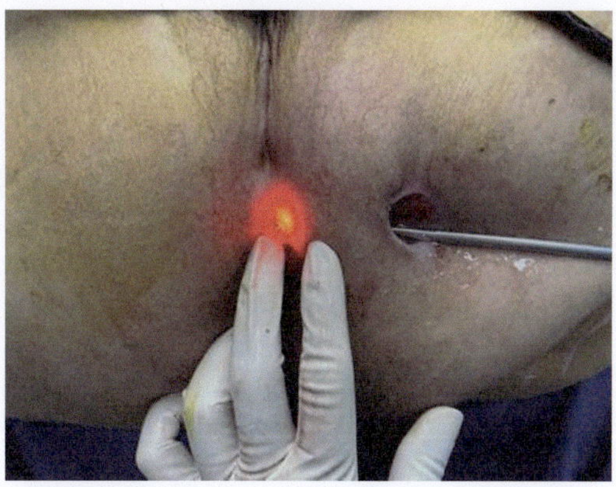

Fig. 15.18 Bright light guides the site of internal opening

- Abscess are located and drained out, seton is optional.
- For complete 360-degree clearance of the tract, ablate all the unhealthy tract, stop the flow if tract is dilated and electrode cannot reach the side walls.
- Closing the internal opening by suture or stapler is prone for failures, as sutures breakdown.
- We favour to excise the internal opening till intersphincteric space, curette the deep intersphincteric space.
- The fistuloscope is introduced into external anal sphincter (EAS) to intersphincteric space.
- Fulgurate and curette the tract in external sphincter and distal up to EO.
- Close the defect in EAS from within the anal canal with 2.0 PDS. Then marsupialise the mucosa margins to EAS (Fig. 15.19).
- Tube drain can be kept in the external opening for drainage of fluid and prevention of premature closure of external opening.
- VAAFT in itself is not complete treatment. How one closes the IO matters a lot when it comes to prevention of reoccurrence.

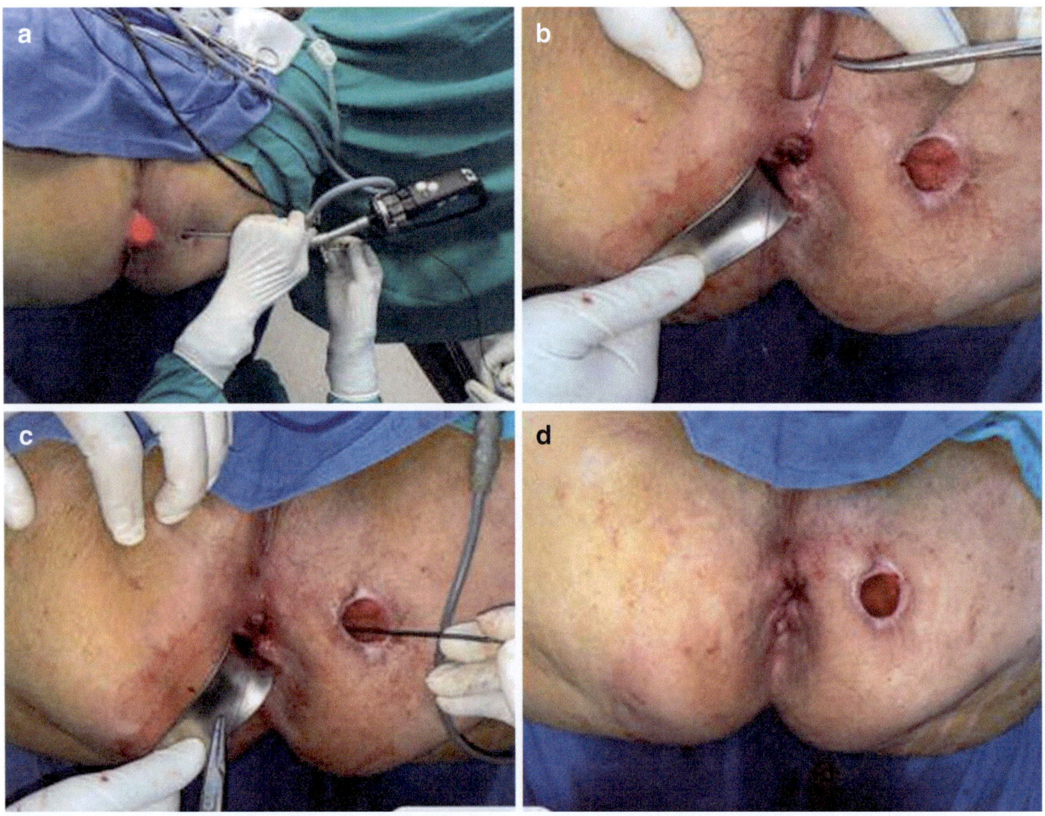

Fig. 15.19 (**a**) Fulgurate part of the tract in external sphincter under vision. (**b**) After excising the internal opening till intersphincteric space, close the defect in EAS from the anal canal with PDS. (**c**) Check the closure by inserting probe. (**d**) Marsupalise the internal wound. External wound is large due to previous drainage of abscess

Algorithm for VAAFT

History-discharging sinus in perianal region and buttocks
Clinical examination, DRE (tract anatomy and sphincter tone)
MRI/endo US (best yield in cases external opening is 2 cm from anal verge, posterior horse shoe fistula, recurrent fistula and complex fistula on DRE)
Make 3d picture of anatomy of fistula in cortex diary
Complex fistula define need for sphincter preserving surgery
Equipment Meinero's scope, set video endoscopic trolley
Spinal/GA, position lithotomy/prone in case of external opening quite high and posterior in gluteal area
Glycin mannitol/saline as irrigant for the procedure—for diagnostic phase
In case of trans sphincteric, supra sphincteric and extra sphincteric fistula, enter from external opening.
For pure intersphincteric fistula going high with only internal opening, enter from inside the anal canal from dentate line
Define the tract, associated abscess and secondary tracts and internal opening
Therapeutic phase-fulgrate the tract with monopolar bug bee or ball point electrode/1470 diode radial LASER fibre
Debride and clean tract with endobrush or Volkman's scoop
Close the internal opening by appropriate method
Our preference is to excise central disease and close the opening in external sphincter from inside the anal canal by 2.0 PDS suture
Minimal external wound to take care by washing and putting a pad
Female sanitary napkin adhered to undergarment on back side suffices

References

1. Meinero P, Mori L. Video-assisted anal fistula treatment (VAAFT): a novel sphincter-saving procedure for treating complex anal fistulas. Tech Coloproctol. 2011;15(4):417–22. https://doi.org/10.1007/s10151-011-0769-2. Epub 2011 Oct 15. Erratum in: Tech Coloproctol 2012 Feb;16(1):111. PMID: 22002535; PMCID: PMC3226694
2. Balciscueta Z, Uribe N, Balciscueta I, Andreu-Ballester JC, García-Granero E. Rectal advancement flap for the treatment of complex cryptoglandular anal fistulas: a systematic review and meta-analysis. Int J Color Dis. 2017;32(5):599–609. https://doi.org/10.1007/s00384-017-2779-7. Epub 2017 Feb 28. PMID: 28247060
3. Ho YH, Tan M, Leong AF, Seow-Choen F. Marsupialization of fistulotomy wounds improves healing: a randomized controlled trial. Br J Surg. 1998;85(1):105–7. https://doi.org/10.1046/j.1365-2168.1998.00529.x.
4. Piercarlo Meinero Video-Assisted Anal Fistula Treatment VAAFT page 406 in C. Ratto et al., editors. Anal Fistula and Abscess, Coloproctology © Springer Nature Switzerland AG 2022.
5. Rojanasakul A, Pattanaarun J, Sahakitrungruang C, Tantiphlachiva K. Total anal sphincter saving technique for fistula-in-ano; the ligation of intersphincteric fistula tract. J Med Assoc Thail. 2007;90(3):581–6.

Suggested Reading

Charalampopoulos A, Papakonstantinou D, Bagias G, Nastos K, Perdikaris M, Papagrigoriadis S. Surgery of simple and complex anal fistulae in adults: a review of the literature for optimal surgical outcomes. Cureus. 2023;15(3):e35888. https://doi.org/10.7759/cureus.35888. PMID:36911578; PMCID: PMC9993441

Piercarlo Meinero Video-Assisted Anal Fistula Treatment VAAFT 391–411 in C. Ratto et al., editors. Anal Fistula and Abscess, Coloproctology © Springer Nature Switzerland AG 20.

Fistula in Ano: Sphincter-Saving Procedures Trans-Rectal Opening of Inter-Sphincteric Space (TROPIS)

16

Abstract

- Fistula in ano of crypto-glandular origin persists due to inadequate drainage of trapped abscess in inter-sphincteric space.
- Like any other abscess to heal, this abscess also needs to be widely laid open and then allowed to heal by granulation tissue from base.
- Concept of opening inter-sphincteric space in the anal canal for drainage of acute abscess presenting inside the anal canal region is well established.
- Pankaj Garg recently applied the same concept in chronic abscess, i.e., fistula in ano and baptised the procedure as trans-rectal opening of inter-sphincteric space (TROPIS). Technique works in more than 85% of cases. Though it was earlier suggested by Eisenhammer and practised by A.G. Parks also.
- Extension of tract through the external anal sphincter (EAS) and ischiorectal fat can be managed by curettage, LASER ablation or tube-drainage till the internal opening heals by granulation tissue.
- It saves the external sphincter from any damage thereby decreasing rate of anal incontinence.

16.1 What One Should Know Before the Procedure Indications

- If peri-anal abscess is acute suppuration, then fistula is a chronic suppuration which has not been drained adequately by nature or surgeon.
- Source of such infection is anal gland in inter-sphincteric space.
- Persistence of this infection is the major source of fistula formation, its maintenance and reoccurrence.
- Basis of this procedure is that if we drain this trapped infection in inter-sphincteric space adequately, then rest is all secondary tracts.
- Trans-anal or trans-rectal route is selected to lay open the inter-sphincteric space (TROPIS), and then it is kept open inside the lumen.
- Tract passing through external sphincter and in ischio-rectal space can be curetted, LASER ablated or drained by putting small tube drains till the central wound heals.
- So this procedure spares the external sphincter from cutting.

Supplementary Information The online version contains supplementary material available at https://doi.org/10.1007/978-981-96-6190-9_16. The videos can be accessed individually by clicking the DOI link in the accompanying figure caption or by scanning this link with the SN More Media App.

S. K. Singla, K. Mital, *Operative Manual of Minimally Invasive and LASER Ano-proctology*,
https://doi.org/10.1007/978-981-96-6190-9_16

- Procedure has been well studied by robust follow-up clinically and radiologically (magnetic resonance imaging (MRI)) by the inventor [1].
- Long duration of healing by secondary intention and persistent tubes in distal tracts is the limitation as of today.
- Of course, around 13–15% of cases fail to heal and need other procedures.

16.2 Indications

- All complex fistulae. Garg classification grade III–V [1].

16.3 Contraindications

- Simple fistulae. Garg classification grade I and grade II are better managed by fistulotomy [1].

16.4 Pre-operative Consideration

- Define the fistulous tract by clinical examination and magnetic resonance imaging (MRI), as in all sphincter-preserving surgeries for fistula in ano in modern practice (Figs. 16.1 and 16.2).

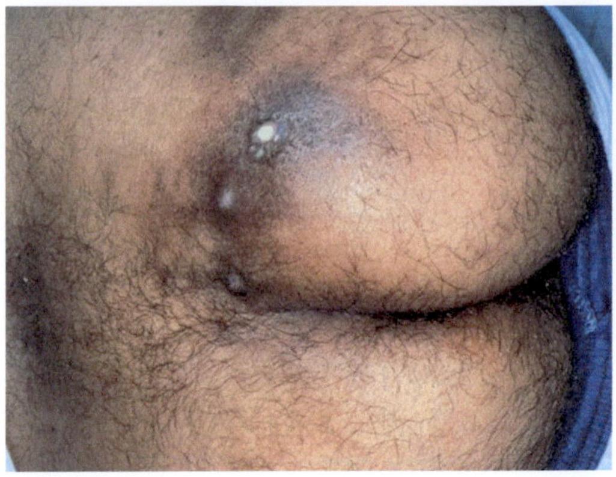

Fig. 16.1 Complex fistula—internal opening post midline and three external openings on right gluteal area almost near sacrococcygeal area

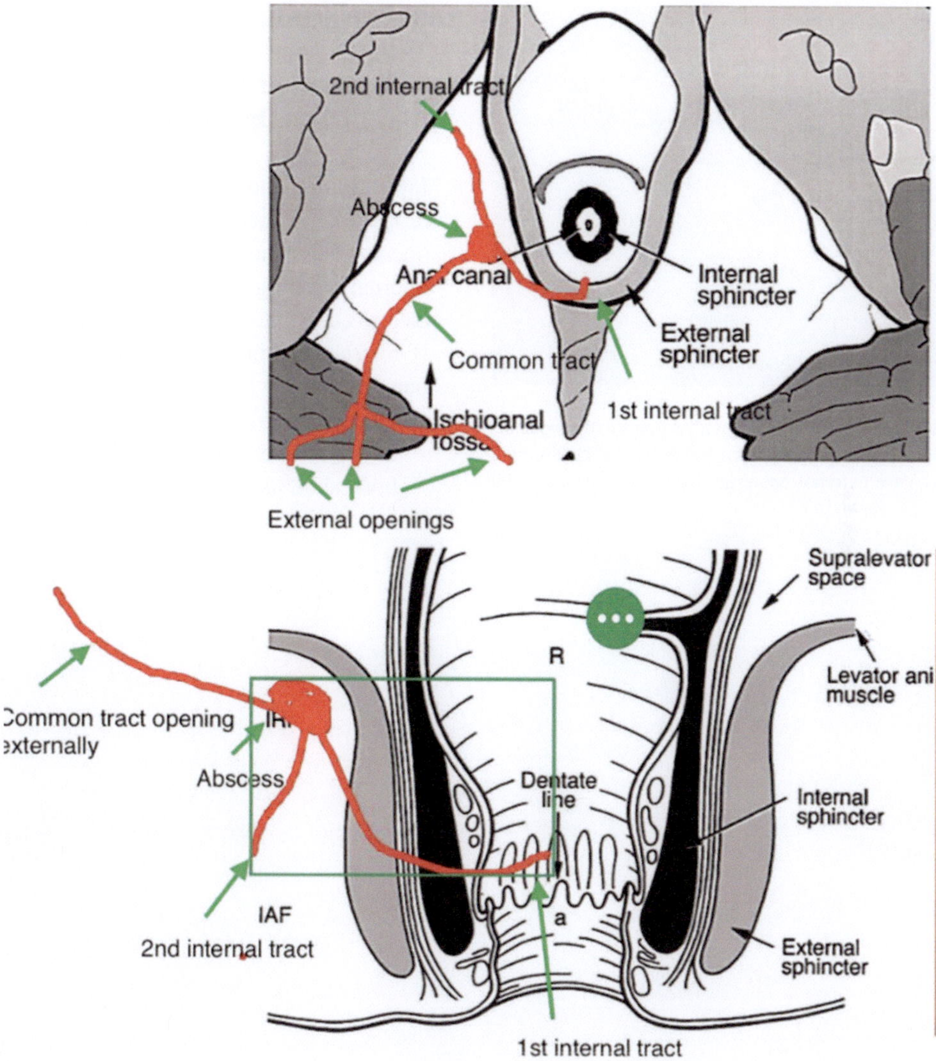

Fig. 16.2 MRI findings of the same patient as in Fig. 16.1

16.5 Equipment

- Operation table with stirrups for lithotomy (Fig. 16.3).
- For prone position, rolled sheets and cushions with tapes for strapping (optional). In case of anterior fistulae, it is easy to work on floor by putting patient in prone position than operating on ceiling in lithotomy.
- Sterile drapes and gowns.
- Povidine iodine solution.
- Xylocaine jelly, surgical gloves, saline-soaked gauge pieces.
- Syringes.
- Normal saline and lignocaine 2%.
- Park's speculum.
- Mosquito artery forceps.
- Electro surgical unit.
- Infant feeding tube.
- Methylene blue diluted.
- Hydrogen peroxide.

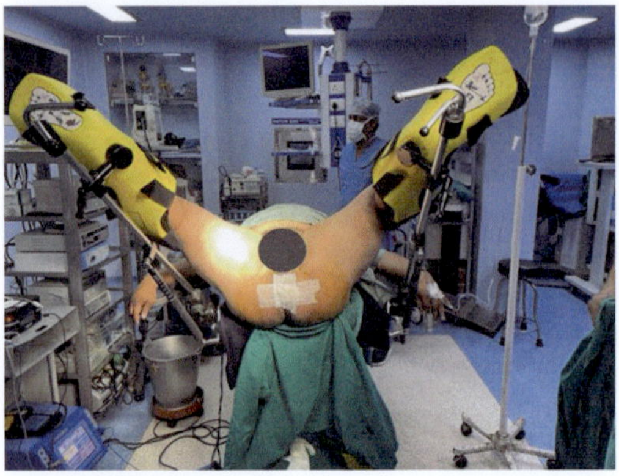

Fig. 16.3 Lithotomy position with Allen stirrups hydraulic sliding rod hyper extended position can be attained easily in case external opening of posterior fistula going cephalic as shown in Fig. 16.1

16.6 Procedure (Fig. 16.4)

16.6.1 Location of Internal Opening (IO) on Operation Table

- Inject dilute methylene blue mixed with a few drops of hydrogen peroxide through external opening (EO) and check for its egress from internal opening. Mark IO with a stroke of electro coagulation by monopolar pencil.
- If internal opening is not readily identified, one can take the help of following modalities:
  - Garg protocol for finding internal opening is (1) reassessment of MRI, (2) in non-horseshoe fistulae, the IO was assumed to be at the point where the fistula tract

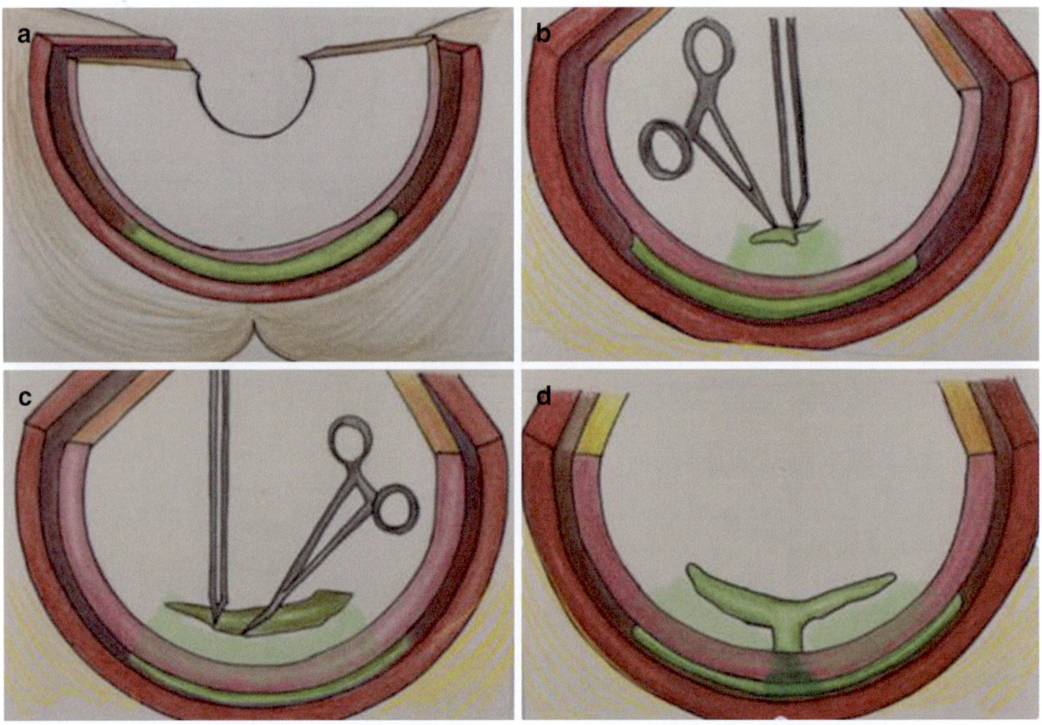

Fig. 16.4 Principle of TROPIS as suggested by Pankaj Garg. (**a**) Abscess in inter-sphincteric space (ISS) horseshoe type. (**b**) Opening ISS at dentate line from site of IO at 6 o' to left side. (**c**) Opening ISS to right side. (**d**) Laid open horse shoe inter-sphincteric fistula

reached closest to the sphincter-complex (3) In horse-shoe fistulae, the IO was assumed to be located in the midline (anterior or posterior as per the horseshoe location) [2].

16.6.2 Trans Rectal/Anal Opening of Inter-Sphincteric Space (TROPIS)

- All primary internal openings are at dentate line, corresponding to the opening of affected anal gland.
- Assess the inter-sphincteric tract, its direction and extent carefully by clinical examination and MRI pictures.
- Engage a curved small mosquito artery forceps in the opening and advance on right or left circumferentially or vertically in deep inter-sphincteric tract depending on situation in a given case.
- Lay open the tract over tip of mosquito artery forceps with monopolar cautery by cutting mucosa and circular fibres of internal sphincter (IS), one can take help of bipolar cautery also in case submucosal cushions are engorged and bleed.
- In case of horse-shoe extension in inter-sphincteric space, one may lay open inter-sphincteric tract on both sides of the midline in circular manner (Fig. 16.4).
- In case extension is vertical, one can lay open in vertical direction but avoid cutting anorectal ring area, it is better to lay open distal part and curette the more proximal tract and keep the distal part wide open for drainage (Fig. 16.5).

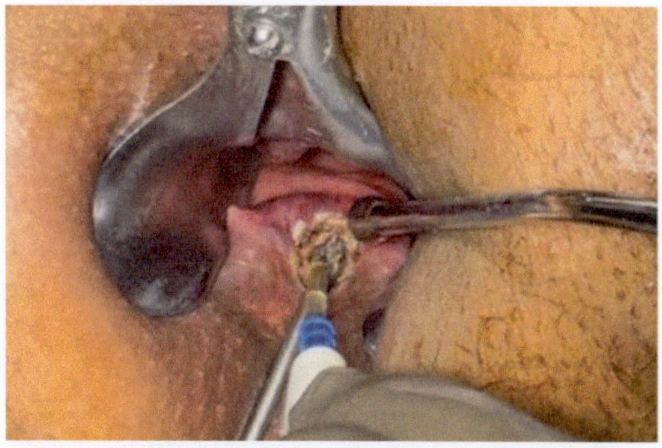

Fig. 16.5 Lay open the vertical deep inter-sphincteric tract over a probe but never cut internal sphincter in ano-rectal ring area

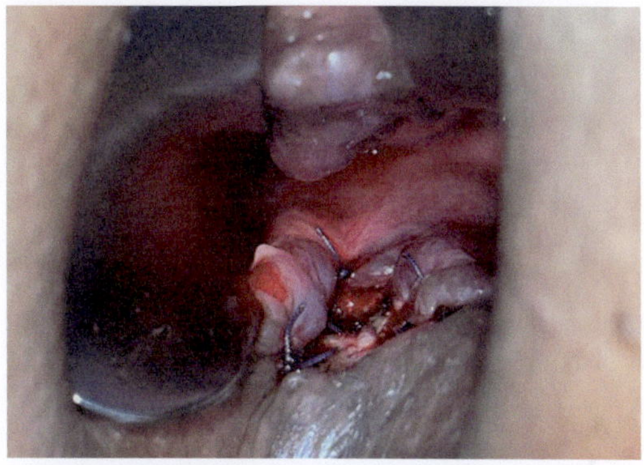

Fig. 16.6 Incise distal internal sphincter to make lower end of the wound saucer shaped for drainage. Marsupialise this wound to avoid premature closure

- Excise small portion of internal sphincter below the dentate line distal to internal opening till anal verge, for keeping space open for drainage and making distal wound saucer shaped (Fig. 16.6).

16.6.3 Managing Distal Tract

- Distal tract from the skin to external sphincter can be curetted or LASER ablated and drained with K 90 catheter or fine abdominal drains in distal tract.
- Small drainage tubes are cut flush with the skin and fixed with 3.0 nylon (Fig. 16.7).

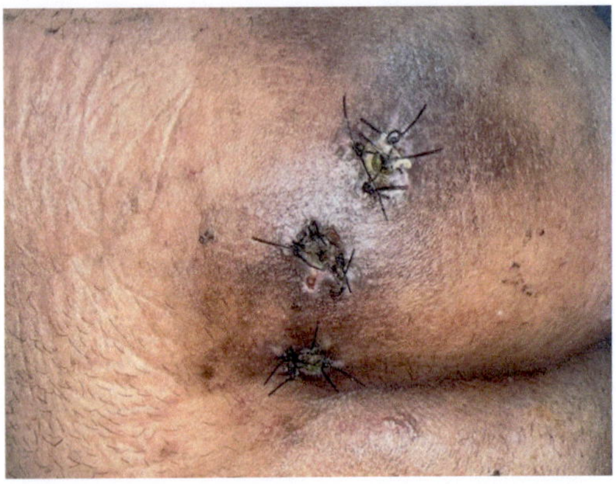

Fig. 16.7 Drainage tubes in distal tracts stitched flushed with the skin

16.7 Stepwise Approach for TROPIS in a Patient with Complex Fistula (Video 16.1)

- Assessment and confirmation of the anatomy of the tract.
- Young male patient with internal opening at 6 0′, inter-sphincteric tract from 6 0′ to 4 0′, breach in external sphincter at mid-anal canal at 4 0′ then tract runs in ischiorectal fossa to open at skin level. His intersphincteric tract as per MRI is as shown in Fig. 16.8.
- Identification of internal opening and establishing connection between IO and EO (Fig. 16.9).
- Laying open inter-sphincteric space (ISS) on curved mosquito or Mixter forceps (Figs. 16.9 and 16.10). Management of distal tract by coring and LASER ablation (Fig. 16.10).

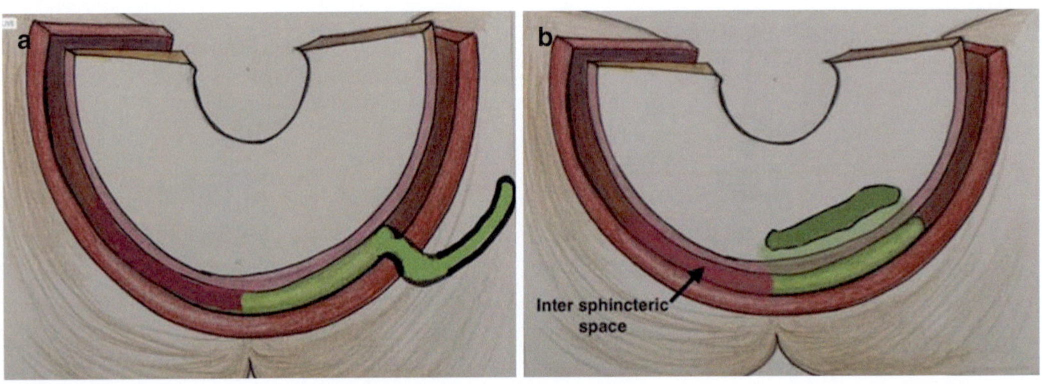

Fig. 16.8 Axial section of inter-sphincteric extension and trans-sphincteric component of a fistula. (**a**) Whole tract in axial view. (**b**) Trans-rectal opening of inter-sphincteric tract (TROPIS)

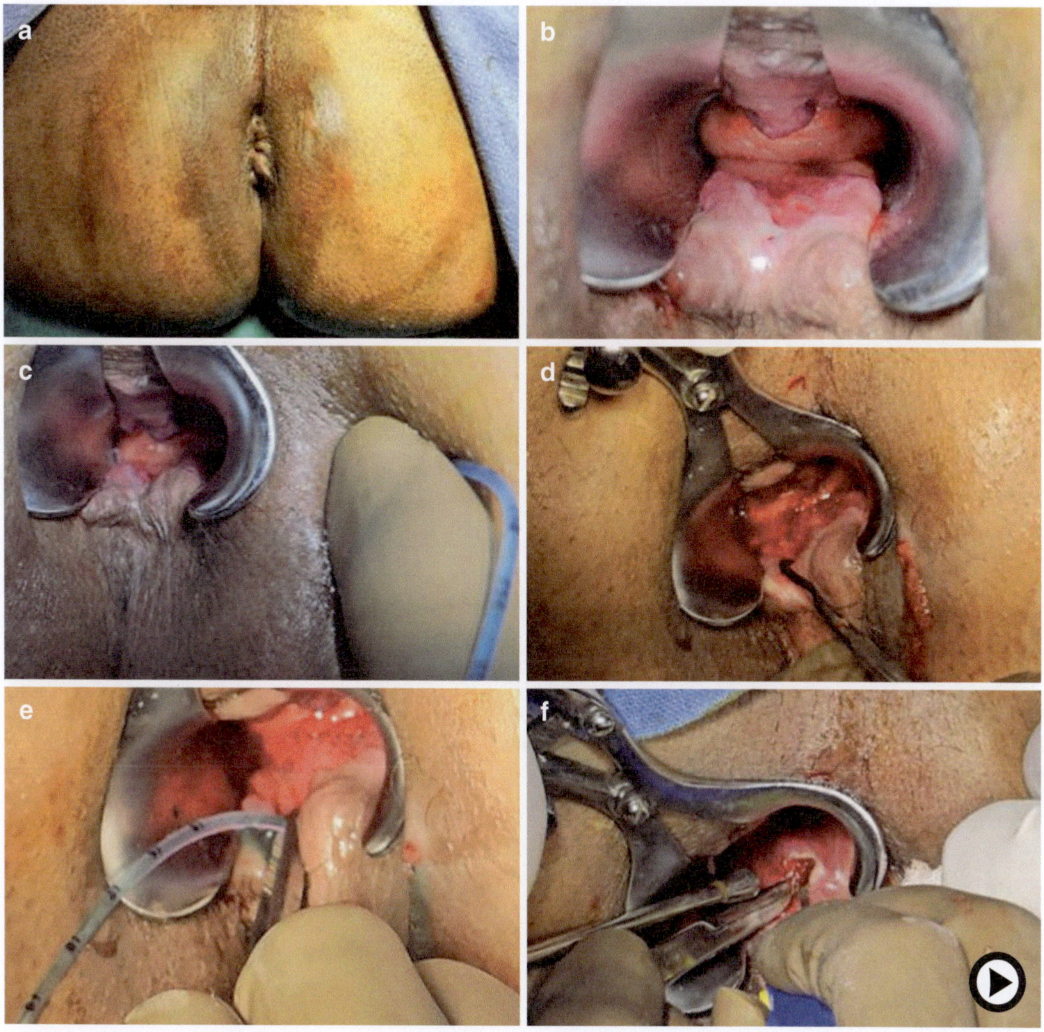

Fig. 16.9 (**a**) Clinical photograph in lithotomy position showing external opening (EO). (**b**) Dimple at 6 0′ clock internal opening (IO). (**c**) Instillation of dye from EO no egress at suspected IO, (**d**) IO reverse probed probe entered easily in IO. (**e**) Dye instilled from IO came out from EO. (**f**) Tip of Mixter forceps engaged in IO and ISS opened over it by incising mucosa and IS circumferentially Video 16.1 Step-wise approach for TROPIS in a patient with complex fistula (▶ https://doi.org/10.1007/000-hqa)

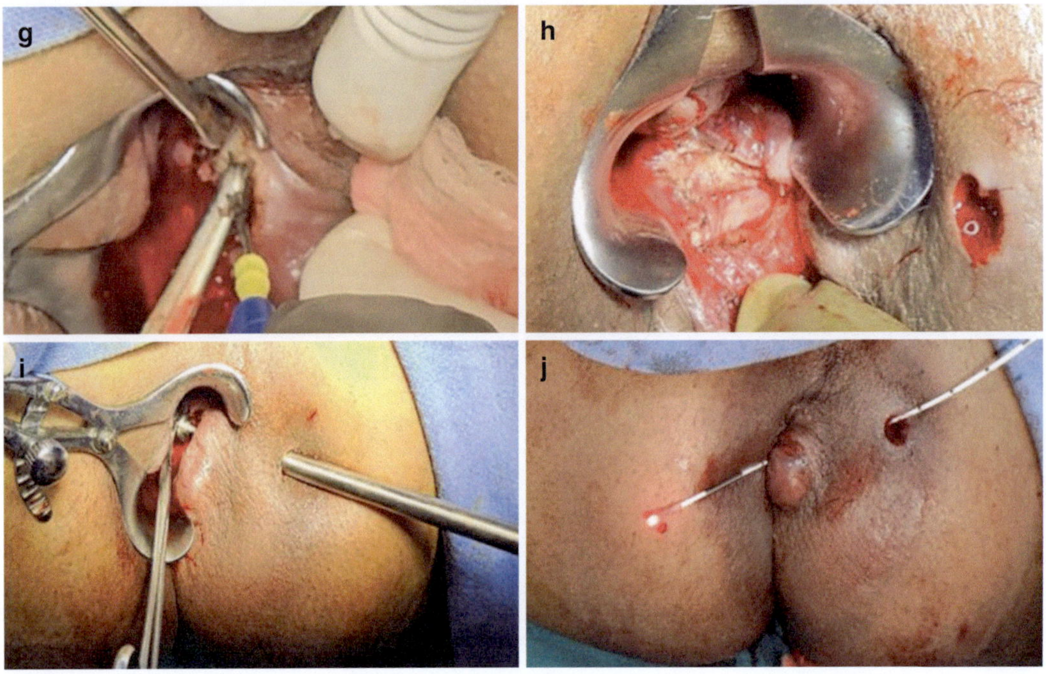

Fig. 16.10 (**g**) ISS opened from 6 0′ to 4 0′ over Mixter with monopolar pencil (**h**) opened ISS. (**i**) Coring done for distal tract by FiXcision device. (**j**) LASER ablation of residual granulation

16.8 Post-operative Care

- Patient's relative is advised to apply ointment to internal opening to avoid its premature closure. We usually marsupialise the internal wound created after trans-rectal opening of inter-sphincteric space.
- No flushing is done from external opening, instead new internal opening created after surgery is allowed to fill by granulation tissue—this process may take few months at times.
- Slowly withdraw external tubes by 1 cm each time at an interval of 10 days, to avoid premature closure of external wound before healing from inside.

16.9 Tips and Tricks

- Pre-operative mapping of fistula tract by MRI is highly desirable.
- On-table assessment of IO is mandatory because that corresponds to infected inter-sphincteric space.
- To open the inter-sphincteric space circumferentially or vertically, it is best to go transanal or transrectal.
- While doing transanal or rectal opening of inter-sphincteric space, in case of engorged submucosal cushions if monopolar pencil dissection leads to bleeding, one can use bipolar coagulation.
- Do not flush tracts from external opening after TROPIS, instead allow internal opening to heal by secondary intention by formation of granulation tissue.

16.10 Complication (Table 16.1)

Table. 16.1 Complications of TROPIS

Complications	Prevention	Management
Spontaneous fall of tubes in distal tracts	Apply monofilament sutures on 3–4 sides	Refixation with the skin
Delayed healing	Meticulous drainage of all tracts, do not flush the tract from EO	
Reoccurrence	Meticulous drainage of inter-sphincteric space	Get MRI done if still there is persistent infection in inter-sphincteric space do TROPIS again. Otherwise adopt other procedure

Algorithm for TROPIS

History and clinical examination
MRI for fistula in ano and perianal spaces
As per Garg classification—complex fistulae grade iii, iv and v are for TROPIS
Identification of internal opening
Injecting methylene blue with few drops of H_2O_2 from external opening
Check egress from internal opening
Primary internal opening (IO) is at dentate line
Check for circumferential or vertical spread of the intersphincteric tract
Engage tip of curved mosquito forceps in the IO and cut mucosa and internal sphincter over the tip of forceps by monopolar cautery
Open intersphincteric space in upper anal canal as per the situation
Go right and left in case of horseshoe tract in intersphincteric space
Curette it well
Incise internal sphincter distal to dentate line in corresponding sector to make the wound at anal verge as saucer shaped
Distal tract through ES and ischiorectal fossa in managed either by curettage, LASER ablation or tube drainage
Tube in distal tract is fixed flush to the skin at external opening by nylon sutures
Relative is advised to do DRE daily to avoid pre mature closure of IO
We usually do marsupialisation of internal wound after TROPIS
Withdraw the tube in distal tract @ 1 cm every 10 days till the internal wound heals completely
No flushing from external wound

References

1. Garg, P. Garg Classification for anal fistulas: is it better than existing classifications?—a review. Indian J Surg. 2018;80:606–8. https://doi.org/10.1007/s12262-018-1788-2.
2. Garg P, Kaur B, Singla K, Menon GR, Yagnik VD. A simple protocol to effectively manage anal fistulas with no obvious internal opening. Clin Exp Gastroenterol. 2021;14:33–44. https://doi.org/10.2147/CEG.S291909. PMID: 33564257; PMCID: PMC7866917

Suggested Reading

Garg P. Transanal opening of intersphincteric space (TROPIS) – a new procedure to treat high complex anal fistula. Int J Surg. 2017;40:130–4. https://doi.org/10.1016/j.ijsu.2017.02.095. Epub 2017 Mar 1. PMID: 28259693

Huang H, Ji L, Gu Y, Li Y, Xu S. Efficacy and safety of sphincter-preserving surgery in the treatment of complex anal fistula: a network meta-analysis. Front Surg. 2022;9:825166. https://doi.org/10.3389/fsurg.2022.825166. PMID: 35211503; PMCID: PMC8861434

Fistula in Ano: Minimally Invasive Procedures
Setons, Ksharsootra
Draining Setons as Definitive Treatment
Rerouting of Setons

17

Abstract

- Setons as treatment of fistula in ano has 2500 years history and is still a resourceful method.
- Many modifications are being tried to make it minimally invasive, sphincter preserving and less painful procedure.
- Fistula is a chronic suppuration which has not been drained well by nature or surgeon, seton ensures drainage if kept for sufficient duration. In Crohn's anorectal fistulae, at times it is left as a prolonged treatment modality (Gold SL, Cohen-Mekelburg S, Schneider Y, Steinlauf A. Gastroenterol Hepatol (N Y), 14(9):521–528, 2018).
- Are setons bail out procedure where one is not sure how much to cut? May be in emergency setting of peri-anal abscess with fistula in ano, not in a nonemergent situation of chronic fistula in ano where one can investigate with magnetic resonance imaging (MRI)/endo-Ultrasound (US).
- Draining setons decrease the height of fistula over time, at times, they spontaneously come out through skin. Can draining setons be used as staged fistulotomy with slow cutting property? Yes.
- Draining setons are used as bridge to definitive sphincter saving surgery like ligation of intersphincteric fistula tract [LIFT].
- Draining setons can be converted to cutting-setons to save another surgery in many situations.
- Surgeons reroute fistula tract and use setons as external sphincter saving, definite treatment for fistula in ano.
- Chemical setons like "Ksharsootra" is being used in India by Auyrvedic surgeons since ages and allopathic surgeons recently for various situation with good results.
- To decrease time of healing and make it less painful, recently a novel method to intercept fistula tract by application of "ksharsootra" has been described (IFTAK).
- Cutting seton is also not bad if used judiciously especially taking care on speed of cutting by decreasing the frequency of tightening it, as incontinence rates are inversely proportional to duration of cutting.
- Long duration for healing and pain experienced while changing "ksharsootra" or tightening a seton are limitations of the procedure as of today.

Supplementary Information The online version contains supplementary material available at https://doi.org/10.1007/978-981-96-6190-9_17. The videos can be accessed individually by clicking the DOI link in the accompanying figure caption or by scanning this link with the SN More Media App.

S. K. Singla, K. Mital, *Operative Manual of Minimally Invasive and LASER Ano-proctology*,
https://doi.org/10.1007/978-981-96-6190-9_17

17.1 What One Should Know Before the Procedure

- When intent is to drain the suppuration, seton is tied loose around the musculature and skin. In such situation, seton is called as draining seton.
- Materials like vascular loops, rolled rubber of surgical gloves, prolene, nylon, silk sutures or "Kshar-sootra" when tied loose can be used as draining seton.
- For any material to cut, seton is tied tight to encircled muscle after incising skin and anoderm. Due to ischemia and crushing effect, cutting setons are painful initially till they become loose.
- All above material used as loose setons can be tightened at intervals to make them cutting. Malleable stainless steel wires have also been used as cutting setons.
- For seton to be tied, internal and external openings should be identified accurately and one should be able to probe whole of the tract.
- Knowledge of anatomical route taken by fistula tract is must before one uses seton otherwise one may make life of the patient more difficult (Fig. 17.1).

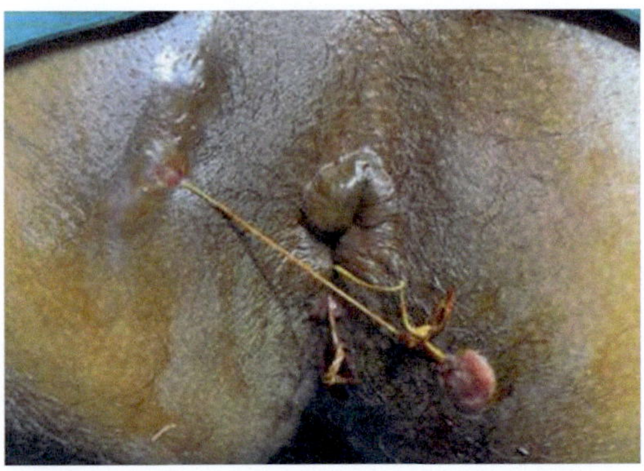

Fig. 17.1 Ignorance about anatomy of fistula tracts led an indigenous physician to create a challenging situation to manage

17.2 Indications

- Peri-anal abscess with fistula.
- Trans-sphincteric, horse-shoe fistulae.
- Inter-sphincteric fistula are better managed by intra-anal fistulotomy or fistulectomy by coring the tract from inside.

17.3 Contraindications

- Extra-sphincteric and supra-sphincteric fistulae.

17.4 Equipment

- Routine trolley for fistula surgery.

Additional equipment required is as follows:

- Fistula probes with hook at the tip (Fig. 17.2)
- Park's speculum (Fig. 17.3).
- Vaginal speculums various size lighted (Fig. 17.3).
- Curettes or Volkman's scoupe.

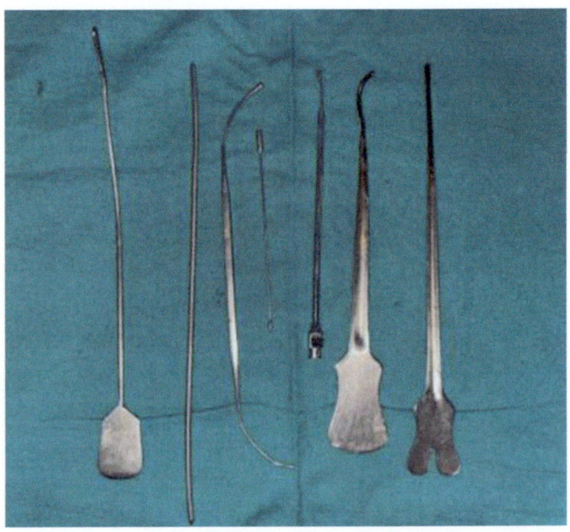

Fig. 17.2 Fistula probes and irrigation needle

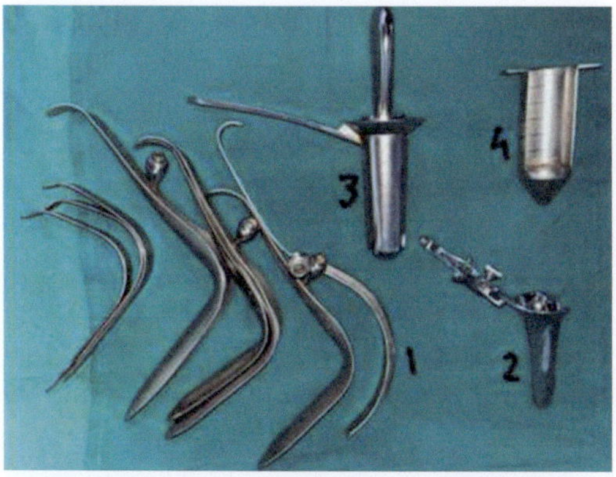

Fig. 17.3 (1) Vaginal speculum lighted various size. (2) Park speculum. (3) Proctoscope. (4) Half split speculum

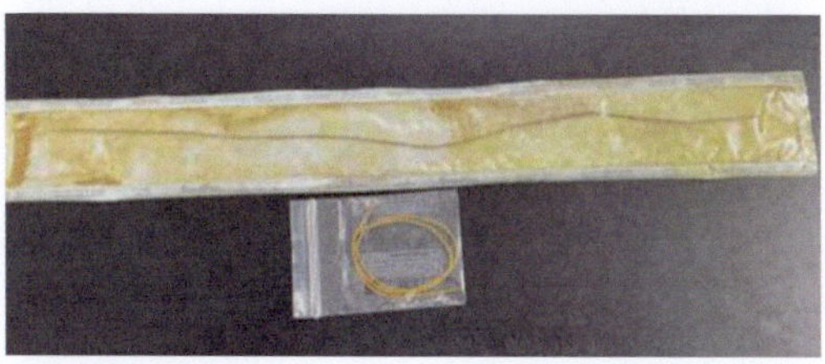

Fig. 17.4 Ksharsootra

- Electrocautery and monopolar pencil and bipolar coagulator.
- Seton to be used, one of the authors (S.K.S.) uses "Ksharsootra" both as drainage seton and cutting seton (Fig. 17.4).
- Polyglactin sutures 2.0 on round body needle.

17.5 Position of the Patient

Lithotomy.

17.6 Anaesthesia

Spinal or general anaesthesia (GA) for any specific requirement by anaesthetist.

17.7 Procedure

- Inspection and palpation of the anal verge and perianal area for external opening and tract route.
- Digital rectal examination (DRE) for palpation of inner part of the tract.
- Ano-proctoscopy and anal speculum examination after putting very diluted methylene blue with help of infant feeding tube (IFT) in external opening.
- Tip of IFT is cut bevelled beyond the side openings for the purpose.
- Identify the internal opening after injecting very diluted dye, at times aided by few drops of hydrogen peroxide mixed in dye.
- We mark the internal opening with the stroke of monopolar pencil.
- Try to negotiate fistula from external opening to internal opening with a malleable fistula probe gently, avoiding any force to prevent formation of any false passage.
- Pass the probe tip beyond the internal opening, assistant takes loop of Ksharsootra near the tip of the hook on the probe, keeping one end of thread in his hand. Surgeon hooks the thread and pulls other end back through the tract. Double-knot is applied loose over the muscle and skin.
- One can use simple probe with eye at the lower end and pass the seton by negotiating whole probe through the internal opening. At times, this becomes difficult and causes more damage to the area.
- At times dye does not show up at the internal opening as it is closed due to debris and is very narrow. Navigate the probe gently up to beneath the mucosa and excise some segment of fistula up to probe under vision and then pass the seton and ligate it.
- In case of pus coming from internal opening and no external opening, one can reverse probe the

internal opening and open the inter-sphincteric space over the probe (Figs. 17.5 and 17.6).

- One of the authors (S.K.S.) frequently ties "ksharsootra" loose around the muscle after drainage of the abscess as in case of perianal abscess with fistula. It helps to mark the fistula as well as drains the cavity (Fig. 17.7).
- Extra length of "ksharsootra" which is coated with 'kshar' (herb alkaloids) is put in the abscess cavity which helps to chemically treat the infected granulation and is anti bacterial in nature. Alkaline effect of Kshar is buffered in 24 h [2].
- After fifteen days, loose seton is changed by new ksharsootra and is snuggly tied around the muscle. Ksharsootra is changed every fortnight till it comes out through the muscle. Usually, it takes three to four changes.
- Do not be in a hurry, slow cutting without crushing is associated with very less pain and preserves the sphincter tone.
- Always incise the skin and anoderm when "Ksharsootra" or any seton is tied snuggly over the muscle with cutting intent. Pain happens due to crushing effect, try to minimise it. Ten to fifteen days later when infected fluid discharge stops, tighten the seton around sphincter complex, converting it in to cutting seton.
- Tissue cut proximally by seton heals in the meantime and this way patient is saved from second surgery for trans-sphincteric fistula, with very low recurrence and almost no incontinence (Figs. 17.8 and 17.9).
- Our only indication for Ayurvedic medicated seton used as cutting seton is when there is associated abscess with trans-sphincteric extension.

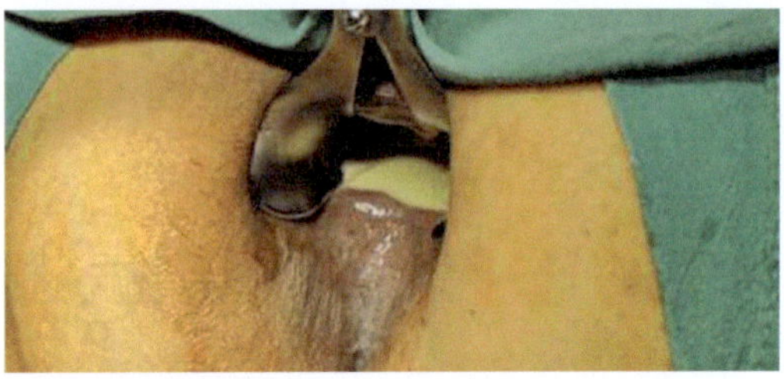

Fig. 17.5 Pus from deep inter-sphincteric space abscess, flowing on opening of parks speculum

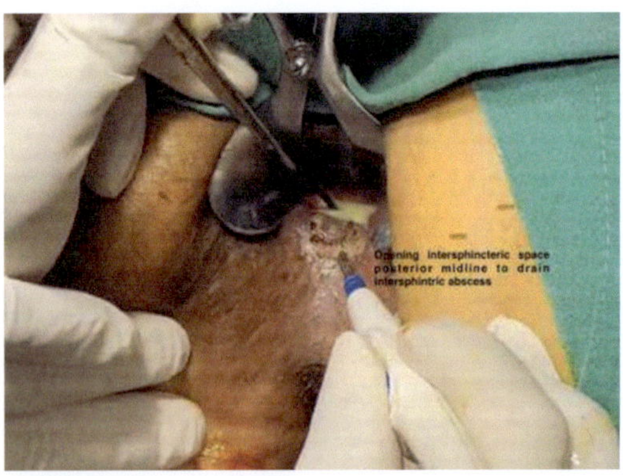

Fig. 17.6 Reverse probe in internal opening at dentate line and opening of inter-sphincteric space on tip of the probe

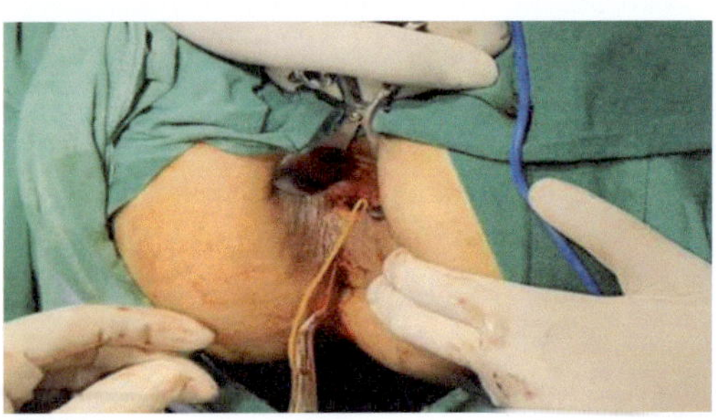

Fig. 17.7 Passing seton to drain the posterior trans-sphincteric extension of the abscess

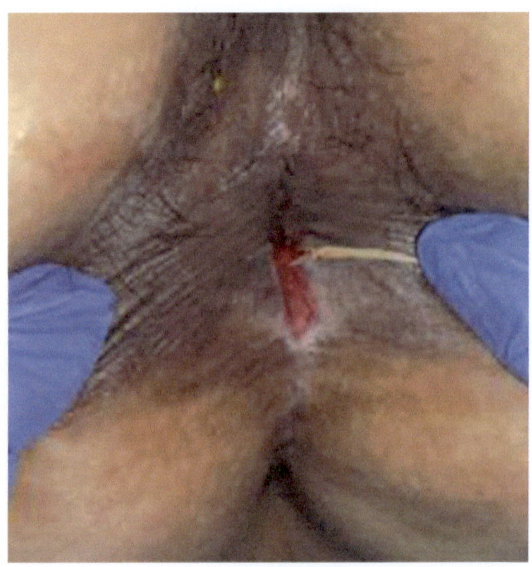

Fig. 17.8 Chemical seton (ksharsootra) tightened to act as cutting seton and changed fortnightly. After 6 weeks seton very near to cut through the muscle which healed along

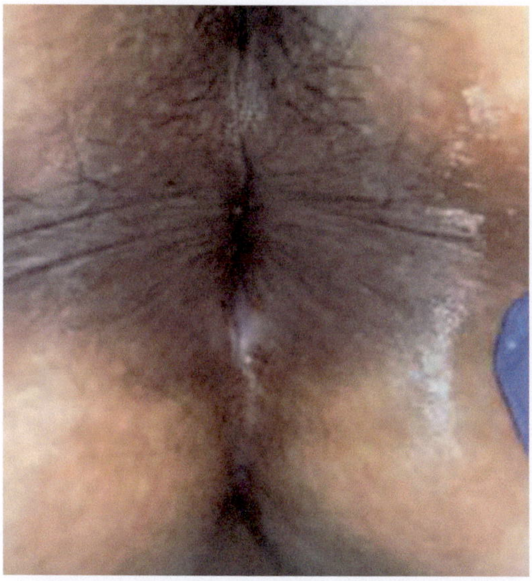

Fig. 17.9 Same patient as in Fig. 17.8 at 2 months—postop

- Marsupialise the wound margins by biodegradable sutures to avoid premature closure and facilitate complete drainage of pus and fluid. Chemical on the thread usually degrades these sutures early.

17.8 Staged Fistulotomy

- All steps of putting a seton are same as described earlier except that after initial drainage when seton comes down and amount of encircled left out external sphincter is very less. Surgeon ensures that cutting of the rest of muscle in one go will not affect the continence. To speed up the process, remaining tissue is cut in one go [3].

17.9 Interception of Fistula Track by Application of "Ksharsootra" [4]

17.9.1 Indication

- Main advantage in cases where the tract is taking curvilinear path and internal opening is either in posterior midline or anterior midline.
- Horse-shoe extensions.

17.9.2 Contraindications

- Simple straight short fistulas can be treated effectively by alternate techniques.

17.9.3 Anaesthesia

- Regional or general, at times local block.

17.9.4 Position

- Lithotomy.
- Extended lithotomy position helps in exploration of the tract in posterior midline.

17.9.5 Procedure (Video 17.1)

- The course of the fistulous track and position of internal opening is assessed by Digital rectal examination (DRE) (Fig. 17.10) and imaging (Fig. 17.11).
- Injecting methylene blue or diluted dye mixed with a few drops of hydrogen peroxide into

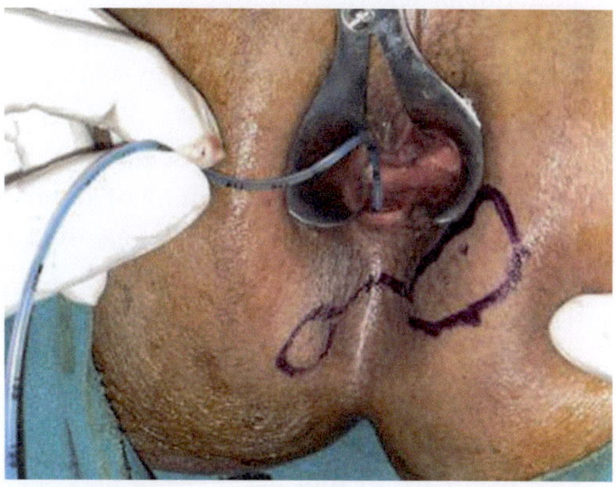

Fig. 17.10 DRE internal opening in midline posterior, horse-shoe-shaped indurations posteriorly as marked

Fig. 17.11 MRI scan (**a**) and (**b**) coronal section, (**d**) sagittal section showing deep post anal tract with collection, (**c**) axial section shows midline opening at 6 0' position and anal canal pushed to right

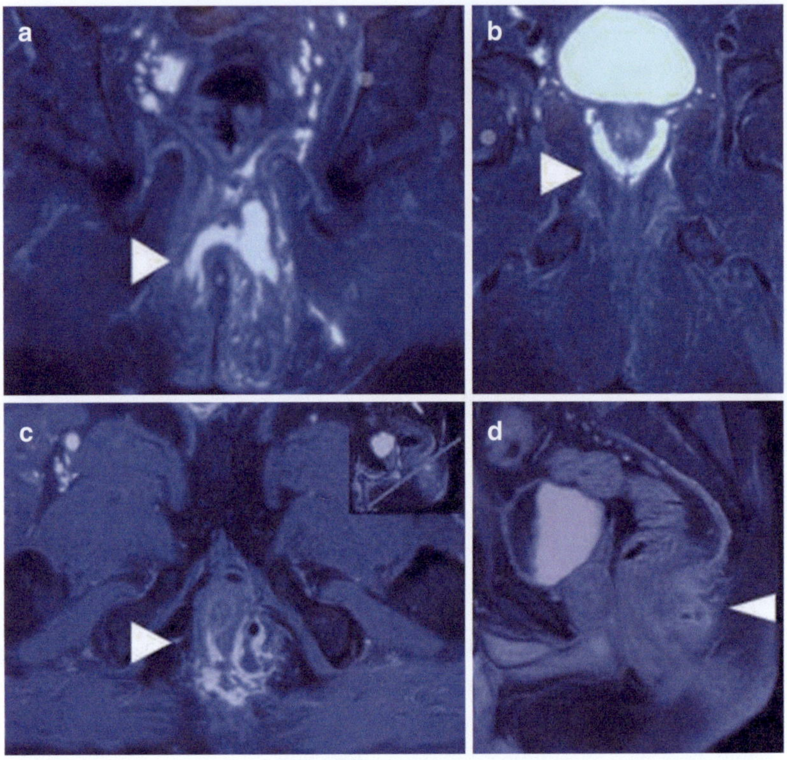

external opening of the fistulous track and checking its egress from internal opening. In present case, as there was no external opening, dye injected in internal opening led to filling of spaces around the anal canal as marked (Fig. 17.10).

- Malleable silver probe can be negotiated gently in curvilinear tracts.
- According to the position of internal opening, posterior or anterior midline, a vertical incision 1–1.5 cm is given either posterior or anterior midline almost 2 cm away from anal verge (Fig. 17.12).
- Be gentle and take care of haemostasis by injecting diluted 1.200000 solution of adrenaline before the incision and judicious use of electrocoagulation.
- The underlying tissue, muscle fibres are separated by using a pair of mosquito artery forceps at the level of the external sphincter until the fistulous track is identified.
- One may have to split the fibres of anococcygeal ligament if the tract or part of collection is in deep postanal space (Fig. 17.12).

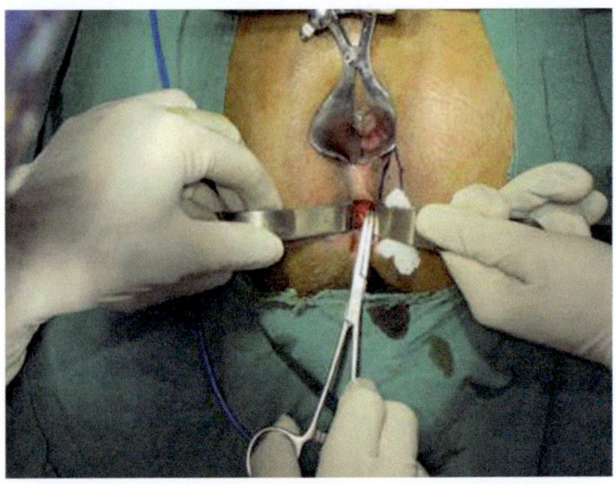

Fig. 17.12 Case of internal opening in posterior midline, vertical incision 2 cm away from anal verge to intercept fistula tract by meticulous splitting of subcutaneous tissue and fibres of anococcygeal ligament in present case

- Fistulous tracks with their whitish, shiny, cord-like character are identified after proper dissection.
- At times in cases of blind fistulas or high trans-sphincteric tracks, guidance by the index finger of the opposite hand placed in the anal

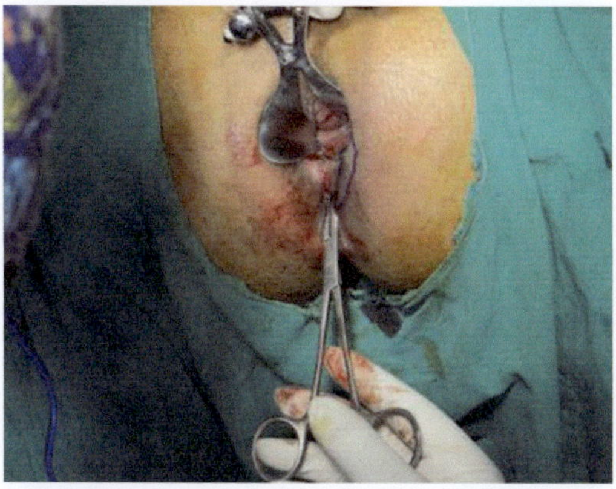

Fig. 17.13 Gap is created in the tract by scissors or blade and proximal tract negotiated with Lahey's forceps up to internal opening at dentate line

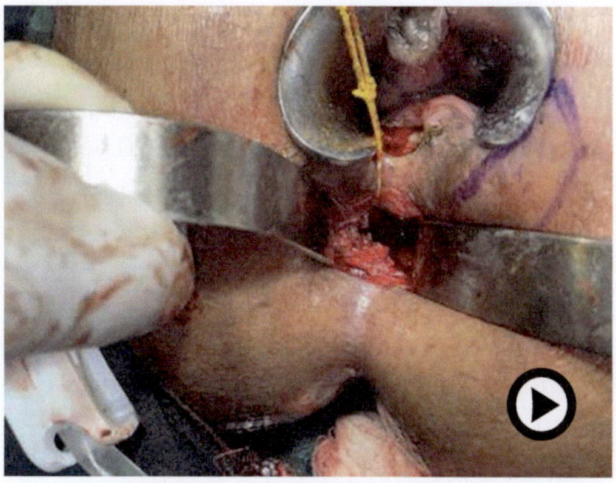

Fig. 17.14 Ksharsootra in the proximal tract and opened deep post-anal space after separating fibres of anococcygeal ligament in posterior midline. Video 17.1 IFTAK (▶ https://doi.org/10.1007/000-hqb)

canal or a malleable probe reverse passed from inside into the fistulous track can help in location of the tract.

- Once the track is identified, it is opened by fine scissors or blade creating a gap between proximal and distal tract.
- Proximal tract is negotiated through the gap, with curved Lahey's forceps (Fig. 17.13) or malleable blunt-tipped silver probe with a notch at the tip (like a cobbler's needle) up to the internal opening at the dentate line and "ksharsootra" is passed and kept loose (Fig. 17.14).
- Gap is widened by using a pair of artery forceps to provide adequate drainage to the primary track as well as to the secondary extensions or abscesses located in adjacent anatomical spaces (Fig. 17.15).
- The distal part of the fistulous track is curetted and biopsy is taken for histopathology. If it harbours an abscess, then tails of ksharsootra are packed into the cavity.
- The wound is dressed with a sterile pad.
- With high rates of success (96%), relatively low recurrence (3–7%) in two years, follow-up by inventor of the technique and practically negligible chances of complications like incontinence, IFTAK can be opted as the treatment of choice for the management of complex and recurrent fistulae. Simultaneous use of transrectal ultrasonography while performing IFTAK can further add to the accuracy of treatment and its higher success [4].
- It can be concluded that the success in the management of fistula in ano mainly depends upon the correct identification of the site of cryptoglandular infection and its prompt eradication rather than dealing with the track or the branches and this is the main principle behind the IFTAK therapy [4].

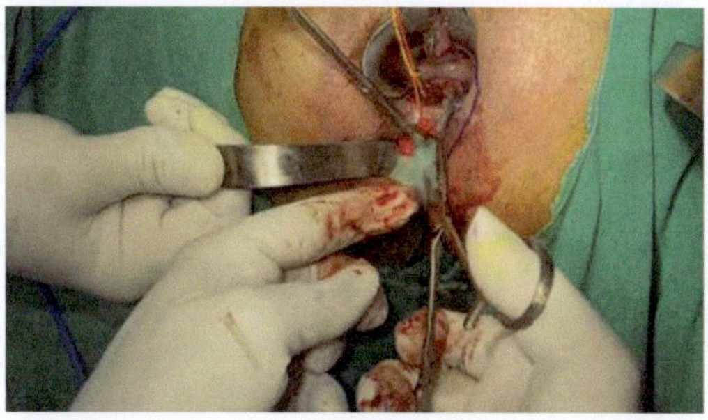

Fig. 17.15 Gap widened in intercepted tract in deep post anal space led to free drainage of pus mixed with dye

17.10 Post-operative Care

- Pain management by oral or injectable nonsteroid anti-inflammatory drugs (NSAIDs).
- Observation for immediate post-operative bleeding.
- In case of associated abscess or cellulitis, we advocate ofloxacin and metronidazole for 5 days.
- Advice to take sitz bath with lukewarm water (40–45 °C) twice daily to keep the wound clean.
- A bowel softener like psyllium husk or lactulose is suggested for smooth bowel movements.
- The patients are advised to visit the outdoor clinic at weekly intervals to assess the patency of the window (site of interception) and the condition of the external opening for any discharge.
- Khasharsootra is changed fortnightly that means on alternate visits.

17.11 Complications (Table 17.1)

Table 17.1 Complications of seton management

Complications	Prevention	Management
Pain	Do not tie the sutures very tight, avoid crushing the tissue. One can replace the seton under local block	NSAIDs
Long duration of treatment	Slow cutting helps to preserve the continence better. Its limitation of the good procedure	
Scarring	While using cutting setons always incise skin and anoderm before tying seton around the muscle	
Incontinence	Incontinence rate is inversely proportional to duration between seton tightening or replacement. More duration less incontinence	Usually it is minor incontinence. Kegel's exercise should be advised
Excessive chemical necrosis	Take Ksharsootra from authentic place or make your own. Remove extra kshara from seton	Wash with good amount of saline or replace with non medicated seton
In case of IFTAK, inadequate drainage due to narrowing of the opening at the site of interception	One can ask the patient to slightly pull the seton periodically	Periodical widening of the intercepted site is required to facilitate proper drainage

17.12 Rerouting of Setons [5]

17.12.1 What One Should Know Before the Procedure

Concept is again to persistently drain intersphincteric space till healing occurs and avoid cutting EAS.

One can reroute seton in two ways:

1. Reroute seton around EAS, spare the internal sphincter and close the internal opening by mucosal advancement flap. Once healing is achieved then remove seton around EAS without allowing it to cut through EAS (Fig. 17.16).
2. Reroute seton around internal sphincter and spare the external sphincter (Fig. 17.17).

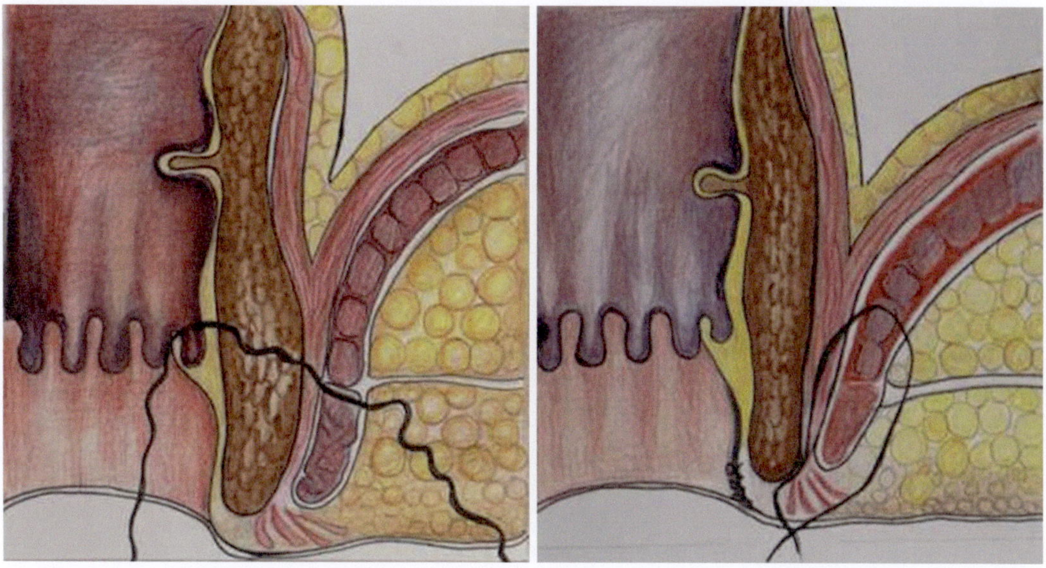

Fig. 17.16 Draining seton rerouted around external sphincter and internal opening closed by mucosal advancement flap

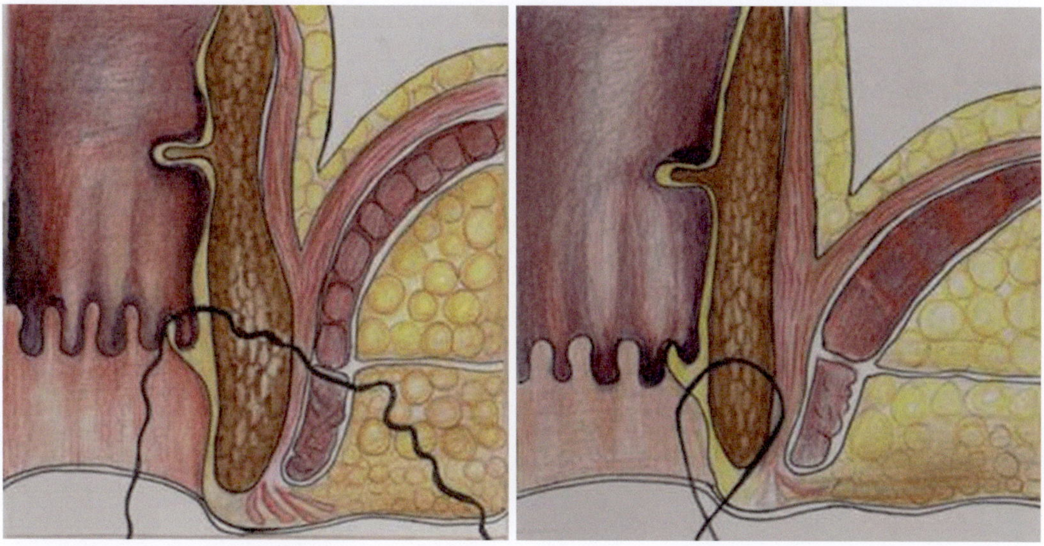

Fig. 17.17 Rerouting seton around IAS

17.12.2 Indications

- High trans-sphincteric fistula
- Rerouting around EAS with mucosal advancement can be done in all cases where endorectal advancement flap (ERAF) can be done.
- We are aware of a surgeon at Sir Ganga Ram Hospital, New Delhi, India, Dr Tarun Mittal who combines VAAFT with rerouting seton around IAS.

17.12.3 Contraindications

- As such no contraindication but simple fistulae are usually treated with other effective and easy ways of treatment.

17.13 Rerouting Around External Sphincter

17.13.1 Pre-operative Assessment

- History
- Clinical examination for anatomy of fistula tracts
- Sphincter tone analysis—resting tone and squeeze pressure and objective incontinence scoring.
- MRI for detailed anatomy and associated abscess.

17.13.2 Equipment

- Routine trolley for fistula surgery.

Additional:

- Park's speculum.
- Vaginal speculums, various size lighted.
- Curettes or Volkmann's scoupe.
- Electrocautery and monopolar pencil and bipolar coagulator.
- Fistula probes.
- Seton to be used, in a published report the author used silk.
- Polyglactin sutures 3.0 on round body-needle for suturing advancement flap.

17.13.3 Anaesthesia

- Spinal.

17.13.4 Position

- Lithotomy.

17.13.5 Procedure

- We usually give combination of ofloxacin and metronidazole as prophylactic antibacterial in all our anorectal cases.
- Identification of internal opening by injecting very diluted methylene blue with few drops of hydrogen peroxide mixed in it.
- Mark the internal opening by stroke of monopolar pencil.
- Negotiate a malleable fistula probe gently from external opening till tip comes out of internal opening.
- Skin between external opening and external anal sphincter (EAS) is incised with monopolar pencil. Extra sphincteric extensions in ischiorectal fossa are laid open and curetted well.
- Silk suture 1.0 is passed as seton.
- Inter-sphincteric plane is opened by electrocautery.
- Seton is rerouted to tie the EAS loosely and sparing the IAS.
- Internal opening is excised by taking 5 mm margins.
- Mucosal advancement flap is created without taking any internal sphincter fibres.
- Internal opening is covered by the flap by polyglactin 3.0 sutures without any tension.

17.13.6 Post-operative Case

- Stool softeners like lactulose for 4 weeks.
- Patient advised to avoid squatting.
- Ofloxacin and metronidazole for 5 days.
- No DRE examination before 4 weeks.
- Examination with the help of small vaginal speculum to ensure healing of flap is done at four weeks.
- Loose seton around EAS snipped off with scissors without cutting any fibres of EAS.

17.14 Rerouting Seton Around Internal Anal Sphincter (IAS)

- All steps are same as in previous procedure till the creation of inter-sphincteric space.
- Seton is rerouted around IAS and was tied tightly around the IAS, sparing the EAS (Fig. 17.17). The seton was kept in place until it fell spontaneously after cutting through the IAS fibres.

17.14.1 Post-operative Care

- Stool softeners.
- Pain relief by NSAIDs.
- Examination every week till silk sutures falls.
- Patients are examined every month for any early failure.
- Objective incontinence scoring is done.

According to the published literature, the drained mucosal flap technique was associated with significantly lower incidence of faecal incontinence, yet longer operative time and longer time to complete healing compared to rerouting seton around the IAS. The success rate of both techniques was comparable [5].

17.15 Tips and Tricks

- Before applying any seton with cutting intent always incise anoderm and skin. Apply seton around musculature only.
- Tighten cutting seton at increased interval to allow cutting at a slow speed to maintain continence.
- In IFTAK periodical widening of the intercepted site is required to facilitate proper drainage.

Algorithm

Seton Management

History, clinical examination

Imaging MRI endo US

On table define internal opening, tract and external opening

Pass malleable probe from external opening up to internal opening

Put seton in the tract and tie loose around the skin and muscle

In case one wants to change it into cutting seton

Incise skin and anoderm and tie seton only around musculature

Periodic tightening or replacement of the seton every 15 days

For Staged Fistulotomy

After periodic tightening when seton comes down and amount of uncut sphincter is small enough to cause any incontinence, if cut in one go

Left out muscle is cut to decrease the duration of treatment

For IFTAK

Define the tract after clinical examination and MRI or endo US

For complex fistulae in ano especially curvilinear tracts opening anterior mid line or in posterior midline

Give 2 cm vertical incision in posterior or anterior mid line as per fistula presentation

Dissect subcutaneous tissue and muscle fibres to locate the fistula by its white shining cord-like appearance

Give a cut on tract with a pair of scissors or blade, widen the opening and pass fis-

(continued)

tula probe with a hook at the tip like cobblers needle or Lahey's forceps from created window

Pass probe up to internal opening at dentate line, hold ksharsootra in the tip of hook or in Lahey's forceps and bring it out from external wound created to intercept the fistula

Incise the anoderm and skin over the sphincter muscle and tie ksharsootra snuggly fit on the muscle

Wide open the side tracts from the window

Curette the secondary tracts and leave them to heal by themselves

Then continue to drain the intercepted track and tighten the seton periodically every fortnight to cut and heal the sphincter gradually and simultaneously

For Rerouting Around EAS/Mucosal Advancement Drained Flap

Best suited for high transphincteric fistula define the tract by dilute methylene blue

Probe the tract, incise skin and tract in ischiorectal fossa

Pass the seton like silk thread

Open intersphincteric space

Reroute the seton only around EAS and tie it loose

Leave the IAS spared medially

Raise anal mucosal flap meticulously in area of IO

Debride the opening in IAS and cover it with flap

Once complete healing of flap is ensured in 4 weeks, snip off the seton around EAS

Rerouting Around IAS

Steps same as of rerouting around EAS, till openings of intersphincteric space

Now reroute the seton around internal anal sphincter and spare the EAS laterally

Snuggly tighten the silk seton around IAS just curette the lateral tract

Let this thread drain the intersphincteric space and fall off its own

References

1. Gold SL, Cohen-Mekelburg S, Schneider Y, Steinlauf A. Perianal fistulas in patients with Crohn's Disease, Part 2: Surgical, endoscopic, and future therapies. Gastroenterol Hepatol (N Y). 2018;14(9):521–8.
2. ICMR Collaborating Centers, Central Bio-statistical Monitoring Unit, Madras. Multicentric randomized clinical trial of Kshara Sutra (Ayurvedic Medicated thread), in the management of fistula-in ano. Indian J Med Res (B). 1991;94:77–185.
3. Ho KS, Tsang C, Seow-Choen F, Ho YH, Tang CL, Heah SM, Eu KW. Prospective randomised trial comparing ayurvedic cutting seton and fistulotomy for low fistula-in-ano. Tech Coloproctol. 2001;5(3):137–41. https://doi.org/10.1007/s101510100015.
4. Management of Complex Fistula-in-ano by Interception of Fistula Track with Application of Ksharasutra (IFTAK). A novel technique Manoranjan Sahu1 Ashish Sharma1. J Coloproctol. 2022;42(4):2793285.
5. Abdelnaby M, Emile S, El-Said M, Abdallah E, AbdelMawla A. Drained mucosal advancement flap versus rerouting Seton around the internal anal sphincter in treatment of high trans-sphincteric anal fistula: a randomized trial. Int J Surg. 2019;72:198–203. https://doi.org/10.1016/j.ijsu.2019.11.008. ISSN:1743-9191. https://www.sciencedirect.com/science/articlepiiS1743-9191

Suggested Reading

Balciscueta Z, Uribe N, Balciscueta I, Andreu-Ballester JC, García-Granero E. Rectal advancement fiap for the treatment of complex cryptoglandular anal fistulas: a systematic review and meta-analysis. Int J Colorectal Dis. 2017;32(5):599–609. https://doi.org/10.1007/s00384-017-2779-7.

Burney, Richard E. Invited commentary on "Drained mucosal advancement flap versus rerouting seton". Int J Surg. 2020;73:25. https://doi.org/10.1016/j.ijsu.2019.11.028.

Freeman C, Martin ST, et al. The role of loose seton in the management of anal fistula: a multicenter study of 200 patients. Tech Coloproctol. 2014;18(10):9153919.

Kelly ME, Heneghan HM, McDermott FD, et al. The role of loose seton in the management of anal fistula: a multicenter study of 200 patients. Tech Coloproctol. 2014;18:9153919. https://doi.org/10.1007/s10151-014-1186-0.

Kristo I, Stift A, Staud C, Kainz A, Bachleitner-Hofmann T, Chitsabesan P, Riss S. The type of loose seton for complex anal fistula is essential to improve perianal comfort and quality of life. Colorectal Dis. 2016;18(6):O194–8. https://doi.org/10.1111/codi.13335.

Omar W, Alqasaby A, Abdelnaby M, Youssef M, Shalaby M, Anwar Abdel-Razik M, Emile SH. Drainage seton versus external anal sphincter-sparing seton after rerouting of the fistula tract in the treatment of complex anal fistula: a randomized controlled trial. Dis Colon Rectum. 2019;62(8):980–7. https://doi.org/10.1097/DCR.0000000000001416.

Rosen DR, Kaiser AM. Definitive seton management for transsphincteric fistula-in-ano: harm or charm? Colorectal Dis. 2016;18(5):488–95. https://doi.org/10.1111/codi.13120.

Sahu M, Sharma A. Management of complex fistula-in-ano by Interception of Fistula Track with Application of Ksharasutra (IFTAK): a novel technique. J Coloproctol. 2022;42(4):2793285.

Schrader L, Brandstrup B, Olaison G. Slowly cutting, loose seton ligature and staged fistulotomy for healing of idiopathic perianal fistula and infiuence on anal continence. Langenbecks Arch Surg. 2023;408(1):352. https://doi.org/10.1007/s00423-023-03005-0.

Subhas G, Gupta A, Balaraman S, Mittal VK, Pearlman R. Non-cutting setons for progressive migration of complex fistula tracts: a new spin on an old technique. Int J Colorectal Dis. 2011;26:793–8. https://doi.org/10.1007/s00384-011-1189-5.

Sungurtekin U, Ozban M, Erbis H, Birsen O. Loose seton: a misnomer of cutting seton. Surg Sci. 2016;7(2193):225. https://doi.org/10.4236/ss.2016.75030.

Zbar AP, Ramesh J, Beer-Gabel M, Salazar R, Pescatori M. Conventional cutting vs. internal anal sphincter-preserving seton for high trans-sphincteric fistula: a prospective randomized manometric and clinical trial. Tech Coloproctol. 2003;7(2):89–94. https://doi.org/10.1007/s10151-003-0016-6.

18 New Concepts in Minimally Invasive Approach for Fistula in Ano and Futuristic Approach

Abstract

- Key questions faced by surgeons and investigators in anal fistula management like understanding spread of sepsis, assessment and imaging are addressed.
- Importance of two deep posterior anal spaces in posterior horse-shoe fistulas has been explained with sketches and evidence.
- Based on enhanced understanding of magnetic resonance imaging (MRI) and its critical role in complex fistulae, suggestions have been made on ways to do MRI, read and report MRI.
- A versatile method of management of all fistula in ano based on rule of skeletal muscle in drainage of ano rectal sepsis has been suggested.
- Do we really need to cut external sphincter to manage a small portion of fistula passing through it? We have tried to elaborate on this important question.
- To achieve the goal of eradicating all chronic sepsis in inter-muscular spaces, we stress upon dealing all components of fistula separately instead of doing fistulotomy or fistulectomy thereby decreasing morbidity without effecting success rate.
- We propose combining all available resources like VAAFT, LASER, FiXcision, coring and TROPIS to achieve desired results by minimally invasive methods without damaging external sphincter.
- These principles can be applied even in straight low fistulas, fistula-associated abscess with obvious advantages.
- Following pages clear our futuristic approach towards management and research in fistula in ano.

18.1 Understanding Pathological Anatomy of Fistula in Ano of Crypto-glandular Origin

- If perianal abscess is acute suppuration, then fistula in ano is chronic suppuration which has been drained inadequately either by nature or surgeon.
- Source of such infection is the anal gland in inter-sphincteric space.
- Persistence of this infection is the major source of fistula formation, its maintenance and reoccurrence.
- To eradicate source, this infection which is trapped in inter-sphincteric space, knowledge of anatomy of anal canal and perianal musculature is of paramount importance.

For better understanding of how one can address the problem and save the sphincter's integrity without jeopardising the continence mechanism, we propose the following way to understand anatomy.

S. K. Singla, K. Mital, *Operative Manual of Minimally Invasive and LASER Ano-proctology*,
https://doi.org/10.1007/978-981-96-6190-9_18

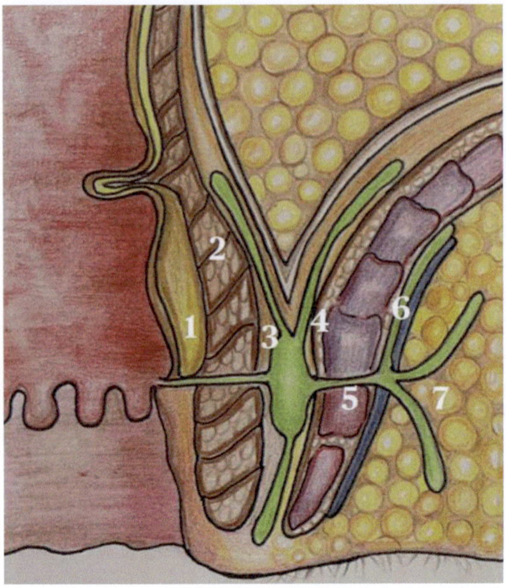

Fig. 18.1 Possible routes of spread of perianal sepsis inner to skeletal muscle 1, 2, 3, 4. Skeletal muscle 5. Outer to skeletal muscle 6, 7

- One can divide the musculature and perianal spaces around the anal canal into three components (Fig. 18.1).

18.2 Inner Component

Medial to skeletal muscle, i.e., external sphincter

- Mucosa, submucosa (Fig. 18.1 '1').
- Internal sphincter (Fig. 18.1 '2').
- Inter-sphincteric space, a plane of embryonic fusion and comprises of actually two spaces.
- Space between internal sphincter and conjoint longitudinal muscle (Fig. 18.1 '3').
- Space between conjoint longitudinal muscle and external sphincter (Fig. 18.1 '4').

Disease in this component is labelled as central disease.

18.3 Middle Component

- External anal sphincter, puborectalis and levator ani complex (all skeletal muscle) (Fig. 18.1 '5').

18.4 External Component

- Space between external sphincter levator ani complex and a fascia outside it (Fig. 18.1 '6') [1].
- Perianal and ischiorectal space up to the skin (Fig. 18.1 '7').

Important Anatomical Information Regarding Spread of Sepsis and Fistula Formation in Posterior Spaces, Specially Relevant to Understand Posterior Horse-shoe-Shaped Fistulas (Fig. 18.2)

- Posteriorly, there are two planes for circumferential spread of sepsis and formation of fistula [2].
- Deep posterior intersphincteric space (DPIS)
- Deep posterior anal extrasphincteric space (DPAS)

Seventy-five percent of the time sepsis first spreads in DPIS circumferentially and then breaches ES at two places and spreads in both ischiorectal spaces, respectively, before opening at skin level (Fig. 18.2b) [2].

Its only 25% of the time that sepsis from the gland in intersphincteric space breaches external sphincter in post-midline and then sepsis spreads in extra sphincteric space towards both right and left ischiorectal spaces (Fig. 18.2a) [2].

In anterior horse-shoe-shaped fistula there is breach in external sphincter at one place and the tract bifurcates in extra sphincteric space (Fig. 18.3).

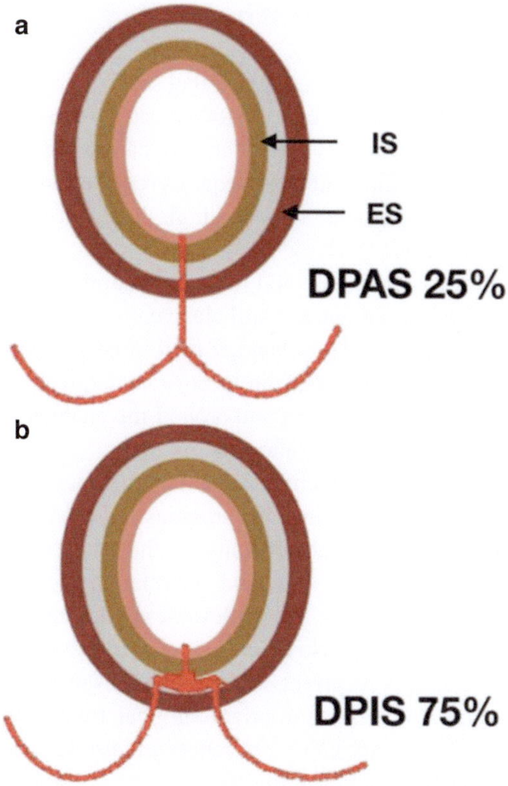

Fig. 18.2 Two deep posterior anal spaces. (**a**) Deep posterior extrasphincteric space. Breech in external sphincter (ES) in midline at one place then bilateral spread in deep post anal space to present as posterior horse-shoe-shaped fistula, 25% cases. (**b**) Deep posterior intersphincteric space. Sepsis spreads first in intersphincteric space. Breech in ES at two places to present as posterior horse-shoe fistula, 75% cases [2].

18.5 How to Assess Each Area

Assessment by Clinical Examination (Figs. 18.4, 18.5 and 18.6)

Be very gentle, with well-lubricated finger-check following:

- Internal opening may feel like depression or induration on dentate line.
- Deep inter-sphincteric supralevator extensions as induration extending cranial from dentate line.
- Spasm of perianal muscles.
- Swap finger all around for any fibrosis.

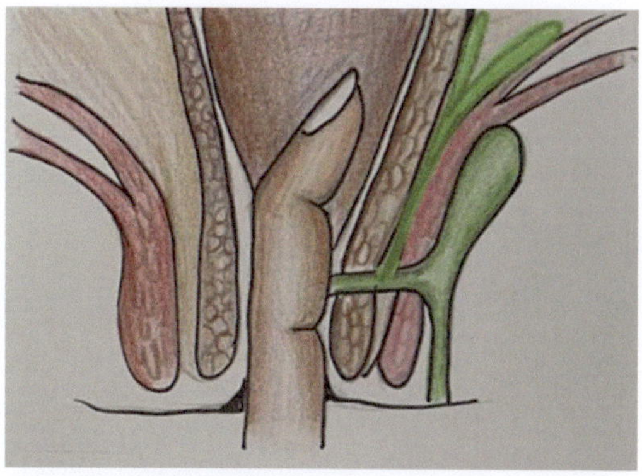

Fig. 18.4 DRE to check vertical spread of infection by feeling buldge/induration

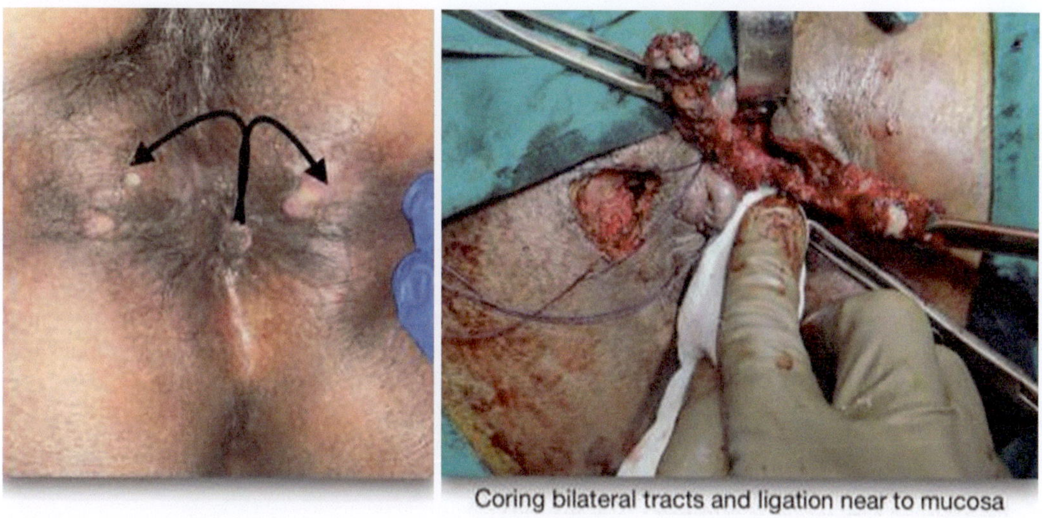

Fig. 18.3 Anterior horse-shoe fistula in a female patient, lithotomy position

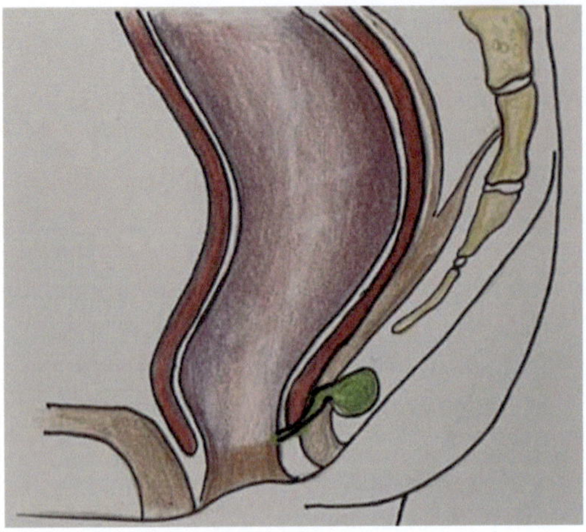

Fig. 18.5 DRE to check spread of infection in posterior deep space by feeling buldge/induration posterior midline

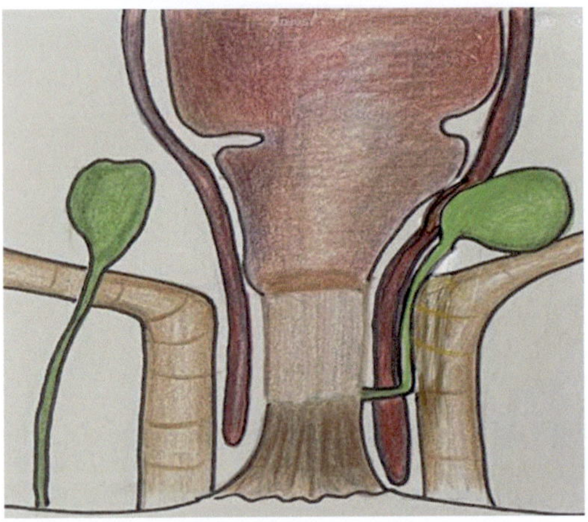

Fig. 18.6 DRE to check circumferential spread near puborectalis sling by feeling buldge/induration or fibrosis at anorectal ring

- Check for circumferential spread at the level of dentate line as well as higher up near puborectalis sling.
- Check sphincter tone.
- Palpate from external opening towards anal canal in all sectors. Low tracts can be felt as cord like structure. Feel for any abscess or cavity under skin in area of ischiorectal fossa.

18.6 Assessment by Imaging

Role of MRI in imaging perianal sepsis

Perianal sepsis in acute form as an abscess and in chronic form as fistulae in ano, causes significant morbidity and often requires repeated surgical management due to high incidence of recurrence.

Best surgical method to avoid recurrence and maintain continence is still elusive.

With resources at hand, it is of utmost importance to know about the location and spread of the fistulous tracks in and around the anal canal before going to operation room (OR).

After thorough clinical examination, magnetic resonance (MR) imaging provides more precise information on the anatomy of the anal canal, spread of fistula tract and its relation to anal sphincter complex and the levator ani muscle.

MR imaging also defines secondary fistulas or abscesses in recurrent cases. It provides required information for appropriate surgical treatment, thereby decreasing recurrence of fistula and avoiding faecal incontinence.

Radiologists familiar with the anatomic and pathologic findings of perianal sepsis should classify fistulae using the St James's University Hospital MR imaging-based grading system. As we have already mentioned in the previous chapter on relevance of classification of fistula in ano, the St James classification needs revision to make it more relevant for surgeons.

18.7 How to Take MRI to Make It More Informative

Anal canal has a forward tilt at ano-rectal angle.

Imaging planes are to be correctly aligned with respect to the anal canal.

It is suggested to take sagittal section of MRI first and then equivalent to anorectal angle or anal tilt at ano-rectal angle, take oblique axial and coronal images to get better information in one section (Fig. 18.7) [3].

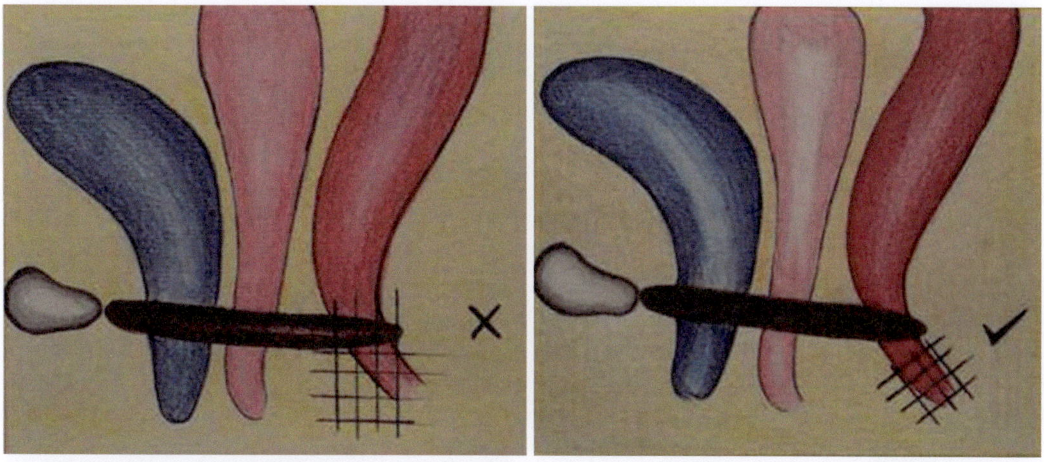

Fig. 18.7 Depicting correct grid (right side picture) to obtain oblique axial and coronal images in MRI: pubic bone (grey), pelvic hiatus (black), urinary bladder (blue), vagina (pink), anorectum (red)

Considering importance of MRI in the treatment of fistula in ano, we propose following.

18.8 Reporting Checklist MRI for Fistula in Ano

Start reporting from inside out that is as disease starts and spreads.

- Like collection or tract in intersphincteric space, breach in internal sphincter and internal opening if traceable.
- Distance from anal verge of internal opening and top of the tract.
- Then any intersphincteric spread either circumferential or vertical (along the wall of rectum in between the circular and longitudinal muscles of the rectum or supralevator).
- Level of vertical breach in external sphincter (LOVE) from anal verge signifying extent of external sphincter involvement height wise.
- Any second breach in ES circumferentially as in a case of posterior horse-shoe fistula (Fig. 18.2) [2].
- Type of fistula-sphincter involvement.
- Recently suggested—any spread between external sphincter-levator ani and their supporting fascia.

Inferolaterally, i.e., RIFIL fistula/roof of ischiorectal fossa in levator ani [1].

- Spread in ischiorectal fossa:
  - going towards the skin
  - Going superior but below levator.
  - Trans-levator extension if any.
  - Associated abscess
- Muscle oedema
- Involvement or fistulisation with any organ.
- Supralevator component.
- Recently an interdisciplinary Delphi consensus on template of anal fistulas reporting by MRI and endo-anal US (SMART) has been published [4].

18.9 A Versatile Treatment for All Fistulas Based on This Information

Either excise the whole tract in each component or drain the each component separately while saving external sphincter and minimal skin cutting to decrease the wound size and subsequently healing time without jeopardising continence mechanism.

18.10 Concept of Skeletal Muscle to Drain the Perianal Abscess

- It is an established fact that perianal abscess medial to (inner to) skeletal muscle is drained inside and perianal abscess outside or (external to) skeletal muscle is drained from outside.
- We advocate to treat fistula in ano in the same way.

18.11 Prevalent Concepts to Treat Fistula

In treatment of fistula in ano to prevent incontinence, whole stress is on the extent of external sphincter which can be cut, without causing practical effects on anal continence mechanism.

But this is also relative and depends on preoperative sphincter strength.

Do we really need to cut external sphincter to treat fistula efficiently?

Components of a given fistula can be either treated from inside the anal canal or from outside the anal canal except part of the tract passing through the external sphincter. Now the question is Can we find ways to eradicate infection in the middle component (tract through the external sphincter or levator ani) without cutting whole external sphincter below it?

Answer is "yes", why not?

Combine the already available resources.

If one knows pathological anatomy precisely, one can ablate that middle component of the tract passing through external sphincter by VAAFT, LASER, coring or FiXcision device.

FiXcision and coring-with small wound becomes technically difficult as fistula goes high, in such cases it is better to use VAAFT and endo luminal ablation of fistula lining by LASER under vision.

Then one can close the defect in ES or iliococcygeus by PDS suture.

Yes at times, though rarely application of that stitch is technically difficult in case of high trans-sphincteric or suprasphincteric fistula. One can use transanal minimal invasive surgery (TAMIS) platform in such situation.

In any case, while operating for supra sphincteric fistula, one cannot cut ES or puborectalis at any cost. One with sound knowledge of anatomy and good operative skills can manage this tricky situation by dealing all three components of fistula without cutting the external sphincter, puborectalis and levator ani (Figs. 18.8, 18.9, 18.10 and 18.11). Operated by Dr. Parvez Sheikh, Mumbai-India.

To achieve this goal by minimal access, we can core out the tracks in internal and external components and ablate the trans-sphincteric

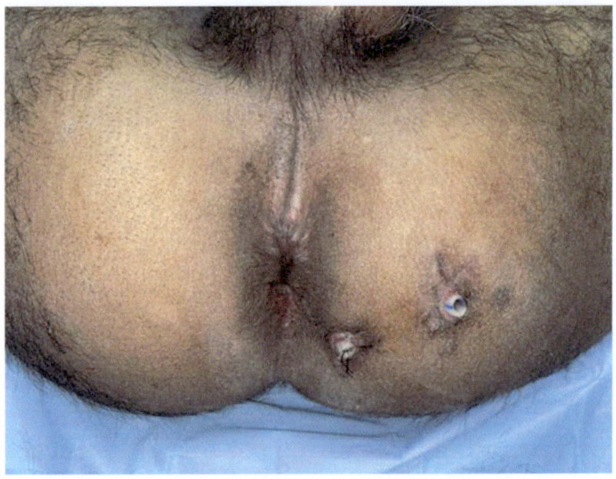

Fig. 18.8 Supralevator abscess drained through ischiorectal fossa leading to suprasphincteric fistula

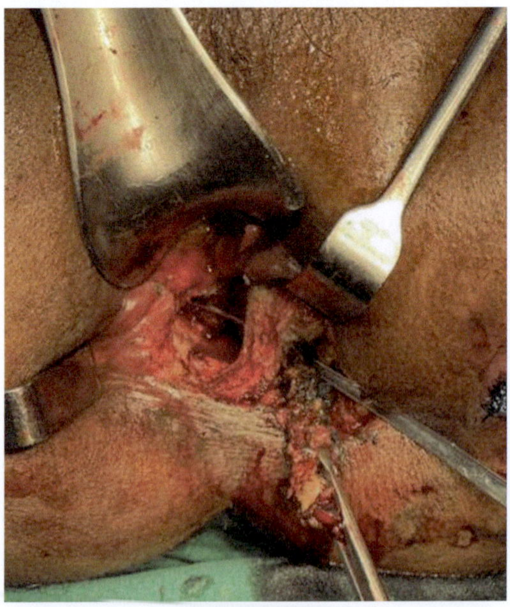

Fig. 18.9 Inner component excised and outer and middle component cored out

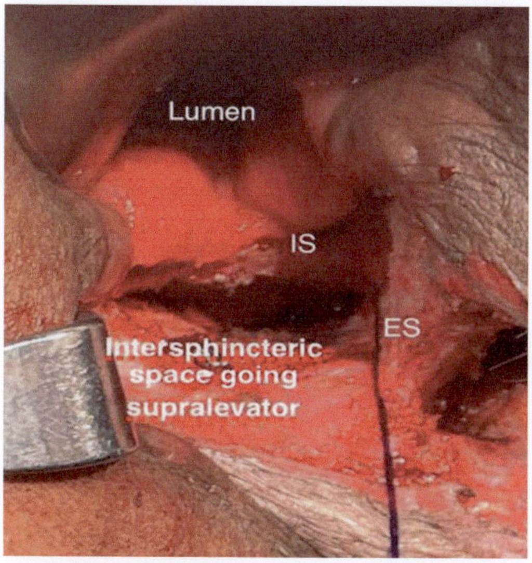

Fig. 18.10 Preserved external sphincter and puborectalis. All diseased components excised coring the part of tract through levator ani. Note transanal closure of a hole in iliococcygeus by stitch

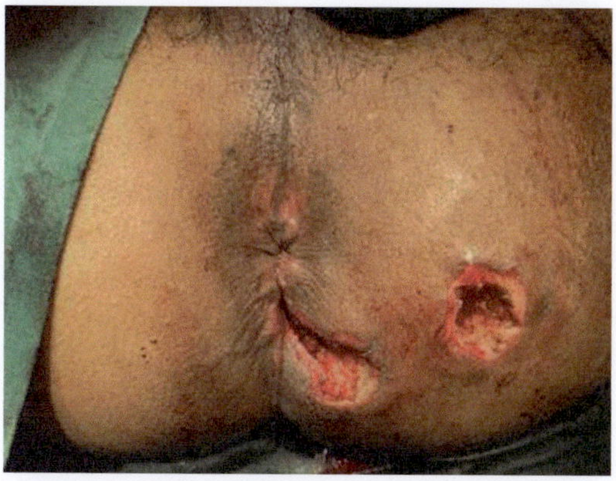

Fig. 18.11 Final picture after coring suprasphincteric tract and then applying PDS stitch to opening in levator ani, external sphincter and puborectalis preserved

component by LASER or we can do FiXcision of the middle and external components. Internal components and any extension in intersphincteric space is excised or laid open in the ano rectum (IAF or TROPIS). If external component is not a mature tract but an abscess, then better to lay it open and drain.

LIFT is good for a linear mature trans-sphincteric tract. One is to perform either excision or laying open of internal component if there is extension in inter-sphincteric space. Similarly, if there is extension in external component one is to either excise that or lay it open and drain.

18.12 What We Do in Fistulotomy

We lay open the whole tract and drain it.

Cutting both internal and external sphincter and incising the skin there by making large wounds and destroying part of external sphincter.

18.13 What We Do in Fistulectomy

We are excising the whole tract again cutting both internal and external sphincter and perianal skin covering ischiorectal fossa. We can add primary closure by suturing the sphincters.

One should never cut the anorectal ring.

One should not cut external sphincter at two different places as in case of horse-shoe extension instead it is advised to core out.

18.14 What We Are Suggesting

Core out or drain internal and external components, separately.

Middle component passing through the skeletal muscle can be ablated with LASER, VAAFT, FiXcision and/or curettage. Defect in external sphincter can be sutured with PDS.

This way excision or drainage of the whole tract and involved spaces is done with minimal trauma to the external sphincter and the skin as well.

This method cures the disease or at least decreases recurrence, maintains sphincter integrity and faecal continence. At the same time, it decreases healing time and pain.

One such procedure combining all available resources has been described in Chap. 14 of this book with the name E-PARK Tech.

These principles can be utilised in the management of low straight fistula as well as treating associated fistula in perianal abscess (Fig. 18.12, 18.13, 18.14 and 18.15).

Leaving a small bridge of the skin and even sparing few fibres of subcutaneous external sphincter, maintains shape of the anal canal, decreases pain, hastens recovery and preserves continence better. If central disease is tackled carefully, recurrence decreases automatically.

Future research on management of fistula in ano should be to refine the application of this knowledge and resources, to help patients and standardise the surgery for fistula in ano.

In this whole discussion, we have written about the perianal fistulas of crypto-glandular origin. Fistulas due to specific inflammatory diseases such as Crohn's disease, tuberculosis and diverticulitis need management of respective disease. Similarly, fistulas due to trauma, malignancy and radiation need specific management beyond the scope of the present discussion.

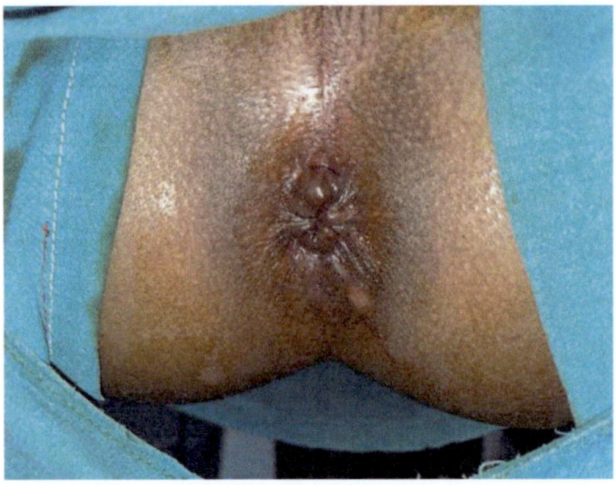

Fig. 18.12 Low straight trans-sphincteric fistula

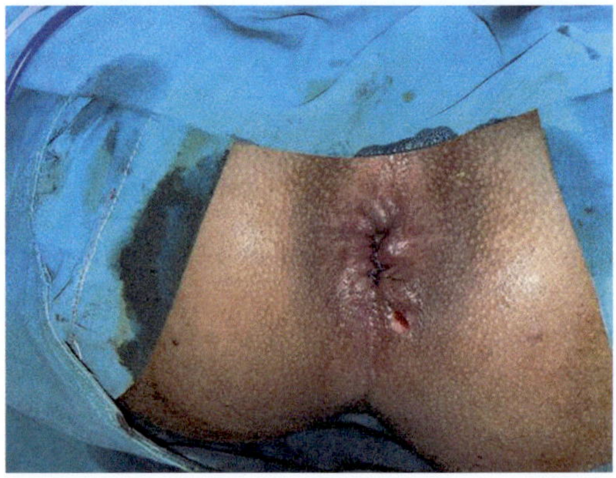

Fig. 18.13 Managed by central disease excision and coring by FiXcision device and LASER ablation and defect in ES closed with PDS. Note anal opening contour, no cutting of ES and minimal skin cutting

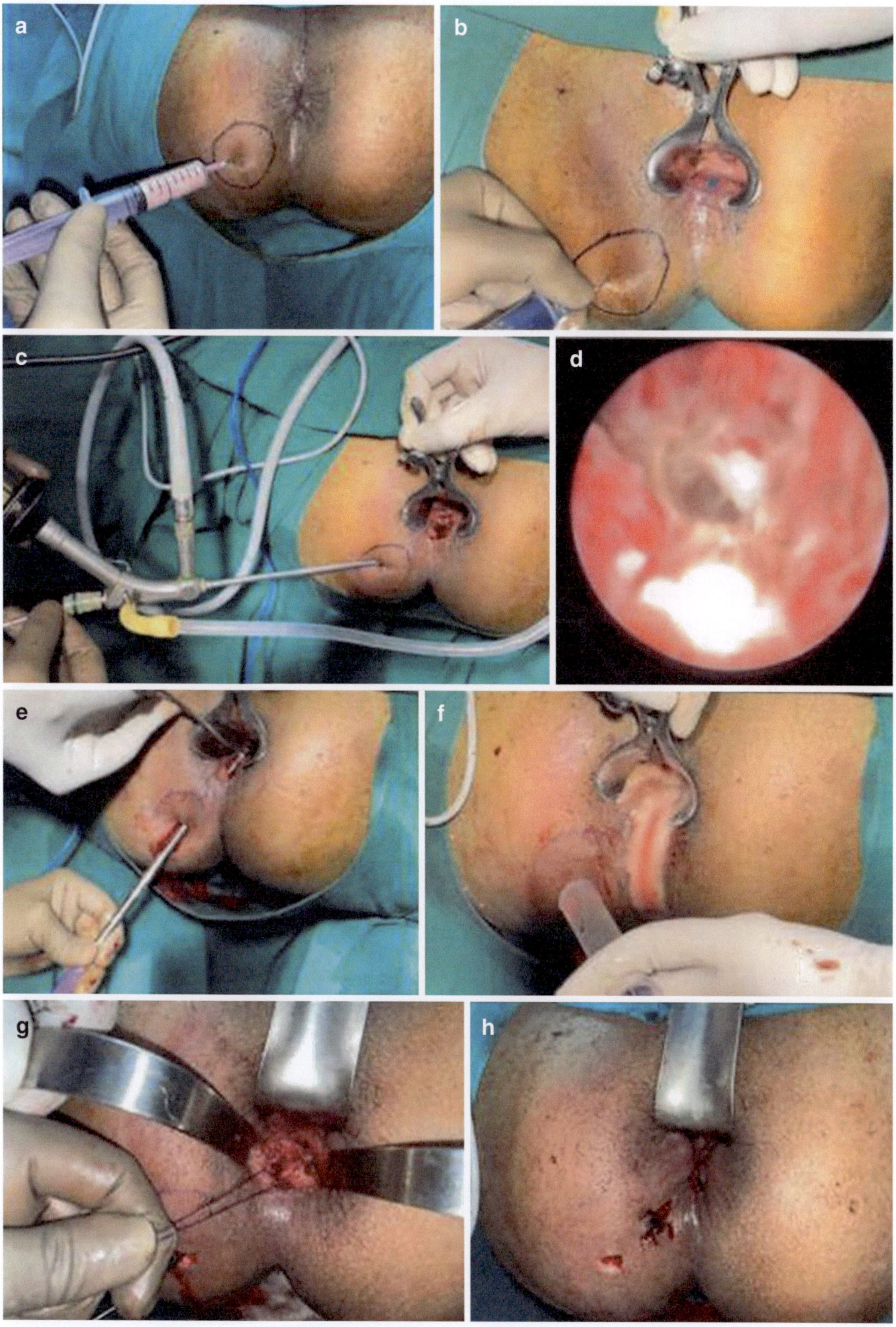

Fig. 18.14 Perianal abscess with trans-sphincteric fistula managed by E-PARK Tech. (**a**) Needle aspiration of pus. (**b**) Internal communication at dentate line. (**c**) Central disease excision and fistuloscope insertion with LASER fibre. (**d**) Internal view of abscess cavity-fulguration by LASER. (E) FiXicision. (**f**) Lavage with H_2O_2 and saline. (**g**) Closure of internal opening in external sphincter by PDS 2.0. (**h**) Drain in abscess cavity

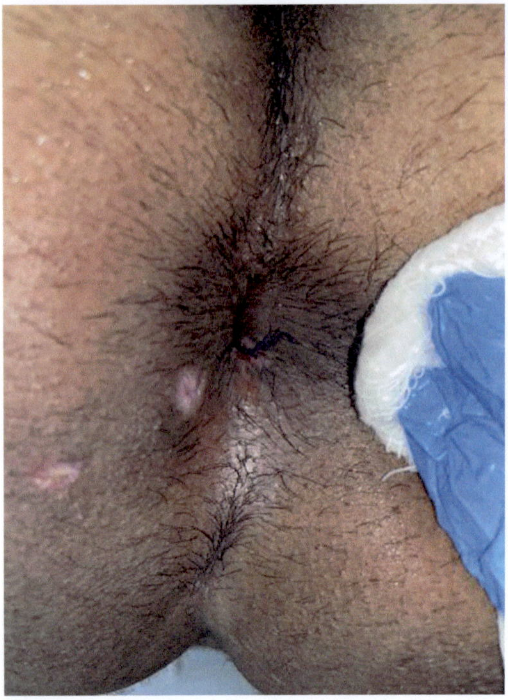

Fig. 18.15 Follow-up picture of a patient shown in Fig. 18.14, healed fistula and abscess after 2 weeks

References

1. Pankaj G, Sushil D, Yagnik VD, Baljit K, Menon GR. Anal fistula at roof of ischiorectal fossa inside levator-ani muscle (RIFIL): a new highly complex anal fistula diagnosed on MRI. Abdom Radiol NY. 2021;46(12):5550–63. https://doi.org/10.1007/s00261-021-03261-y.
2. Zhang H, Zhou ZY, Hu B, Liu DC, Peng H, Xie SK, Su D, Ren DL. Clinical significance of 2 deep posterior perianal spaces to complex cryptoglandular fistulas. Dis Colon Rectum. 2016;59(8):766–74. https://doi.org/10.1097/DCR.0000000000000628.
3. de Miguel CJ, del Salto LG, Rivas PF, del Hoyo LF, Velasco LG, De Las Vacas MI, Marco Sanz AG, Paradela MM, Moreno EF. MR imaging evaluation of perianal fistulas: spectrum of imaging features. Radiographics. 2012;32(1):175–94. https://doi.org/10.1148/rg.321115040.
4. SudoC-SzopiEska I, Garg P, Mellgren A, Spinelli A, Breukink S, Iacobellis F, KoCodziejczak M, Ciesielski P, Jenssen C, SMART Collaborative Group, Santoro GA. Structured magnetic resonance imaging and endoanal ultrasound anal fistulas reporting template (SMART): an interdisciplinary Delphi consensus. World J Gastrointest Surg. 2024;16(10):3288–300. https://doi.org/10.4240/WJGS.V16.I10.3288.

19 Sacrococcygeal Pilonidal Sinus Disease: Why Minimally Invasive Surgery in Pilonidal Sinus Disease (MIS in PNS)

Abstract

- Pilonidal sinus disease (PNS) is an acquired disease of pilosebaceous gland origin. Based on Bascom's hypothesis and the Karydakis theory, factors which initiate, propagate and maintain the disease are explained with sketches.
- From all surgical methods employed so far in the treatment of PNS, flaps have minimum recurrence but with significant wound morbidity at times.
- Traditional and modern minimally invasive methods have comparable short- and long-term outcomes without much wound morbidity. Reasons favouring minimally invasive surgery (MIS) including endoscopic surgery and use of LASER have been enumerated along with their limitations as of today.
- The need to standardise the procedure with endoscopic and LASER application is emphasised, along with the requirement of more comparative studies and robust data from different surgeons around the globe.

19.1 Introduction

- Pilonidal sinus disease (PNS) is an acquired disease of pilosebaceous gland origin, manifesting as subcutaneous infection in sacrococcygeal region, i.e., natal cleft area.
- It may manifest as an acute abscess, chronic discharging sinus in midline or laterally on gluteal areas, non-healing midline ulcer or an indolent ulcer after excision of the disease.
- There is no definitive research-based evidence of its aetiology.

If we believe in Bascom's hypothesis (Fig. 19.1) [1].

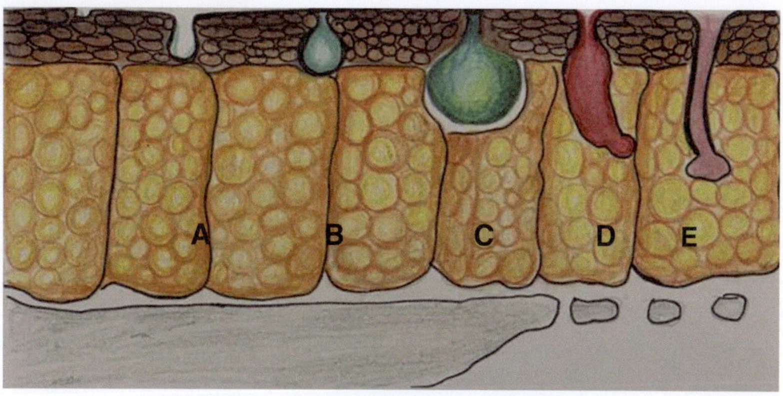

Fig. 19.1 Bascom's hypothesis for formation of pits. (**a**) Stretched hair follicle (HF). (**b**) Infected HF. (**c**) Acute abscess. (**d**) Chronic abscess. (**e**) Epithelial tube or pit

S. K. Singla, K. Mital, *Operative Manual of Minimally Invasive and LASER Ano-proctology*,
https://doi.org/10.1007/978-981-96-6190-9_19

- Pits form from normal hair follicles in midline which get stretched due to midline stretch of movement and then get infected.
- Infection leads to formation of acute abscess which leads to incomplete drainage leading to formation of chronic abscess.
- Opening of abscess cavity gets lined by skin epithelium and forms an epithelial tube or called as pit, which keeps it communicating with the skin surface.
- Loose hair in the area which may come from distant parts like occiput or hair in environment (hair of beard or even of pets in house), gets sucked in those pits (Fig. 19.2).

Karydakis had opinion that

- Skin of the area is vulnerable due to depth and moisture.
- Broken hair enters it with a force and creates foreign body granuloma.

He proposed a simple formula Pilonidal disease = Hair (H) × Force (F) × Vulnerability (V)2 [2].

"H" represents hair, the invader (number of hair, kind of hair–tough or silky, and shape)
"F" A force resulting in hair penetration—depends upon the depth and shape of the natal cleft.
"V" Skin vulnerability—depends upon whether the skin is soft, macerated, excoriated or has wide pores.

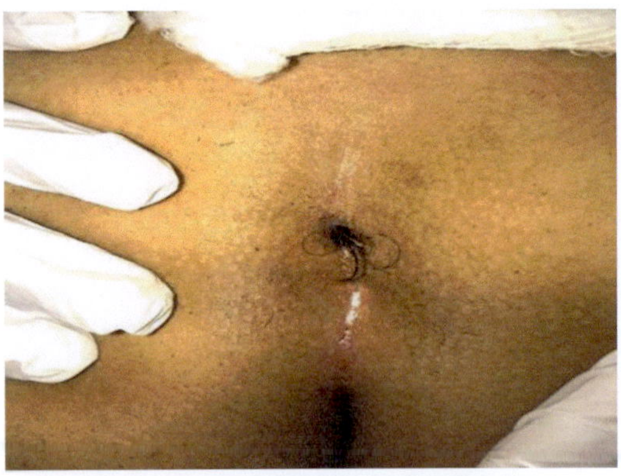

Fig. 19.2 Loose hair entering the preformed pit

The hair's keratin flakes allow the loose hair to move unidirectional.

19.2 Why MIS in PNS

- Significant morbidity and recurrence of PNS still occurs after traditional invasive surgical techniques (Fig. 19.3 and Table 19.1).

Although a meta-analysis of eight randomised control trails (RCTs) done in 2018 shows no sig-

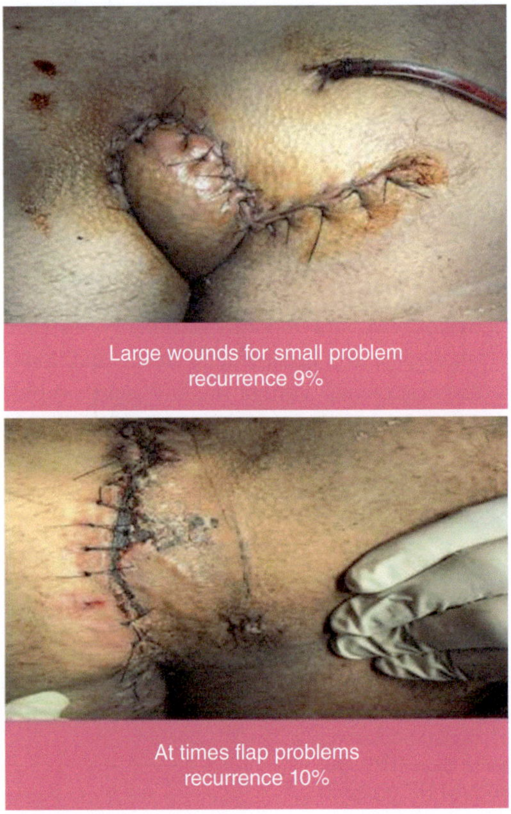

Fig. 19.3 Wound morbidity after flap surgery (Limberg and BASCOM 2) for PNS

Table. 19.1 Morbidity after flap surgery [3]

Flap	Karydakis	Limberg	Modified Limberg
Recurrence	11%	6.3%	1.9%
Seroma	19.8%	5.2%	7.4%
Wound failure	15.4%	2.1%	3.7%

nificant difference in wound healing between Karydakis and Limberg flap but seroma formation is less after Limberg flap [4].

- MIS reduces the morbidity arising from excisional surgery.
- MIS results comparable to traditional surgery as far as early recurrence is concerned.
- MIS scores over traditional excision and flap closure as far as comfort, days off the work is concerned [5, 6].
- MIS demonstrates efficacy in eliminating factors driving the disease process like pit and hair [1, 7, 8].
- In a 5-year follow-up in a meta-analysis, incidence of recurrence after excision and leaving open is 17.9%, after midline closure is 16.8% and after off the midline closure is 10% [9].
- Treatment with LASERS is also quite effective in short term at least and healing time is 2–3 weeks a.c.t. 5–6 weeks after sinusectomy [10].
- MIS combined with endo-vision still improves the results in form of assurance of complete removal of hair and granulation tissue under vision, which should translate into rapid healing and low recurrence a.c.t traditional MIS procedures. On an average recurrence rate is 4–17%.
- One of the studies reports only 4% recurrence [11].
- Another study with longer follow-up of 5 years reports 17% recurrence, which is still comparable to excision surgery outcomes in long term [12].
- Surgeons may find it difficult to understand navicular area, anal triangle and flap-formation (Figs. 19.4 and 19.5).
- Due to learning curve and morbidity associated with flaps, surgeons choose excision of the disease and open management or midline closure.
- Instead one should learn minimally invasive ways to manage pilonidal sinus disease.

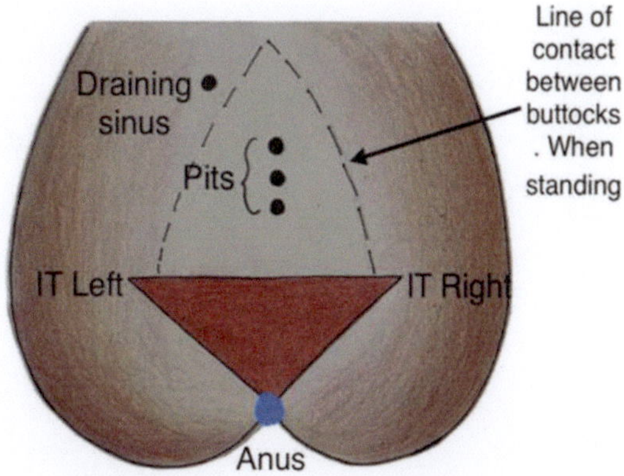

Fig. 19.4 Navicular area and anal triangle

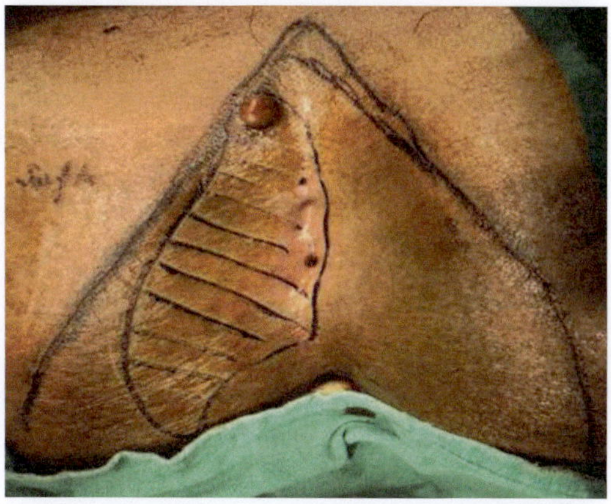

Fig. 19.5 Navicular area and markings for the area to be excised in case of BASCOM cleft closure operation

- Moreover, in MIS for PNS and especially endoscopic management, there is no consideration for navicular area or anal triangle. Longer the tracts, more advantage of endoscopic methods.
- Even in case of recurrence of the disease, endoscopic method can treat the underlying cause of recurrence like missed PIT or retained hair in the sinus [13, 14] (Fig. 19.6).
- Desired goal for success should be that procedure be simple, without much pain, efficient in rapid healing with minimal or no recurrence. MIS in PNS full-fills all except duck recurrence.

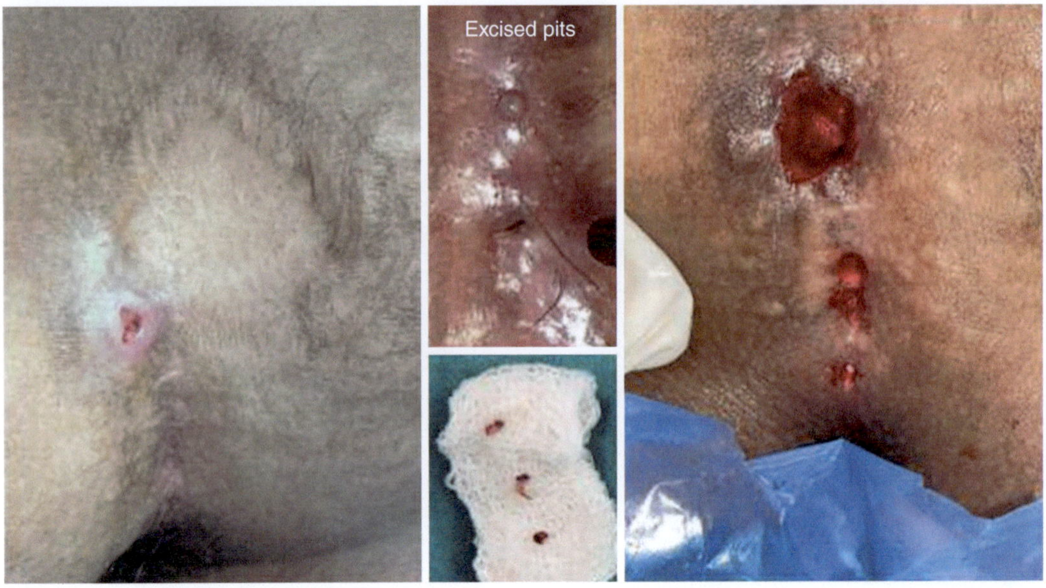

Reoccurrence after LIMBERG flap. Is it really the soar point

Missed or new formed pits in the mid line

Fig. 19.6 Missed pits or newly formed pits removed and endoscopic clearance verified

19.3 Limitations

- Not all patients are fit for MIS.
- There is no standardisations of procedures as of today.
- One of the suggested causative factors, i.e., deep natal cleft is not addressed by minimally invasive techniques. Instead, it is suggested to keep the area clean and epilated to avoid reoccurrence.
- Most of the clinical evidence is presented by few centres.
- Cost and learning-curve involved in endoscopy is another barrier for its universal application.
- Selection of suitable cases for MIS in PNS is yet another problem.
- In the following chapters, we have tried to present steps involved in different minimally invasive procedures and have proposed a novel classification of pilonidal sinus disease which may help one to differentiate between cases suitable for MIS or the cases which need, off the midline flap closure. This classification guides management and further research in the field.

References

1. Bascom J. Pilonidal disease: origin from follicles of hairs and results of follicle removal as treatment. Surgery. 1980;87(5):567–72.
2. Karydakis GE. Easy and successful treatment of pilonidal sinus after explanation of its causative process. Aust N Z J Surg. 1992;62(5):385–9. https://doi.org/10.1111/j.1445-2197.1992.tb07208.x.
3. Arslan K, Said Kokcam S, Koksal H, Turan E, Atay A, Dogru O. Which flap method should be preferred for the treatment of pilonidal sinus? A prospective randomized study. Tech Coloproctol. 2014;18(1):29–37. https://doi.org/10.1007/s10151-013-0982-2.
4. Prassas D, Rolfs TM, Schumacher FJ, et al. Karydakis flap reconstruction versus Limberg flap transposition for pilonidal sinus disease: a meta-analysis of randomized controlled trials. Langenbecks Arch Surg. 2018;403:5473554. https://doi.org/10.1007/s00423-018-1697-7.

5. Garg P, Menon GR, Gupta V. Laying open (deroofing) and curettage of sinus as treatment of pilonidal disease: a systematic review and meta-analysis. ANZ J Surg. 2016;86(1-2):27–33. https://doi.org/10.1111/ans.13377.
6. Soll C, Dindo D, Steinemann D, Haufle T, Clavien PA, Hahnloser D. Sinusectomy for primary pilonidal sinus: less is more. Surgery. 2011;150(5):996–1001. https://doi.org/10.1016/j.surg.2011.06.019.
7. Lord PH, Millar DM. Pilonidal sinus: a simple treatment. Br J Surg. 1965;52:298–300. https://doi.org/10.1002/bjs.1800520413.
8. Nordon IM, Senapati A, Cripps NPJ. A prospective randomized controlled trial of simple Bascom's technique versus Bascom's cleft closure for the treatment of chronic pilonidal disease. Am J Surg. 2009;197(2):189–92. https://doi.org/10.1016/j.amjsurg.2008.01.020.
9. Milone M, Velotti N, Manigrasso M, Anoldo P, Milone F, De Palma GD. Long-term follow-up for pilonidal sinus surgery: a review of literature with metanalysis. Surgeon. 2018;16(5):315–20. https://doi.org/10.1016/j.surge.2018.03.009.
10. Pappas AF, Ref Christodoulou DK. A new minimally invasive treatment of pilonidal sinus disease with the use of a diode laser: a prospective large series of patients. Colorectal Dis. 2018;20(8):O207–14. https://doi.org/10.1111/codi.14285.
11. Azhough R, Azari Y, Taher S, Jalali P. Endoscopic pilonidal sinus treatment: a minimally invasive surgical technique. Asian J Endosc Surg. 2021;14(3):458–63. https://doi.org/10.1111/ases.12893.
12. Foti N, Passannanti D, Libia A, Campanile FC. A minimally invasive approach to pilonidal disease with endoscopic pilonidal sinus treatment (EPSiT): a single-center case series with long-term results. Tech Coloproctol. 2021;25(9):1045–54. https://doi.org/10.1007/s10151-021-02477-w.
13. Meinero P, La Torre M, Lisi G, Stazi A, Carbone A, Regusci L, Fasolini F. Endoscopic pilonidal sinus treatment (EPSiT) in recurrent pilonidal disease: a prospective international multicenter study. Int J Colorectal Dis. 2019;34(4):741–6. https://doi.org/10.1007/s00384-019-03256-8.
14. Manigrasso M, Velotti N, Sosa Fernandez LM, Vertaldi S, Maione F, Gennarelli N, Dinuzzi VP, Musella M, De Palma GD, Milone M. Endoscopic approach to recurrent pilonidal sinus: a retrospective analysis. J Laparoendosc Adv Surg Tech A. 2021;31(1):1–5. https://doi.org/10.1089/lap.2020.0252.

Sacrococcygeal Pilonidal Sinus Disease: Conventional MIS Procedures Pit-Picking and Debridement

20

Abstract

- Minimal invasion surgery for pilonidal sinus disease is not new, Lord and Miller reported their method of pit-picking in 1965 (Lord PH, Millar DM. Br J Surg, 52:298–300, 1965).
- Indications and contraindications of the procedure are explained by clinical photographs.
- Use of punch biopsy forceps to excise a pit taking 1–2 mm margin precisely around the pit has been shown.
- Role of brush with nylon bristles in removing the stubborn hair in the tract has been mentioned.
- Complications have been compiled in the table form.
- Tips and Tricks section may help the reader to improve results.
- "References" and "Suggested Reading" sections enhance knowledge and provide information about methods used by other operators to treat pilonidal sinus disease.

20.1 What One Should Know Before the Procedure [1]

- Pilonidal sinuses are foreign body sinuses in which the foreign body is hair.
- If the hair is removed and free drainage allowed, the sinus will heal.
- Midline pits have been found in association with a pilonidal sinus and it is suggested that these must be removed to avoid recurrence.

20.2 Indications

- PNS cases Tezel type III, IV except midline wounds larger than 1 cm.

20.3 Contraindications (Fig. 20.1)

- Midline non-healing wounds larger than 1 cm.
- Midline wound failure after previous surgery.
- Unusual cases as shown are better managed with flaps as of today.

S. K. Singla, K. Mital, *Operative Manual of Minimally Invasive and LASER Ano-proctology*, https://doi.org/10.1007/978-981-96-6190-9_20

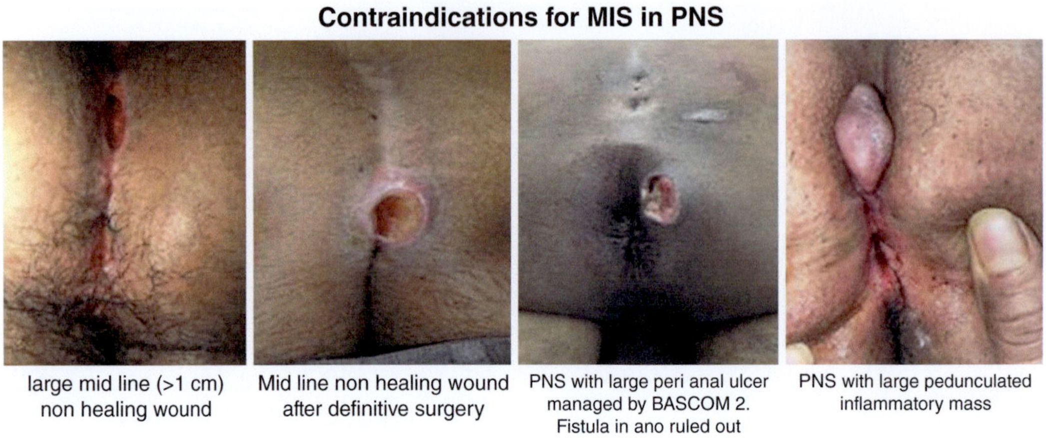

Fig. 20.1 Cases of PNS, which need skin cover—not fit for pit picking alone or any type of minimally invasive method of treatment

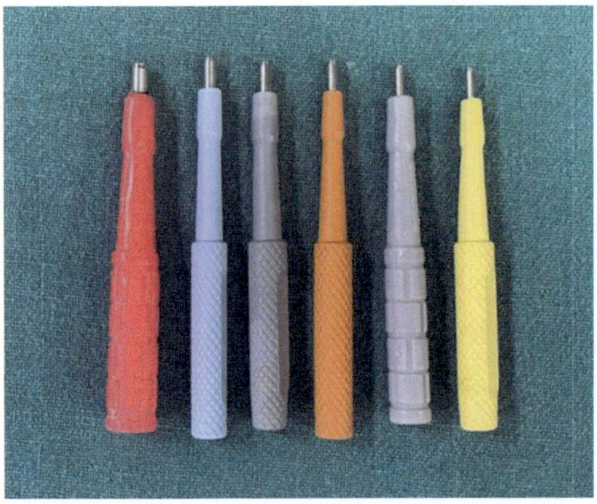

Fig. 20.2 Skin biopsy punches of various diameters to punch out the pits

20.4 Equipment

- Pads and sheets to make prone position.
- Sterile sheets.
- Local anaesthetic agents.
- Syringes and needles.
- Number 11 surgical blade or skin biopsy punch (optional) (Fig. 20.2).
- Volkman's scoupe.
- Fine bottle brush with bristles (Fig. 20.3; Lord and Millar mentioned brush used for cleaning electric razors.)
- Saline and hydrogen peroxide solution.
- Sterile dressing material.

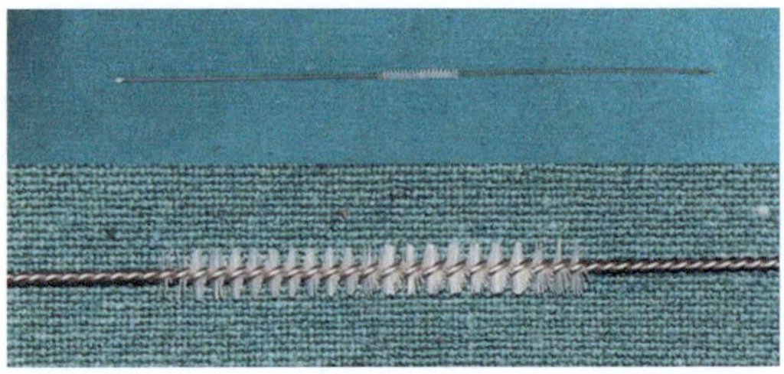

Fig. 20.3 Brush with nylon bristles to remove hair from pilonidal sinus

20.5 Procedure

- Pre-op. epilation by epilatory cream.
- We always check for any hypersensitivity to cream by application of cream on inner side of the forearm of non-dominant hand(patch test).
- Patient lies prone with buttocks strapped to wide open the natal cleft.
- Parts cleaned and draped.
- Take a photograph of the area on mobile phone and then enlarge the picture to see all pits (Fig. 20.4).
- Local anaesthesia is instituted with combination of lignocaine 2% and adrenaline in 1:200000.
- Instillation of saline mixed with few drops of methylene blue shows communicating pits with exit opening through underlying cavity (Fig. 20.5).

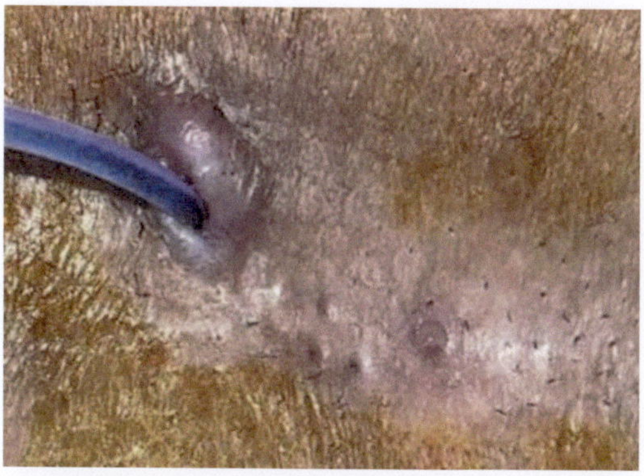

Fig. 20.4 Note three pits close together and one pit with drop of diluted dye in the centre

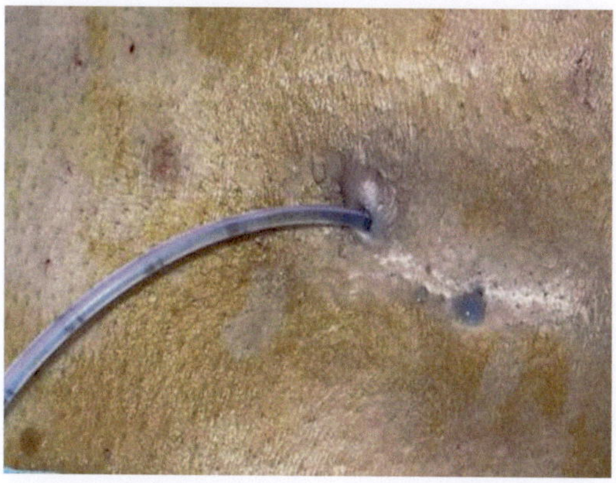

Fig. 20.5 Instillation of very diluted methylene blue in saline, shows communication of pits through underlying sinus cavity

- Hair removed from pits and side opening by curved haemostat (Fig. 20.6).
- Small bottle brush with nylon bristles is used and rotated inside the cavity to remove the hair completely till no more hair come out. Lord and Miller used brush being applied to clean electrical razors in their time (Fig. 20.7).
- Tracts are curetted.
- Pits are excised by number 11 blade by taking margins not more than 2 mm all around.
- When skin biopsy punches of various diameters are used to remove pits, it makes it essentially, Gips procedure.
- Initially, punch is kept perpendicular to skin and after initial penetration through the skin, its axis is aligned with axis of the tract.

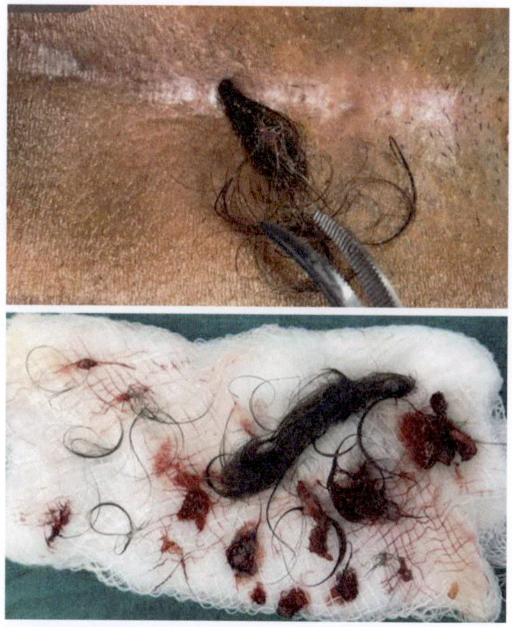

Fig. 20.6 Hair removed from the pit, pulling the nidus gently with mosquito forceps

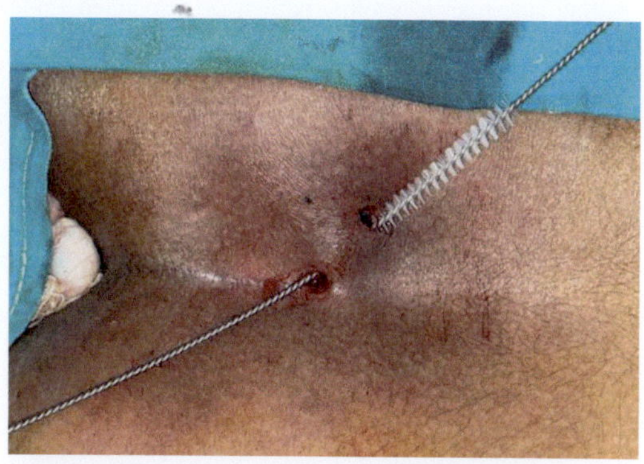

Fig. 20.7 Bottle brush with nylon bristles in use to remove hair, similarly now a days endobrush is used under vision

- Excised pit is removed with curved mosquito forceps.
- To remove the mid-line pit, use smallest size punch adequate to take 2 mm margins all around, while to lay open the side-tract, use large size punch to keep mouth of side tract wide open to prevent premature closure (Fig. 20.8).

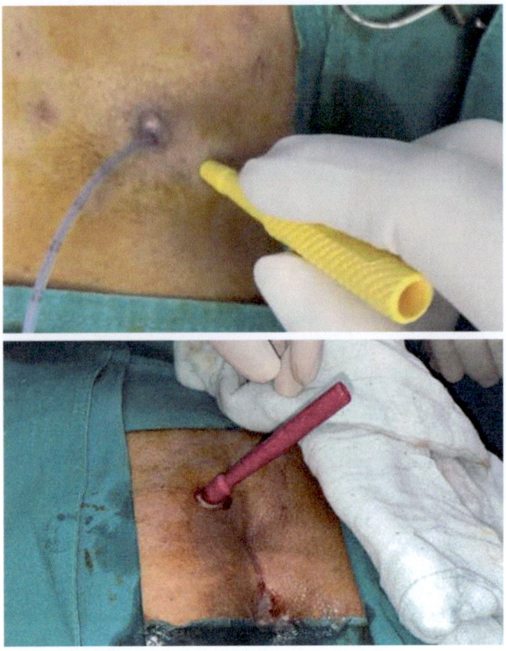

Fig. 20.8 Yellow punch with 2 mm diameter for very small midline pit, red punch with 9 mm diameter for opening side tract in another patient of associated acute infection

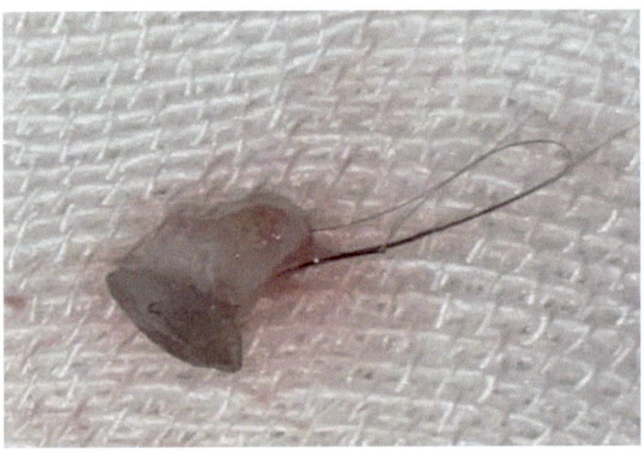

Fig. 20.9 Excised pit showing attached hair which entered through this pit

- At times when pit is punched out, one can observe the hair which entered the pit attached to its inner end (Fig. 20.9).
- At times tuft of hair which are removed from the cavity are quite long and can come from faraway places like occiput, beard of the patient (Fig. 20.10).

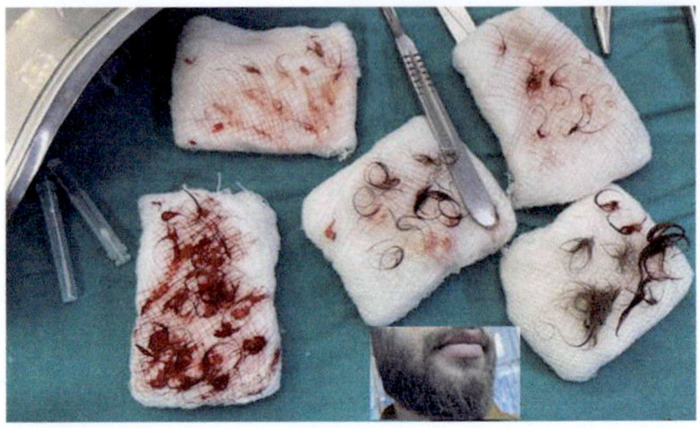

Fig. 20.10 Note some of the hair removed from the pilonidal sinus cavity resembles hair of the beard of the patient

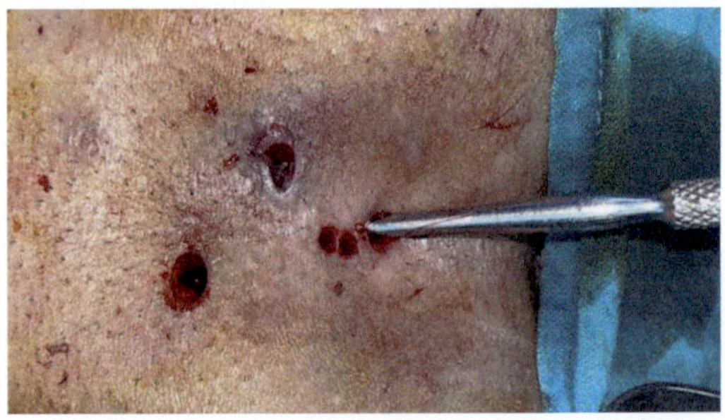

Fig. 20.11 Curette/Volkman's scoupe in sinus cavity to scrape the lining of the cavity and debridement, also note the precise excision of pits by the skin biopsy punch

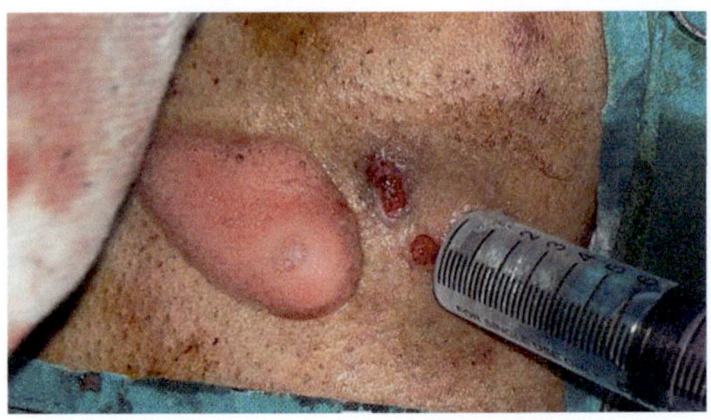

Fig. 20.12 Flush clean the cavity, use saline mixed with few drops of H_2O_2

- Tracts are curetted with Volkman's scoupe thoroughly (Fig. 20.11).
- Tracts are flushed with hydrogen peroxide and saline solution (Fig. 20.12).
- All openings in midline and on sides are left open for drainage.

20.6 Post-operative Advise

- Patient is encouraged to resume normal activity as soon as possible—it helps in draining any fluid in cavity.
- Patient to lie down supine to help obliterate the cavity.

20.7 Complication of Pit Picking (Table 20.1)

Table 20.1 Complications of pit picking and debridment

Complications	Prevention	Management
Bleeding		Local pressure
		Packing
		Bipolar cautery
Delayed healing	Debridement should be thorough	Flush and clean the cavity Local instillation of phenol in the sinus cavity
Retained hair	Use endoscope to remove hair under vision	Repeated brushing
		Use endoscope to clean the cavity under vision

20.8 Tips and Tricks

- No doubt, bottle-brush or endo-brush are very effective in removing even buried stubborn hair in the sinus cavity.
- In modern day practice, we always use endoscope to remove all hair and debris under vision.
- While excising epithealised pits in midline, do not remove more than 1–2 mm skin all around.
- Excised pits and lateral secondary wounds are left open for free drainage.

Algorithm for Pit Picking Procedure

History/clinical examination

Define the need to treat pilonidal sinus disease by minimal invasive method of pit picking

Anaesthesia local/spinal/GA

Position prone

Straps to open the natal cleft

Take photograph of the area and zoom in locate all pits and secondary openings may use diluted

Dye to locate opening pits and their communication with underlying sinus cavity

Remove hair from mid line pits with curved mosquito forceps and brush

Excise all mid line pits with skin biopsy punches

Excise secondary tract openings with skin punch

Curette the tracts and wash them with saline and hydrogen peroxide solution

Leave all openings open to heal by secondary intention

References

1. Lord PH, Millar DM. Pilonidal sinus: a simple treatment. Br J Surg. 1965;52:298–300. https://doi.org/10.1002/bjs.1800520413.

Suggested Reading

Bascom J. Pilonidal disease: long-term results of follicle removal. Dis Colon Rectum. 1983;26(12):800–7. https://doi.org/10.1007/BF02554755.

Doll D, Petersen S, Andreae OA, Matner H, Albrecht H, Brügger LE, Luedi MM, Puhl G. Pit picking vs. Limberg flap vs. primary open method to treat pilonidal sinus disease – a cohort of 327 consecutive patients. Innov Surg Sci. 2022;7(1):23329. https://doi.org/10.1515/iss-2021-0041.

Patey DH. The principles of treatment of sacrococcygeal pilonidal sinus. Proc R Soc Med. 1970;63(9):939–40.

Petersen S. Skin preserving pit excision, so-called pit picking. PSJ. 2017;3(1):1–7.

21 Sacrococcygeal Pilonidal Sinus Disease: Conventional MIS Procedures-Laying Open/Sinusotomy, Sinusectomy and Gips Technique

Abstract

- Pilonidal sinus disease manifests as a chronic discharging sinus in sacrococcygeal area. Usually it harbours broken hair which illicit foreign body reaction and invite infection.
- Sinusotomy or sinusectomy is traditional minimally invasive technique to manage a limited disease without morbidly of complicated flaps.
- Indications and contraindications of sinusotomy (lay open), sinusectomy are enumerated.
- Operative steps are explained by sketches and clinical photographs.
- Skin-sparing sinusectomy with trephines called as Gips technique is shown with clinical photographs in detail.
- How to use Gips philosophy, in acute abscess associated with pilonidal sinus disease is demonstrated well.
- Complications of the procedure are tabulated for ready reference.
- Tips and Tricks are suggested to improve out comes.
- Algorithm of Gips technique is pasted to help brush-up operative steps whenever required.
- "References" and "Suggested Reading" sections are to further enhance understanding of the subject.

21.1 What One Should Know Before the Procedure

- There is wide acceptance that Pilonidal sinus disease is an acquired disease.
- Two major conflicting views on pathogenesis of pilonidal sinus disease are as follows:
  1. Follicular occlusion due to hyperkeratosis, leading to dilatation, infection and finally rupture of a hair follicle makes pits. Entry of broken hair in these preformed pits is a secondary phenomenon.
  2. Perforation of the vulnerable skin by hair that have been shed or cut, leads to these sinuses, as sinuses forming in interdigital clefts of barbers.
- Based on the first view as proposed by BASCOM, removal of hair and excision of these pits should relieve the patient of symptoms and avoid recurrence.
- Sinus-tract forms due to drainage of subcutaneous infection laterally or in midline.
- Laying open (sinusotomy) or excision (sinusectomy) of whole sinus-tract should relieve the patient from this disease.

21.2 Lay Open/Sinusotomy [1]

21.2.1 Indications

Midline pit and sinus-tract going lateral. Disease load, not in midline.

S. K. Singla, K. Mital, *Operative Manual of Minimally Invasive and LASER Ano-proctology*,
https://doi.org/10.1007/978-981-96-6190-9_21

21.2.2 Contra Indications

Disease load in midline. Multiple pits in midline.

Non-healing midline wounds larger than 1 cm.

21.2.3 Equipment

- Pads and sheets to make prone position.
- Sterile sheets.
- Tape to strap buttocks to wide open the gluteal cleft.
- Diluted methylene blue dye to find tract opening.
- Sinus probes.
- Curved haemostats.
- 15 no. Surgical blade on handle.
- Volkman's scoupe.
- Scissors to trim the margins.
- Local anaesthetic agent.

21.3 Procedure

- The sinus opening is probed gently to check the direction and length of the tract (Fig. 21.1).
- The local anaesthetic agent (2% lignocaine with adrenaline 0.005%) is infiltrated around the tract which helps in analgesia as well as keeping the surgery field relatively blood less.
- The tracts are identified with the help of mosquito (small artery) forceps and are laid open, base and side walls of the tract are not excised (Fig. 21.2).
- If there are more than one tract, then all the tracts are opened at the same time.
- Hair and debris are removed from the tracts. Granulation tissue is curetted with Volkman's scoupe.
- Overhanging skin margins are trimmed.
- Any extensions sideways, cranial or caudal are checked and laid open.
- The bleeding points are controlled by bipolar forceps.
- Wound dressed with gauge soaked in povidine iodine.

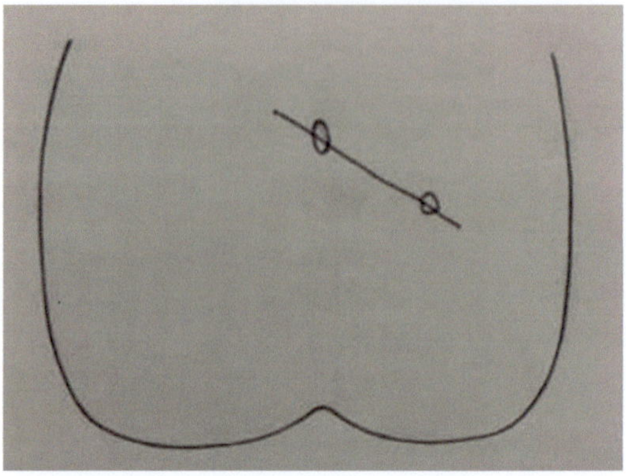

Fig. 21.1 Midline pit and side tract probed

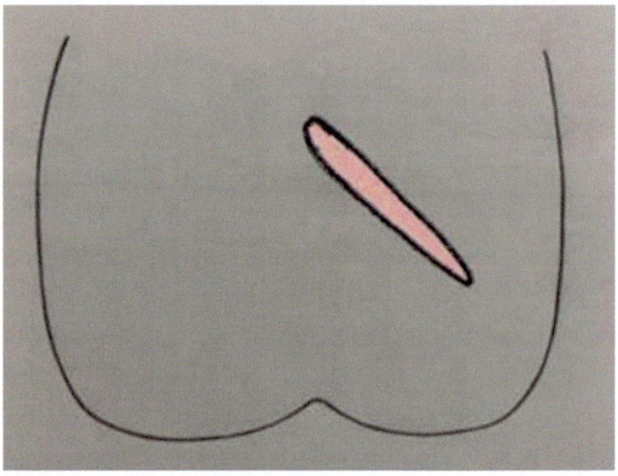

Fig. 21.2 Sinus tract laid open and cavity cleaned and margins trimmed

21.4 Post-operative care

- Dressing change—packed gauge is removed after 24 h. Instead loose dressing is applied.
- Regular dressings under supervision.
- Keep the area epilated till the wound heals.
- Usual healing time is 6 weeks. Its little longer than healing time taken by coring the tracts and LASER treatment.
- Thereafter, LASER epilation of 5 cm radius all around the area is done to decrease the reoccurrence.

21.5 Complications (Table 21.1)

Table 21.1 Complications of laying open the sinus

Complications	Prevention	Management
Hyper granulation tissue pouts over margins		Apply silver nitrate or phenol
Margins close prematurely	Trim the skin from margins	Reopen the bridge and allow healing from base

21.6 Skin-Sparing Sinusectomy

- Circumferential incision of the pilonidal orifices is done, avoiding wide excision of skin margins.
- Subcutaneous extirpation of the sinus without incising skin is done, it makes a subcutaneous tunnel which is left open on both sides and is allowed to heal by granulation tissue.

21.7 Other Variations

21.7.1 Gips Technique/Sinusectomy Is Done by Trephine

Gips technique is an ambulatory surgical treatment for pilonidal disease which integrates the principles suggested by both Lord–Millar and Bascom and introduces the use of skin trephines (Fig. 21.3) for the easy excision of pilonidal pits and debridement of underlying cavities and tracts. Gips did not use brush to remove hair, instead deep cavity walls were shelved by trephines [2].

21.7.2 Indications

Midline pit and sinus-tract going lateral.

21.7.3 Contra Indications

Complex cases with skin loss.

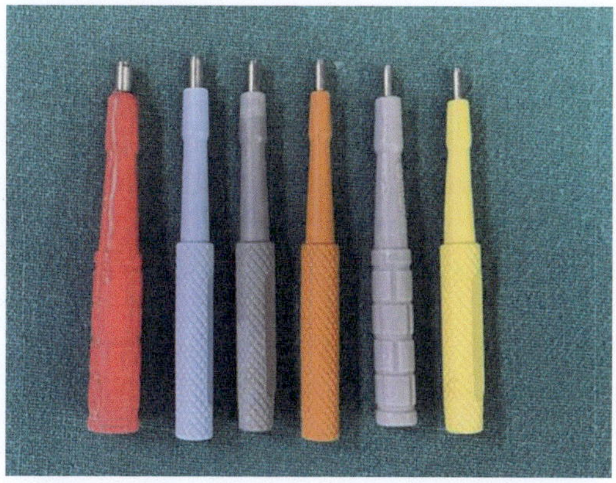

Fig. 21.3 Skin biopsy punches used as trephines

21.7.4 Equipment

- Pads and sheets to make prone position.
- Sterile sheets.
- Tape to strap buttocks to wide open the gluteal cleft.
- Diluted methylene blue dye to find tract opening.
- Sinus probes.
- Curved haemostats.
- Skin trephines or punch biopsy disposable kit (Fig. 21.3). Gips used Keyes and Elliot type skin and ophthalmic trephines for pit excision [2].

We use disposable skin punches of various diameters for the purpose of pit excision and sinusecotomy over the probe (Fig. 21.3).

21.7.5 Position of the Patient

Prone with buttocks strapped to wide open the natal cleft.

21.7.6 Anaesthesia

Local anaesthesia is employed with 2% lidocaine solution with adrenalin.

21.7.7 Procedure

- Buttocks are strapped to wide open the natal cleft area.
- Each visible pit and secondary tract are probed gently to judge the depth and direction.
- At times oedema and inspissated debris obscure the opening.
- One may instil a diluted dye in saline with few drops of hydrogen peroxide from one opening, which may show the obscured openings.
- All openings and tracts are then cored out, utilizing disposable skin punches/trephins 2.0–9.0 mm in diameter.

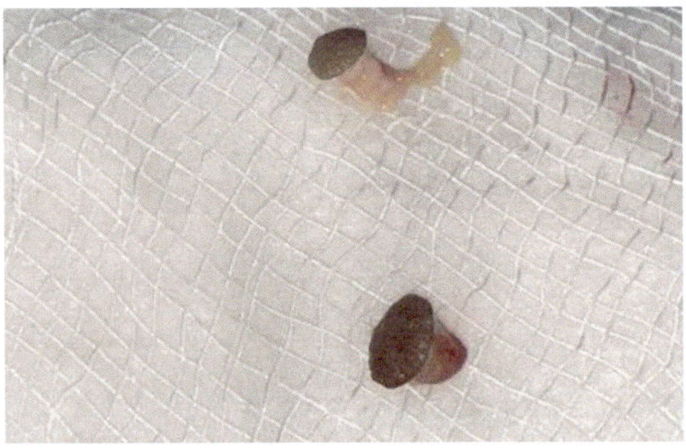

Fig. 21.4 Small pits and short tracts removed with skin punch

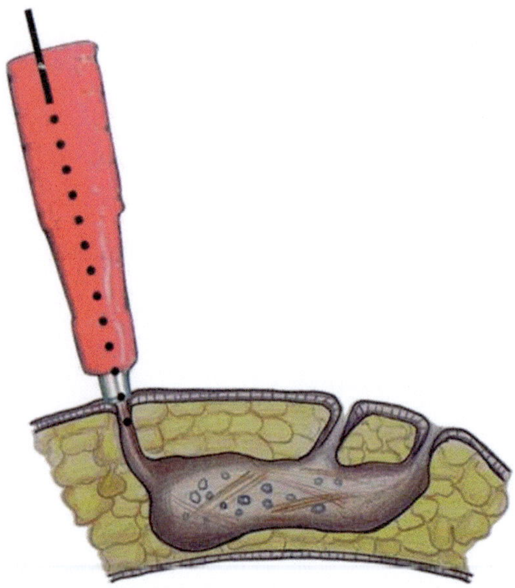

Fig. 21.5 Coring the tract over a probe by punch

- Small pits with short tracts are removed with 2.0–3.0 mm trephines (Fig. 21.4).
- Pits leading to subcutaneous cavities are then excised down to the cavity, using 4.0–5.0 mm trephines over a probe (Fig 21.5, 21.6 and 21.7).
- Openings of fistulas and drainage openings for acute suppurations are excised using 6.0–9.0 mm trephines (Fig. 21.8).

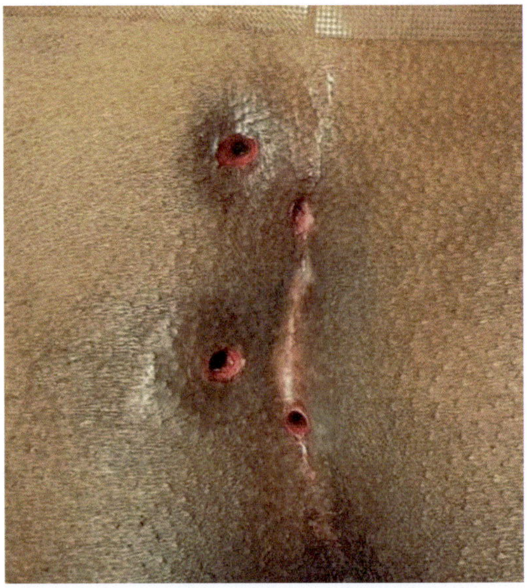

Fig. 21.6 Natal cleft of a patient with PNS after pits and side tracts punched out and cavities cleaned

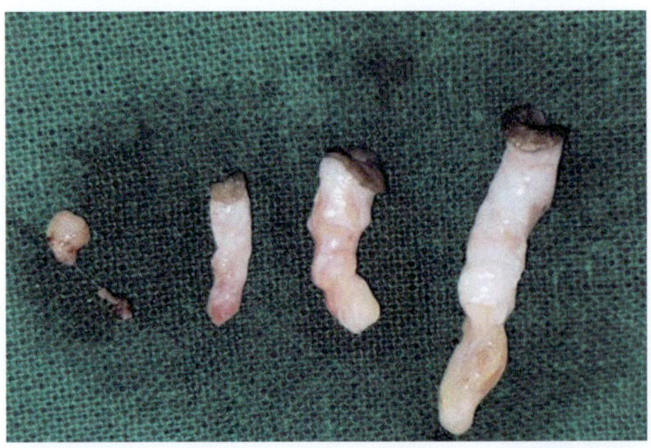

Fig. 21.7 Excised pits with small punch and sinus tracts trephined with punch over a probe, note the whole length of the tract is excised

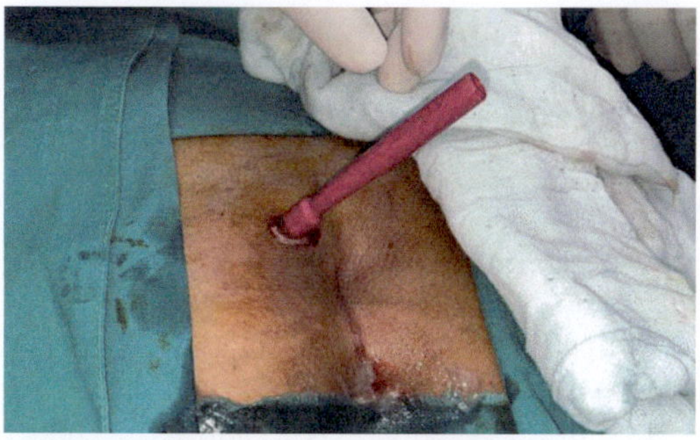

Fig. 21.8 Drainage of acute suppuration with 9 mm punch

- To lay open the abscess, instead of long para median incision, punch out overlying skin at two places. It effectively drains the abscess without application of drain or packing gauge wick. Curette the cavity well (Fig. 21.9).
- Midline pit may be obscured in an abscess which becomes visible after 4–5 days and can be punched out under local anaesthesia (Fig. 21.9).

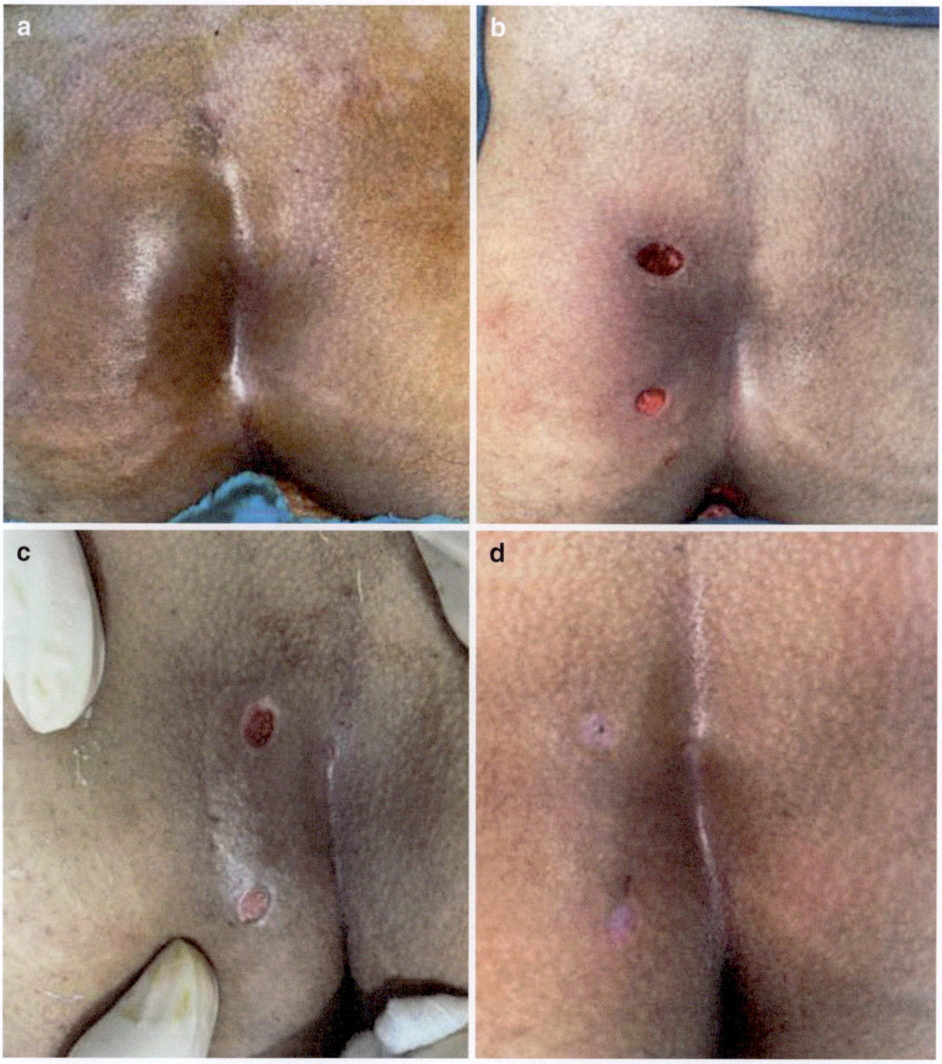

Fig. 21.9 Gips procedure in case of abscess associated with pilonidal sinus. (**a**) Abscess swelling of same patient as shown in Fig. 21.8. (**b**) Over lying skin punched out at two extreme ends of cavity, pus drained and cavity curetted. (**c**) Midline pit visible on day 4 was punched under local anaesthesia. (**d**) Healed cavity and midline pit wound. Note: With the availability of scope we now a days always ensure complete debridement under vision

- Groups of 2 or 3 adjacent pits are punched out separately or at times removed together if they are very close, using 4.0–6.0 mm trephine (Fig. 21.10).
- For each opening, skin biopsy punch is first advanced perpendicularly to the skin. Once it enters the skin, it is aligned in direction of the tract (judged earlier by probe) up to sinus cavity and whole tract can be cored out sparing the over lying skin.
- It helps in removing the epithelised pits and fibrous tract thus ensures early closure.

- Small and large curettes are used to debride the whole cavity to remove the hair debris and granulation tissue (Fig. 21.11).
- Cavity is flushed with hydrogen peroxide solution with saline.
- Bleeding which is usually minimal can be controlled by pressure over the excised tract.

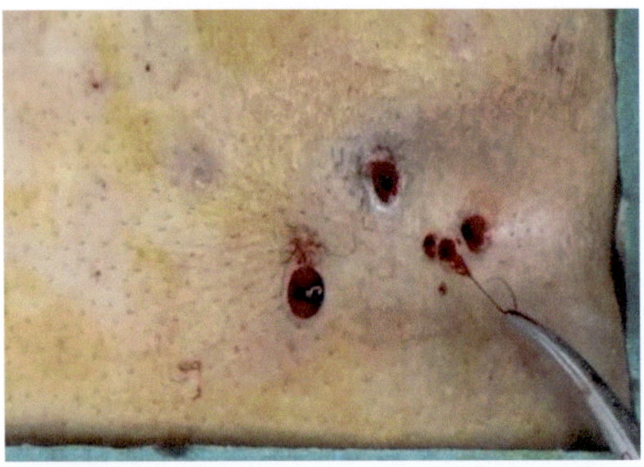

Fig. 21.10 Group of three pits close by, punched out separately and precisely

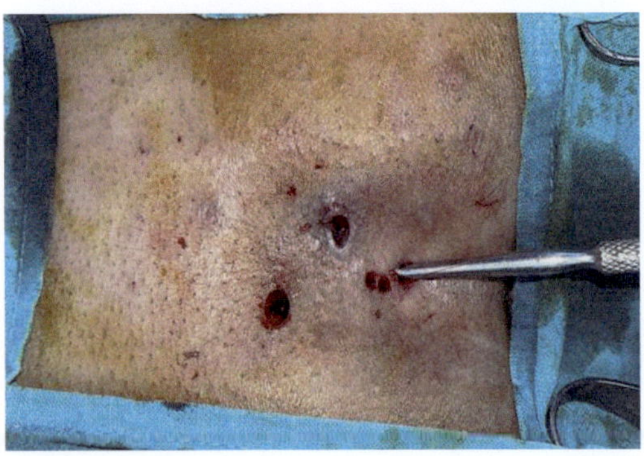

Fig. 21.11 All the tracts are curetted with small and large curettes depending on size of opening

- All openings are left open for drainage.
- Inter-gluteal dressing with small pads to occlude the cleft is done.

21.8 Post-operative Care

- All patients are encouraged to lie supine to help occlude the tract further.
- Routine activity is allowed rather encouraged.
- Post-operative antibiotics for immunocompromised patients or patients with acute abscess and cellulitis.
- First post-operative visit is after four days to check the wound for any collection or haematoma in the tract.
- Follow-up visits are usually at 1–2 week intervals until the wounds heal.
- On each visit, wounds are superficially cleaned with sterile ear buds to prevent premature closure.
- Epilation of the area till wound heals.

21.9 Tips and Tricks

- Selection of cases suitable for lay-open or skin-sparing sinusectomy/Gips technique with trephines, is very important.
- Disposable trephines (punches) are good for excision of skin pits.

- For long tract, either punches can be used over a probe or long coring devices available to core fistula tracts can also be used.

- Debridement with curettage and pulsed lavage with saline—hydrogen peroxide solution is very important.
- Keep all openings open otherwise one can close midline openings and keep side tract open for drainage.
- Cleft-occlusive dressings are essential to prevent any collection in the tracts.

21.10 Complications of Gips Technique (Table 21.2)

Table 21.2 Complications of Gips procedure

Complication	Prevention	Management
Fever	Pre-operative control of infection	Drainage of pus, antipyretics, antibiotics
Infection	Intravenous (I/V) antibiotics with application of anaesthesia	Debridement, saline lavage and antibiotics
Bleeding		External packing
		Local pressure

Algorithm for Gips Procedure

History and clinical examination
Indication and contraindications
Prone position
Strap buttocks to wide open the natal cleft
Local anaesthesia
Punch out mid line pits
Core outside tracts from secondary lateral opening with punch over the probe
Curette cavity well to remove hair and debris
Flush with saline mixed with few drops of H_2O_2
Leave all openings open for adequate drainage
With availability of scope, we now a days ensure complete removal of hair and debride under vision

References

1. Garg P, Garg M, Gupta V, Mehta SK, Lakhtaria P. Laying open (deroofing) and curettage under local anesthesia for pilonidal disease: An outpatient procedure. World J Gastrointest Surg. 2015;7(9):214–8. https://doi.org/10.4240/wjgs.v7.i9.214.
2. Gips M, Melki Y, Salem L, Weil R, Sulkes J. Minimal surgery for pilonidal disease using trephines: description of a new technique and long-term outcomes in 1,358 patients. Dis Colon Rectum. 2008;51(11):1656–63. https://doi.org/10.1007/s10350-008-9329-x.

Suggested Reading

Aydede H, Erhan Y, Sakarya A, Kumkumoglu Y. Comparison of three methods in surgical treatment of pilonidal disease. ANZ J Surg. 2001;71(6):362–4.

Doll D, Novotny A, Rothe R, et al. Methylene Blue halves the long-term recurrence rate in acute pilonidal sinus disease. Int J Colorectal Dis. 2008;23:18137.

Patey DH. The principles of treatment of sacrococcygeal pilonidal sinus. Proc R Soc Med. 1970;63:939340.

Soll C, Hahnloser D, Dindo D, Clavien PA, Hetzer F. A novel approach for treatment of sacrococcygeal pilonidal sinus: less is more. Int J Colorectal Dis. 2008;23(2):177–80. https://doi.org/10.1007/s00384-007-0377-9.

Soll C, Dindo D, Steinemann D, Hauffe T, Clavien PA, Hahnloser D. Sinusectomy for primary pilonidal sinus: less is more. Surgery. 2011;150(5):996–1001. https://doi.org/10.1016/j.surg.2011.06.019.

Sacrococcygeal Pilonidal Sinus Disease: Conventional MIS Procedures BASCOM 1

22

Abstract

- A minimally invasive treatment for pilonidal sinus disease by pit-picking was described initially in 1965 by Lord and Millar.
- In 1980, Bascom increased awareness that the pits play a key-role in the pathogenesis of pilonidal disease. Mechanism of formation of pits as suggested by Bascom is explained with sketch.
- After removal of pits to clean the sinus cavity of hair and debris, Bascom suggested an incision of 1–2 cm over the secondary lesions (fistulous openings, scars, indurations, subcutaneous cavities lateral to the natal cleft).
- He further suggested to detach midline pits from post-sacral fascia by making a flap of fibro fatty tissue from posterior medial wall of sinus cavity.
- Procedure is done under local anaesthesia and steps are thoroughly explained by text and sketches. Technical details may vary across published medical literature, but the basic principles remain the same.
- Common complications encountered during Bascom's procedure are put in a table form.
- Tips and Tricks section will help the reader to improve the results.
- "References" and "Suggested Reading" sections are to make the reader more aware about what others say about this procedure.

22.1 What One Should Know Before the Procedure

- In formation and propagation of pilonidal sinus disease, who is the culprit?
  - Pits
  - Hair
  - Deep natal cleft
- If one believes in Bascom's hypothesis (Fig. 22.1) [1].
- Pits form from normal hair follicles in midline which get stretched due to midline stretch of movement and then get infected.

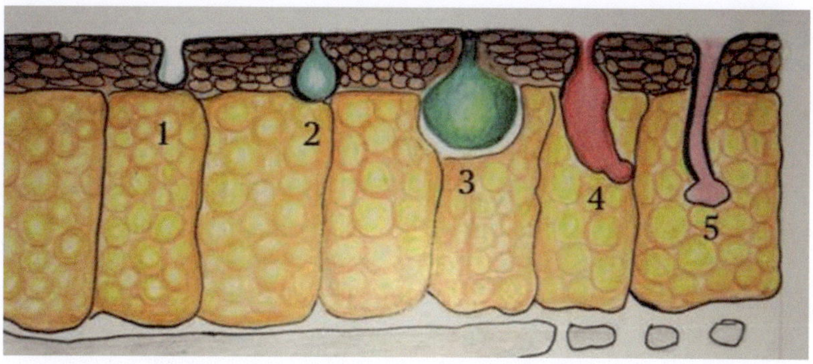

Fig. 22.1 Five stages of pit formation from normal hair follicle to stretching (1), inflammation (2), abscess formation (3), chronic abscess and (4) epithealised tract (5)

S. K. Singla, K. Mital, *Operative Manual of Minimally Invasive and LASER Ano-proctology*,
https://doi.org/10.1007/978-981-96-6190-9_22

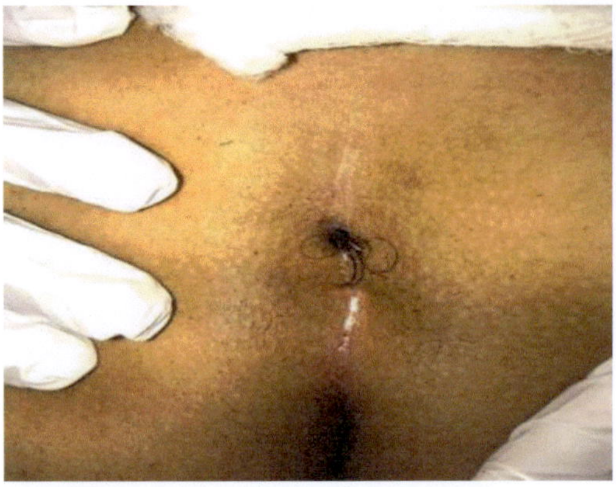

Fig. 22.2 Loose hair entering the preformed pit

- Infection leads to formation of acute abscess which leads to incomplete drainage leading to formation of chronic abscess.
- Opening of abscess cavity gets lined by skin epithelium so-called epithelial tube or pit which keeps it communicating with skin surface.
- Loose hair in the area which may come from distant parts like occiput or hair in environment (hair of beard or even of pets in house), then gets sucked in those pits (Fig. 22.2). Deep natal cleft facilitate towards creation of that sucking force.

- It is akin to abdominal hair and fibres of under shirt found in naval pit next morning.
- Bristles on hair make it a one way entry, hair bury in soft tissue under the skin to make chronic abscess and migrate to come out either in midline cephalad (93% of cases) or caudal (in less than 7%) of cases [2].
- Exit tract may go lateral in one or both gluteal areas.
- Lateral tracts usually limit within navicular area but may extend beyond the navicular area.

22.2 Principles of Bascom Procedure/Bascom 1/Pit Picking

- Distended hair follicles (presenting as small pits not yet communicating with sinus cavity) are removed individually from the natal cleft in the midline. Similarly, already epithealised tracts (pits communicating with the sinus cavity) are excised down to the cavity by taking 1–2 mm skin around their margins.
- In addition, an incision of 1–2 cm over the cavity of the chronic abscess lateral to natal cleft is made to debride the sinus cavity. Lateral incision may include previous scars and indurations or fistulous openings.
- Similarly, the acute abscess is drained by an incision—1 cm off the midline.
- Cavity walls are not excised, instead are allowed to fall closed and to heal. One or two stitches, to approximate skin flap to a flap of fibro-fatty tissue from base of the cavity, may facilitate early closure and detaches midline pits from post sacral fascia.
- An epithelial tube or secondary tract is dissected out through para-median incision.

22.3 Indications

- Chronic abscess with pits in the midline.
- Midline pits with lateral fistulous tracts, close to midline.
- Acute abscess.

22.4 Contraindications

- Large midline wounds are better managed by Bascom cleft lift/Bascom 2 procedure.
- Lateral discharging sinus wide away from midline.

22.5 Equipment

- Pads and sheets to make prone position.
- Sterile sheets.
- Local anaesthetic agent with 1.200000 adrenaline.
- Number 11 surgical blade or skin biopsy punch (optional).
- Volkman's scoupe.
- Normal saline and hydrogen peroxide solution.

- 10-ml syringes and suction.
- Tooth forceps and needle holder.
- 4.0 nylon suture on cutting needle.
- Sterile dressing material.

22.6 Procedure

- Position of patient prone with buttocks strapped.
- Pre-operative antibiotic is given. We prefer Amoxy clav three shots. One at induction of anaesthesia and two more post-operative shots 12 hourly.
- Local anaesthesia suffice in majority of the cases.
- Spinal or GA as per temperament of the patient and anaesthesiologist preference in special cases.

- Take a photograph on your mobile and zoom in to look for pits, we err on side of excising all suspicious pits than leaving any pit behind.

- In acute abscess cases, one can look for pits after 5 days when oedema subsides and pits can be excised after 5 days.

22.7 Bascom's Technique in Pilonidal Abscess (Figs. 22.3 and 22.4)

- Give an incision over acute or chronic abscess cavity 1–2 cm off the midline.
- Curette well, do not excise wall of the cavity.
- Curette medially up to midline to raise a skin flap up to pits.
- Excise pits with number 11 blade taking 1–2 mm margin with minimal amount of tissue equivalent to grain of rice as suggested by Bascom.
- One may use skin biopsy punch to excise the pits precisely with minimal tissue loss.

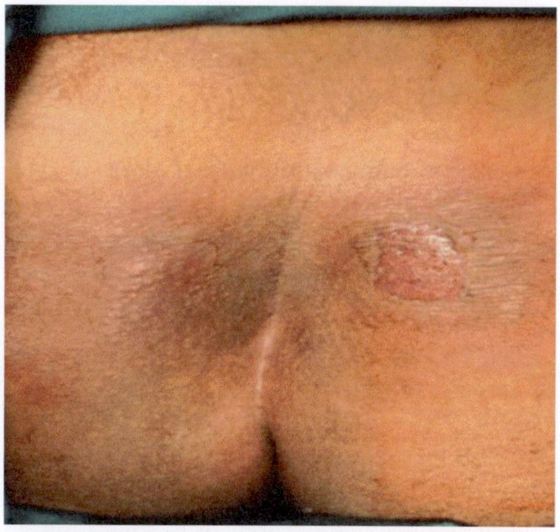

Fig. 22.3 Bilateral chronic abscess with midline pits

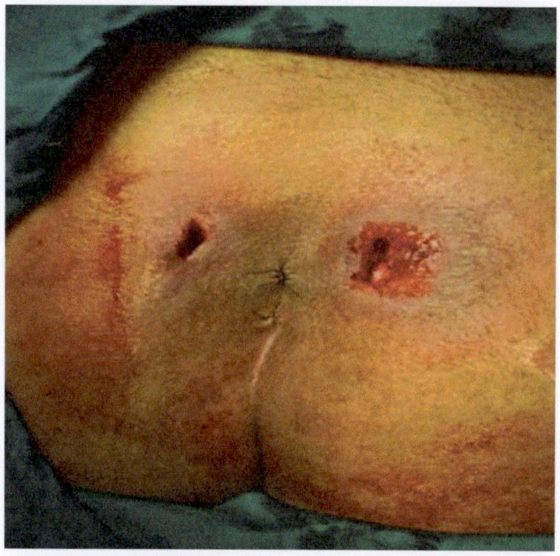

Fig. 22.4 Abscess cavities drained and curetted by incision 1 cm off the midline. Pits excised and closed with vertical mattress sutures

- Lavage the sinus cavity thoroughly with saline—hydrogen peroxide solution.
- Close midline pits with 4.0 nylon vertical mattress sutures.
- Keep lateral wound open for drainage.
- Epithelial tube if present can be completely dissected from lateral wound.
- Dress with ointment over gauge.

22.8 Bascom's Technique for Chronic Pilonidal Sinus Disease

- Cover the procedure with a dose of pre-operative antibiotic (Amoxy clav 1.2 Gm) and it is repeated twice 12 hourly.
- Local anaesthesia by infiltration of a mixture of equal volumes of 1% lignocaine, 0.5% bupivacaine with 1: 200000 adrenaline and normal saline.

- Carefully identify each pit by taking a photo of cleft after strapping and stretching the post-anal skin caudally. Zoom in to figure out all pits.
- We err on the side of removing all suspicious pits rather than leaving any pit behind.
- Midline pits are excised, removing a minimal amount of tissue equivalent to a grain of rice (Fig. 22.5).
- Underlying sinus cavity is then drained laterally to the most convenient side of the midline, or if on any side there is old scar of drainage or any induration, then select that side. Give a para-median incision parallel and 1–2 cm off the midline (Fig. 22.6).

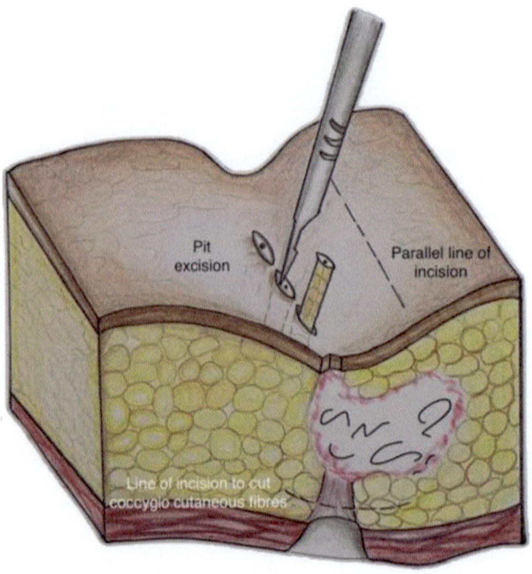

Fig. 22.5 Midline pit excision and parallel line of incision lateral to midline

- The sinus cavity is curetted to remove all infected granulation tissue and hair.
- An incision is given below the sinus cavity to detach it from sacrum. This creates a subcutaneous flap of fibro fatty tissue from posterio-medial wall of the sinus cavity (Fig. 22.7).
- Subcutaneous flap is stitched to the skin bridge between midline pits and para-median incision. It helps to decrease the size of the sinus cavity and divide the fibres anchoring midline cleft to post sacral fascia (Fig. 22.7).

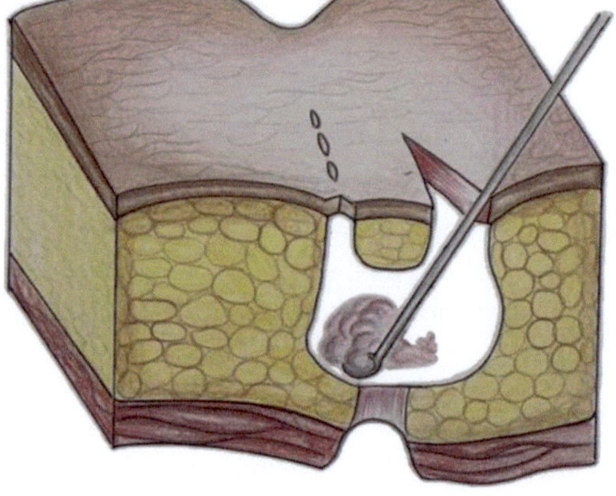

Fig. 22.6 Sinus cavity is curetted from para-median incision

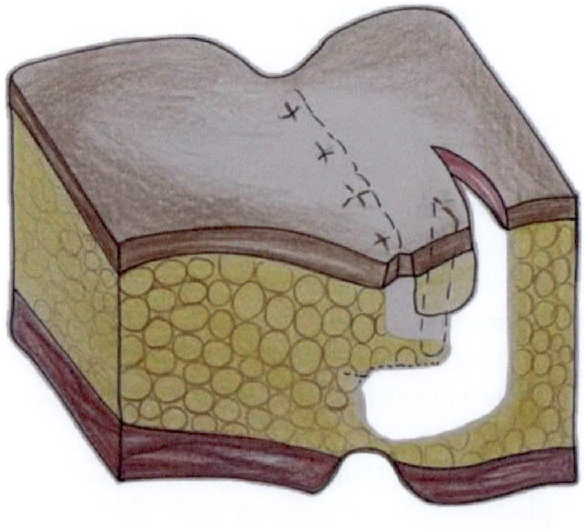

Fig. 22.7 Subcutaneous flap of fibro fatty tissue from posterio-medial wall of the sinus cavity is stitched to the skin bridge between midline pits and para-median incision

- Midline wounds, created after pit excision, are closed with vertical mattress sutures or subcuticular stitch.
- Haemostasis is ensured, bleeding points controlled using biopolar forceps.
- Lateral incision is loosely filled with gauge wick.

22.9 Post-operative Care

- Analgesics, oral nonsteroidal anti-inflammatory drugs (NSAIDs) suffice in most of the cases.
- Antibiotics: If there is cellulitis or the patient is immuno-compromised like in diabetes or having prosthesis.
- Keep lateral wound open to avoid premature closure, before the cavity heals from depth.
- Keep the area epilated till the wound heals (Table 22.1).

Table 22.1 Complication of BASCOM 1

Complications	Prevention	Management
Bleeding	As surgery is done under local infiltration of anaesthetic agent with adrenaline, surgeon should be very meticulous in haemostasis at completion of surgery. Curette the cavity well and application of silver nitrate swab is done to handle the excessive granulation tissue	Pressure, pack with ribbon gauge or bipolar cautery
Abscess	Curette the cavity well and avoid premature closure of lateral opening	Reopen lateral incision and drain the pus and curette

22.10 Tips and Tricks

- Identify all pits on table by stretching skin-caudal to anal-canal and after the application of side straps to wide open the natal-cleft. Take a photograph of the affected area in this position with cell-phone and zoom in, to check for all pits.
- We err on the side of removing all suspicious-pits than to leave any without excision.
- Snap away coccygeo cutaneous attachments, i.e., detach midline skin from post-sacral fascia by creating a flap of fibro-fatty tissue from base of sinus cavity as explained in Fig. 22.7. It may help in decreasing recurrence [3].
- As for any procedure done after infiltration of adrenaline, be fastidious about haemostasis at completion of surgery.

Algorithm for Bascom 1 Procedure

History and clinical examination
Define the indication for Bascom 1 procedure
Prone position with straps on buttocks
Local anaesthesia/with sedation
During local infiltration do pits identification
Removal of pits by taking small tissue around, equivalent to size of rice grain
Incision parallel and 1–2 cm off the mid line
Go deep to sinus cavity from lateral side
Curette and debride the sinus cavity of all granulation tissue and hair
Wash with H_2O_2 saline solution
Make a flap of sub cutaneous fat by incising below the sinus cavity from opposite side of para median incision
Stitch this flap to the underside of skin flap between mid line pits and paramedian incision
Close mid line wounds by vertical mattress sutures or sub cuticular stitch
Ensure haemostasis
Anti-septic dressing

References

1. Bascom J. Pilonidal disease: origin from follicles of hairs and results of follicle removal as treatment. Surgery. 1980;87(5):567–72.
2. Pilonidal Sinus, Michael RB, Williams KNS. Surgery of the anus, rectum & colon, vol. 1. 3rd ed. Philadelphia: Saunders Elsevier; 2008. p. 517.
3. Senapati A, Cripps NP, Thompson MR. Bascom's operation in the day-surgical management of symptomatic pilonidal sinus. Br J Surg. 2000;87(8):1067–70. https://doi.org/10.1046/j.1365-2168.2000.01472.x.

Suggested Reading

Bascom J. Pilonidal disease: long-term results of follicle removal. Dis Colon Rectum. 1983;26(12):800–7. https://doi.org/10.1007/BF02554755.

Iesalnieks I, Ommer A. The management of pilonidal sinus. Dtsch Arztebl Int. 2019;116(1-2):12–21. https://doi.org/10.3238/arztebl.2019.0012.

Koskinen K, Harju J, Hermunen K. Long-term results for pit-picking and flap procedures in primary pilonidal sinus disease. BMC Surg. 2023;23(1):99. https://doi.org/10.1186/s12893-023-02014-6.

Nordon IM, Senapati A, Cripps NP. A prospective randomized controlled trial of simple Bascom's technique versus Bascom's cleft closure for the treatment of chronic pilonidal disease. Am J Surg. 2009;197(2):189–92. https://doi.org/10.1016/j.amjsurg.2008.01.020.

Sacrococcygeal Pilonidal Sinus Disease: LASER Treatment in PNS Sinus LASER Therapy (SiLaT) a.k.a Sinus Laser-Assisted Closure (SiLaC) or Pilonidal Sinus Laser Treatment (PiLaT)

23

Abstract

- Factors required to form and maintain the pilonidal sinus disease are enumerated.
- Importance of pit excision is well-established part of the procedure and is done with skin punch. Methods to remove the hair are explained.
- Pseudo-epithelium of the sinus cavity is ablated with LASER energy. Equipment and LASER fibre required are shown with pictures.
- Steps involved in the procedure are explained fully with clinical photographs and videos.
- Complications of the procedure along with their prevention and management are compiled in a table.
- Tips and tricks are suggested to further make the procedure safe and effective.
- A table to show the results of SiLaC/SiLaT from scientific literature is added.
- "References" and "Suggested Reading" sections are to make the reader aware of the scientific evidence available to date.

Supplementary Information The online version contains supplementary material available at https://doi.org/10.1007/978-981-96-6190-9_23. The videos can be accessed individually by clicking the DOI link in the accompanying figure caption or by scanning this link with the SN More Media App.

23.1 What One Should Know Before the Procedure

- A sinus to persist, there remain following factors:
  - Epithelised tract—pits in this case.
  - Foreign body—hair in this case.
  - Persistent infection—infected granulation tissue and recurrent infection from the skin in this case.
- That is why Lord and Millar, way back in 1965, gave a strong statement that if the hair is removed and free drainage allowed, the sinus will heal. Midline pits have been found in association with a pilonidal sinus and it is suggested that these must be removed to avoid recurrence [1].
- A method is described to achieve desired results. After cleansing hair and debris from the tract, LASER energy fulgurates the granulation tissue or pseudo-epithelium of the tract [2].
- Pits are excised with 1–2 mm skin margin.
- It is a minimally invasive procedure which can be done under local anaesthesia and can be repeated without any skin excision.

23.2 Indications

- PNS cases Tezel type III, IV except midline wounds larger than 1 cm (Fig. 23.1).

S. K. Singla, K. Mital, *Operative Manual of Minimally Invasive and LASER Ano-proctology*,
https://doi.org/10.1007/978-981-96-6190-9_23

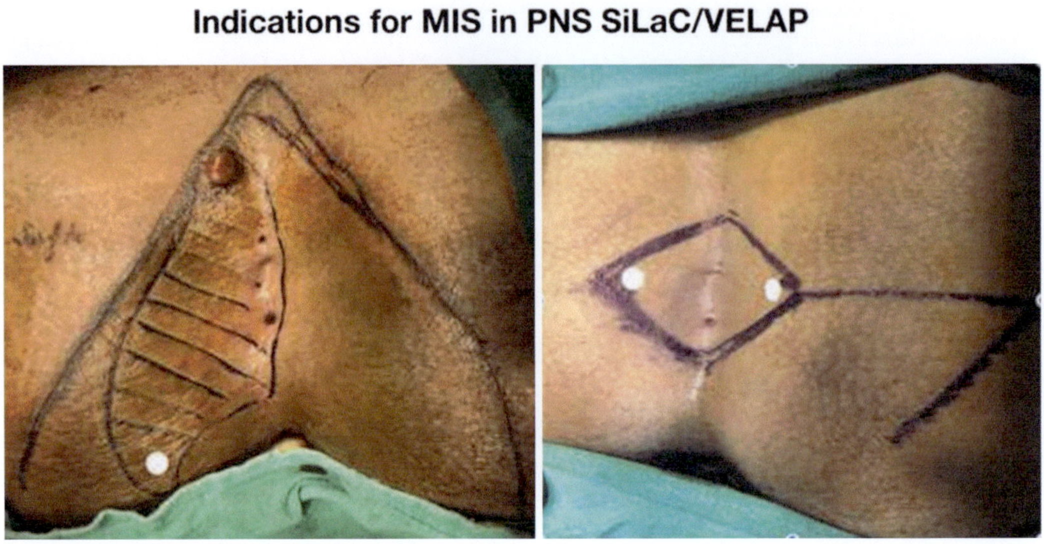

Fig. 23.1 Cases which were earlier managed by flaps can be easily managed with SiLaC/VELAP with decreased morbidity and almost same short-term recurrence VELAP-video endoscopic LASER ablation of pilonidal sinus

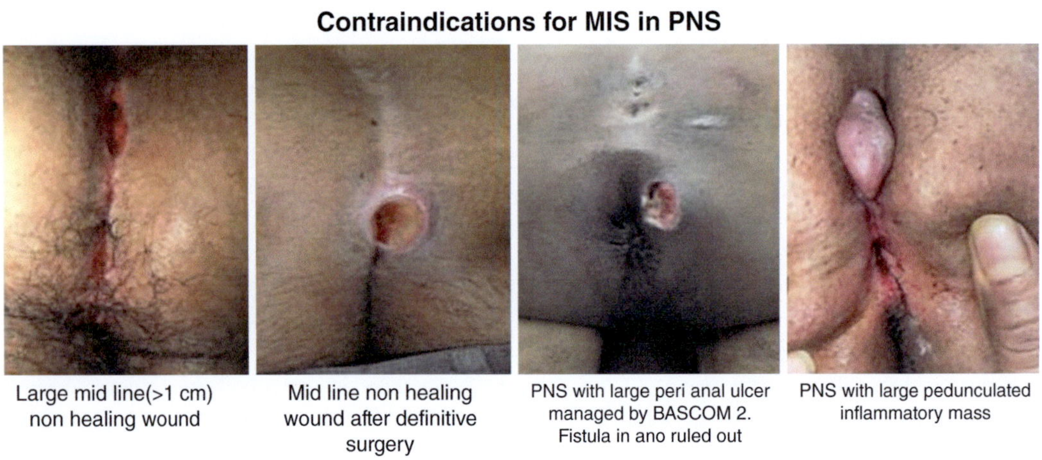

Fig. 23.2 PNS cases which need good skin cover by a flap

23.3 Contra-Indications

- Midline non-healing wounds larger than 1 cm (Fig. 23.2).
- Midline wound failure after previous surgery (Fig. 23.2).
- Unusual cases as shown are better managed with flaps as of today (Fig. 23.2).

23.4 Equipment (Fig. 23.3)

- Pads and sheets to make prone-position.
- Sterile sheets.
- Number 11 surgical blade or skin biopsy punch (optional).
- 1470 nm diode LASER machine and radial fibre.

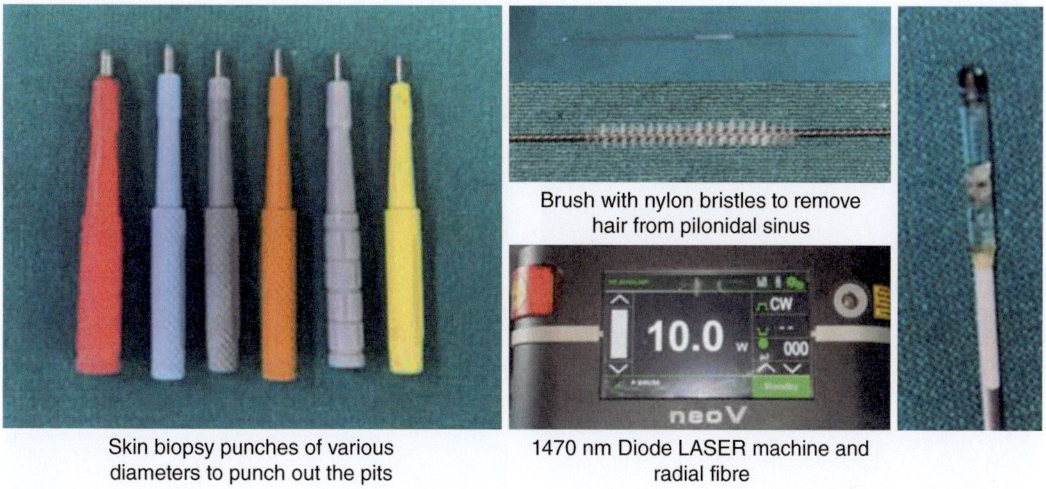

Fig. 23.3 Additional equipment required for SiLAT/SiLaC

- Volkman's scoupe.
- Fine brush with nylon bristles.
- 4.0 nylon suture on cutting needle.

- Tooth forceps.
- Sterile dressing material.

23.5 Procedure (Video 23.1 and 23.2)

- Pre-operative epilation is done by epilatory cream.
- We always check for any hypersensitivity to cream by application of cream on the inner side of forearm of nondominant hand (patch test).
- Take a photograph of the sacrococcygeal area on mobile phone and then enlarge the picture to see all pits.
- Patient lies prone with all bony-prominences padded well.
- Prone jack-knife position is made in case one wants to assess anal opening for any suspicious connection with the anal canal.
- Prophylactic antibiotics ceftriaxone 1 g is given with induction of anaesthesia.
- Strap the area to wide open the natal cleft (Fig. 23.4).

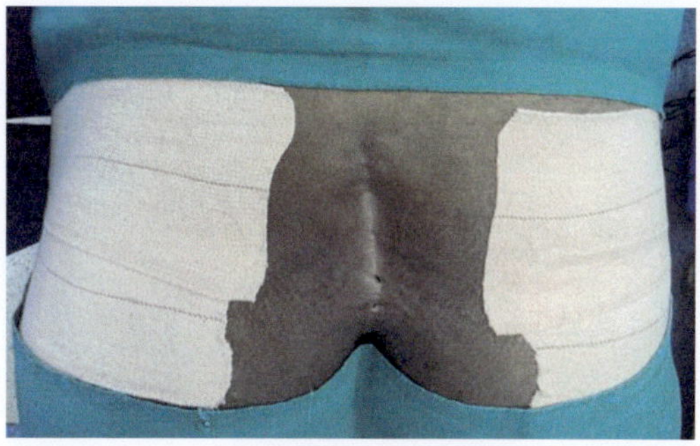

Fig. 23.4 Buttocks strapped to open the natal cleft

- Sterile draping is done.
- Local anaesthesia is instituted with combination of lignocaine 2% and bupivicaine 0.25%.

- Spinal or general anaesthesia can be given as situation demands.
- Planning on table is done as per position of pits and secondary openings. One can instil diluted methylene blue from one opening to check for communicating pits (Fig. 23.5).
- Removal of hair is done with artery forceps (Fig. 23.6).
- Embedded hair can be removed with small bottle brush (Fig. 23.7).
- Excise the pits with 11 no. blade by taking 1–2 mm margin all around.

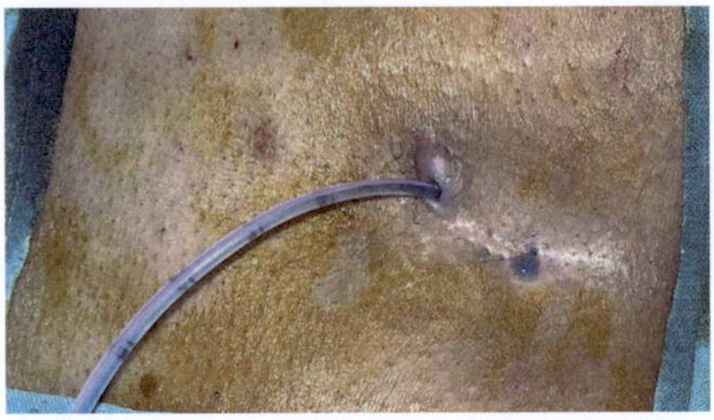

Fig. 23.5 Instillation of diluted dye shows communicating pits

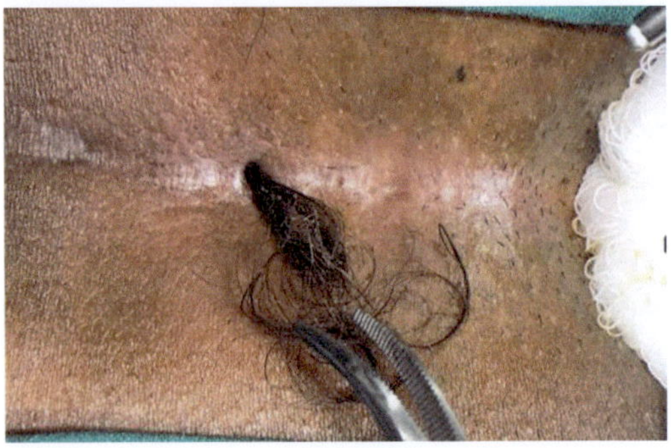

Fig. 23.6 Removal of hair with curved artery forceps

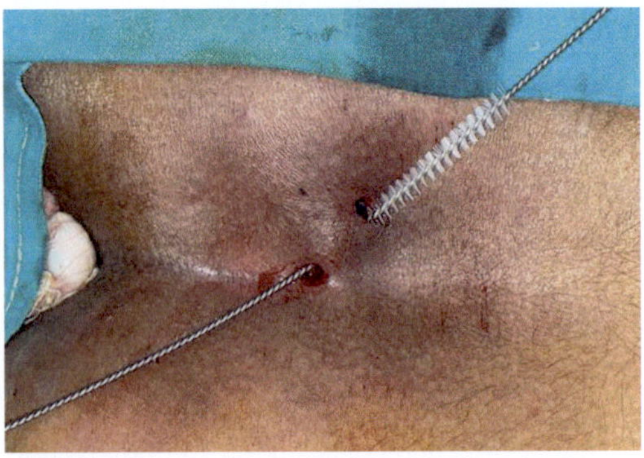

Fig. 23.7 Brush removes the most stubborn hair

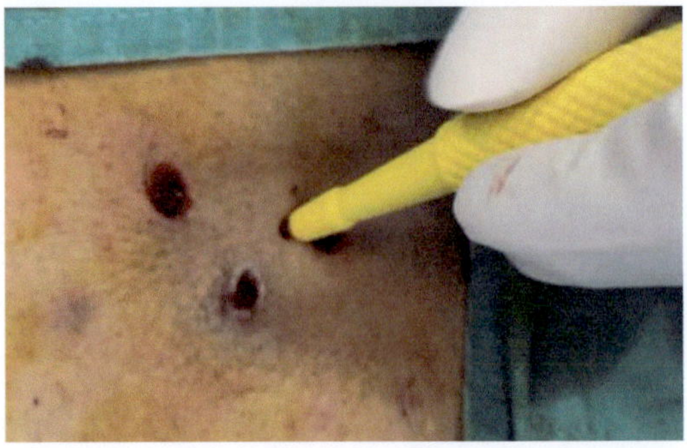

Fig. 23.8 Pit excision with skin biopsy punch

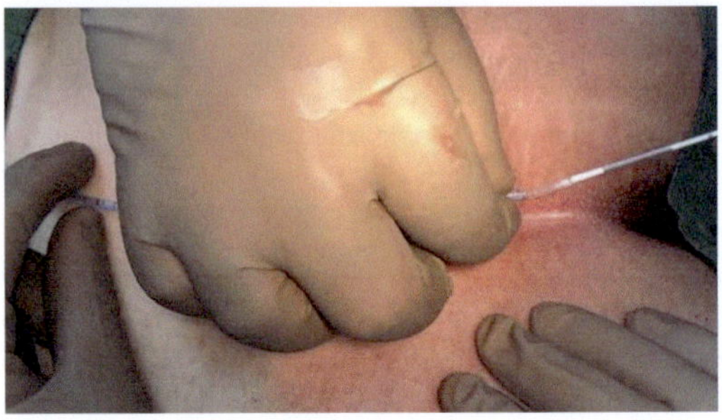

Fig. 23.9 Loading radial LASER fibre in infant feeding tube for protection

- We excise the pits with skin punch of appropriate size (diameter 2 mm more than the pit diameter) (Fig. 23.8).
- Fulgration of pseudo-epithelium of the tract is done by LASER fibre. Always wear LASER protective eye glasses.
- 1470 nm diode LASER radial fibre is inserted in the sinus cavity by rail roading it—in an infant feeding tube of 10 F size (Fig. 23.9). LASER fibre tip is taken to one extreme end.

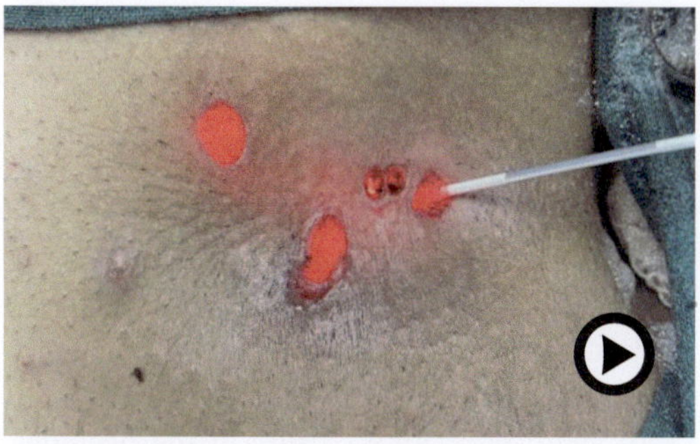

Fig. 23.10 1470 nm diode LASER, radial fibre used to deliver 10 watts in continuous mode fibre withdrawl @ 1 mm/s. Video 23.1 SiLaT/SiLaC procedure (▶ https://doi.org/10.1007/000-hqd)

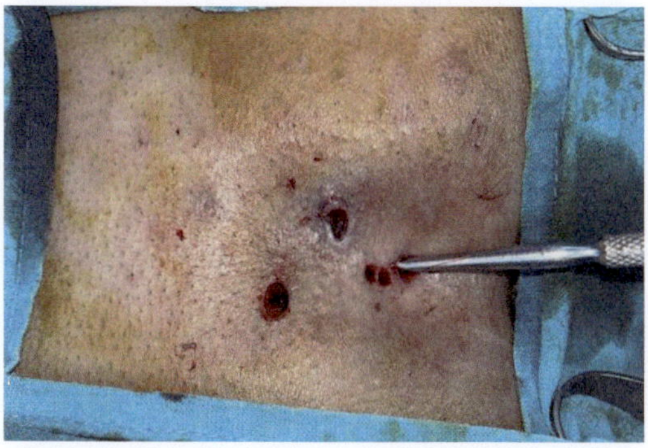

Fig. 23.11 Sinus cavity and tracts curetted with fine Volkman's scoupe

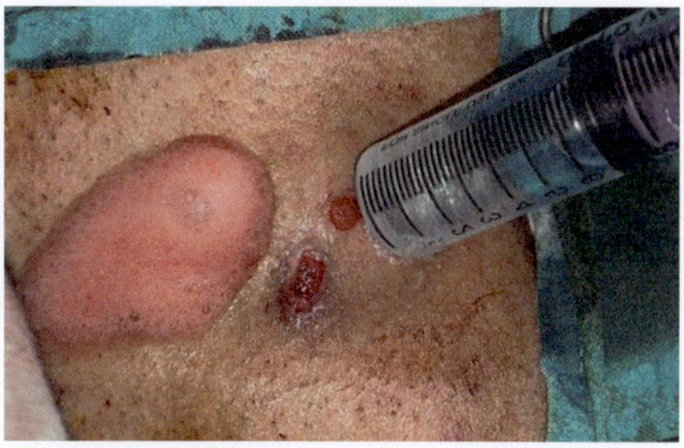

Fig. 23.12 Lavage the tract with normal saline and hydrogen peroxide solution

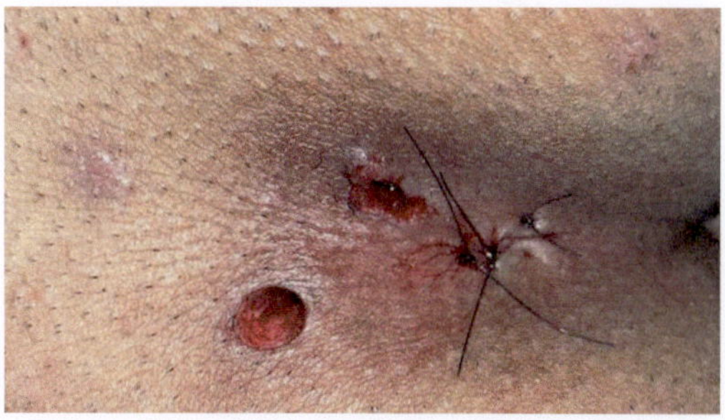

Fig. 23.13 Midline wounds stitched with vertical mattress 4.0 nylon sutures lateral wound left open for drainage

- LASER energy 10 watts is given in continuous mode by withdrawing fibre @ 1 mm/s (Fig. 23.10).
- After ablating pseudo-epithelium with LASERS, the tract is curetted with fine Volkman's scoupe (Fig. 23.11).

- Thoroughly lavage the tract with saline hydrogen peroxide solution and then rinse with normal saline (Fig. 23.12).

- Reinsert the LASER fibre and LASER energy is transmitted with an intent to contract the tract, fine curettage may follow.

- Wash the tract.
- Midline wounds created after excision of the pits are stitched with vertical mattress 4.0 nylon sutures on cutting needle (Fig. 23.13).

- Wound is dressed with sterile pads and covered with water-proof dressing

23.6 Complications (Table 23.1)

Table 23.1 Complications of SiLaT

Complications	Prevention	Management
Thermal damage to skin while fulguration of tract	If skin blanches, stop energy transmission and pour cold saline on the skin	Lavage with cold saline, free flow for 10 min
Premature closure of the opening of the side tract	Keep it patent by ear bud or gentle saline wash	Reopen the mouth of the opening and do mild curettage
Wound infection	Pre-operative antibiotics in case of frank pus in the tract thorough cleansing	Post-operative antibiotics as per culture sensitivity

23.7 Post-operative Advise

- Patient is discharged same evening or as per anaesthesia requirement.
- Patient is encouraged to move around and lie on back.
- We usually prescribe antibiotics for 5 days.
- Post-operative dressing on fourth post-operative day.
- To avoid premature closure of the openings, we use sterile ear buds to clean the openings.
- We press the tracts towards openings to remove any debris or sloughed out tissue.
- Fine curette can be used if debris is more.
- Another dressing on eighth post-operative day.
- Usual healing-time is 14–20 days but a few cases may take a longer time.

23.8 Tips and Tricks

- Identification of all pits is very essential. Stretch skin caudal to the anal canal and sideways by application of side-straps to wide open the natal cleft. Take a photograph of the affected area in this position with cell phone and zoom in, to check for all pits.
- Instil diluted methylene blue in one opening to check communicating pits.
- We err on the side of removing all suspicious pits than to leave any without excision.
- Bottle brush is good for removal of embedded stubborn hair in the sinus tract.
- For midline pit excision, take punch with smallest diameter appropriate for that pit on the contrary for excision of side tracts, use little oversize punch so that lateral tract does not close prematurely.
- Always wear LASER protective glasses before picking LASER fibre.
- Protect tip of radial LASER fibre by loading it in 10 F infant feeding tube (blunt tip of infant feeding tube is cut for the purpose).
- While ablating any sinus tract, use continuous wave LASER energy to avoid skip areas.
- Now a days we use Meinero's endoscope to check complete hair removal under vision before we put LASER fibre in the sinus. That is done to further improve the results (Fig. 23.14; Video 23.2).
- Curette the tract well and use H_2O_2 saline solution to flush the sinus cavity.
- While taking stitches to close the midline wounds, keep the straps and take all stitches, hold the threads in mosquito forceps.

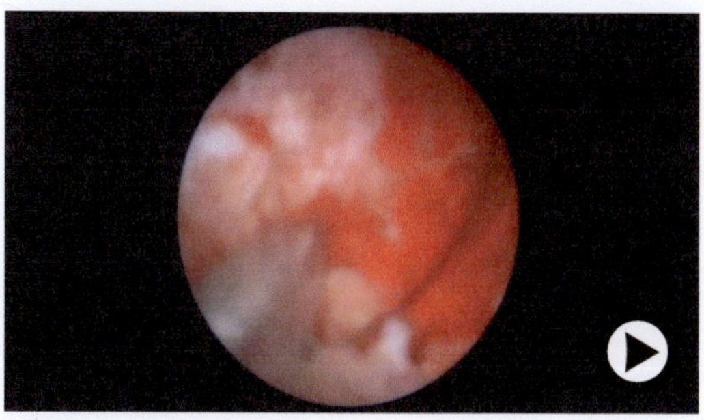

Fig. 23.14 Why do scopy. Video 23.2 SiLaT/SiLaC why do scopy (▶ https://doi.org/10.1007/000-hqc)

- Either take vertical mattress sutures or subcuticular stitch, otherwise margins tend to bend inwards.
- Remove the straps before tying knots to avoid any traction on the stitches.
- Whenever LASER energy is delivered in continuous mode, due to a rise in temperature, carbonisation occurs at the tip of LASER fibre. It increases resistance to further transmission of energy. This carbon deposition should be wiped off by a swab soaked in diluted H_2O_2 by moving the swab from tip to body of the fibre. Wiping in the reverse direction, i.e., from body to tip, may loosen the tip, which may get dislodged from the body of the fibre.
- Check the literature for results before one adapts a new procedure (Table 23.2).

Table 23.2 Comparison of results of LASER in PNS

Author and year	Healing rate	Complications
Pappas et al. (2018). (237 Pt.) [2]	90.3% first session	Wound infection
	97.8% cumulative	7.2%
	After 2 sessions	
De Decker et al. (2023) (226 Pt.) [3]	78.8% first session	Wound infection
	85.4% cumulative	8%
	After 2–3 sessions	
Horesh et al. (2023) (91) [4]	81.3%	Incomplete healing
		8.8%
		Recurrent disease
		9.9%
Sluckin et al. (2022) (311 Pt.) MC cohort study [5]	66% after 1 SiLaC	7% incomplete
	92%–98% 2–3 SiLaC	Wound closure
Comparison with flap		
Tharun Ganapathy Chitrambalam et al. (2024) [6]		8% reoccurrence in
		SiLaC
		12% reoccurrence
		Limberg

Algorithm for Sinus LASER Treatment

History/clinical examination
Define the need to treat pilonidal sinus by minimal invasive method
Anaesthesia local/spinal/GA
Position prone
Straps to open the natal cleft
Take photograph of the area and zoom in
Locate all pits and secondary openings
May use diluted dye to locate opening pits and their communication with underlying sinus cavity
Remove hair from mid line pits with curved mosquito forceps
Excise all mid line pits with skin biopsy punches
Excise secondary tract openings with skin punch
Put radial LASER fibre in the tract
Use 1470 nm diode LASER and deliver 10 watts of energy in continuous wave and withdraw fibre @1 mm/sec delivering 100 joules per cm of the tract
Pour cold saline over the skin
Curette the tracts and wash them with saline and hydrogen peroxide solution

Reinsert LASER fibre and deliver LASER energy with an intent to contract the tract
Fine curettage may be done
Wash with saline
Mid line pits are closed
Lateral openings are left open for drainage
Antiseptic occlusive dressing given

References

1. Lord PH, Millar DM. Pilonidal sinus: a simple treatment. Br J Surg. 1965;52(4):2983300. https://doi.org/10.1002/bjs.1800520413.
2. Pappas AF, Christodoulou DK. A new minimally invasive treatment of pilonidal sinus disease with the use of a diode laser: a prospective large series of patients. Colorectal Dis. 2018;20(8):O207–14. https://doi.org/10.1111/codi.14285.
3. De Decker M, Sels T, Van Hoof S, et al. Does minimally invasive laser-assisted treatment of pilonidal sinus disease live up to its expectations: a multi-center study with 226 patients. Int J Colorectal Dis. 2023;38:33. https://doi.org/10.1007/s00384-023-04324-w.
4. Horesh N, Meiri H, Anteby R, Zager Y, Maman R, Carter D, Meyer R, Nachmany I, Ram E. Outcomes of Laser-Assisted Closure (SiLaC) surgery for chronic pilonidal sinus disease. J Laparoendosc Adv Surg Tech A. 2023;33(6):556–60. https://doi.org/10.1089/lap.2022.0567.
5. Sluckin TC, Hazen SJA, Smeenk RM, Schouten R. Sinus laser-assisted closure (SiLaC®) for pilonidal disease: results of a multicentre cohort study. Tech Coloproctol. 2022;26(2):135–41. https://doi.org/10.1007/s10151-021-02550-4.
6. Chitrambalam TG, George NM, Reddy L, Christopher PJ, Selvamuthukumaran S. Sinus Laser Closure (SiLaC) with pit excision versus Limberg Flap in pilonidal disease: a prospective, randomized study. Surg Open Digest Adv. 2024;13:100126., ISSN:2667-0089. https://www.sciencedirect.com/science/article/pii/S2667008923000484. https://doi.org/10.1016/j.soda.2023.100126.

Suggested Reading

Dessily M, Charara F, Ralea S, Allé JL. Pilonidal sinus destruction with a radial laser probe: technique and first Belgian experience. Acta Chir Belg. 2017;117(3):164–8. https://doi.org/10.1080/00015458.2016.1272285.

Huurman EA, Galema HA, de Raafi CAL, Wijnhoven BPL, Toorenvliet BR, Smeenk RM. Non-excisional techniques for the treatment of intergluteal pilonidal sinus disease: a systematic review. Tech Coloproctol. 2023;27(12):1191–200. https://doi.org/10.1007/s10151-023-02870-7.

Sachin AG, Alçı E. Use of the laser in the pilonidal sinus alone or in combination with phenol. Rev Assoc Med Bras (1992). 2023;69(12):e20230740. doi:https://doi.org/10.1590/1806-9282.20230740

Tyrväinen E, Nuutinen H, Savikkomaa E. Comparison of laser ablation, simple excision, and fiap reconstruction in the treatment of pilonidal sinus disease. Lasers Med Sci. 39(1):202439. https://doi.org/10.1007/s10103-024-03993-5.

Sacrococcygeal Pilonidal Sinus Disease: Endoscopic Pilonidal Sinus Treatment (EPSiT)/Video-Assisted Ablation of Pilonidal Sinus (VAAPS) Variant-Video Endoscopic LASER Ablation of Pilonidal Sinus (VELAPS)/LASER-Assisted Endoscopic Pilonidal Sinus Treatment (LEPSiT)

24

Abstract

Many minimally invasive methods have been described to treat pilonidal sinus disease.

None of them ensures complete removal of hair and debris under vision.

Meinero and Milone described endoscopic method (EPSiT/VAAPS) to manage pilonidal sinus disease under vision (Meinero et al, Color Dis 18(5):O164–O170. https://doi.org/10.1111/codi.13322. PMID: 26946340, 2016; Milone et al, JAMA Surg 151(6):547–553. https://doi.org/10.1001/jamasurg.2015.5233. PMID: 26819186, 2016).

Indications and contraindications of endoscopic method are described and shown with clinical photographs as we observed over the years.

Operative steps of the procedure as we follow today, are elaborated with operative photographs and videos.

Care of the scope and delicate endo-instruments is stressed upon.

Methods to use LASER, instead of monopolar current, are explained.

"Can we combine endoscopic method with a small flap for benefit of the patient?" Is a food for thought and have been demonstrated with clinical photographs of a young lady.

Tips and Tricks will help the operator to achieve desired results and save time and money.

Complications are reported in table form for ready reference.

- "References", "Suggested Reading" and viewing are to further enhance the knowledge and skills.

Supplementary Information The online version contains supplementary material available at https://doi.org/10.1007/978-981-96-6190-9_24. The videos can be accessed individually by clicking the DOI link in the accompanying figure caption or by scanning this link with the SN More Media App.

S. K. Singla, K. Mital, *Operative Manual of Minimally Invasive and LASER Ano-proctology*,
https://doi.org/10.1007/978-981-96-6190-9_24

24.1 What One Should Know Before the Procedure

Minimal invasive procedures without endoscope cannot ensure complete removal of hair and debris from the sinus cavity.

Under vision fulgration of pseudo-epithelium either by monopolar current or LASER ensures complete ablation of sinus cavity lining.

Pit excision by skin punch removes whole epithelial tube (Macroni of BASCOM) connecting skin surface with underlying sinus cavity.

24.2 Indications

- All pilonidal sinus (PNS) cases Tezel type II, III, IV and V except midline wounds larger than 1 cm, can be managed by endoscopic method (Figs. 24.1 and 24.2).
- Cases with secondary pits outside the navicular area, or in-anal triangle can be easily managed with endoscopic means.

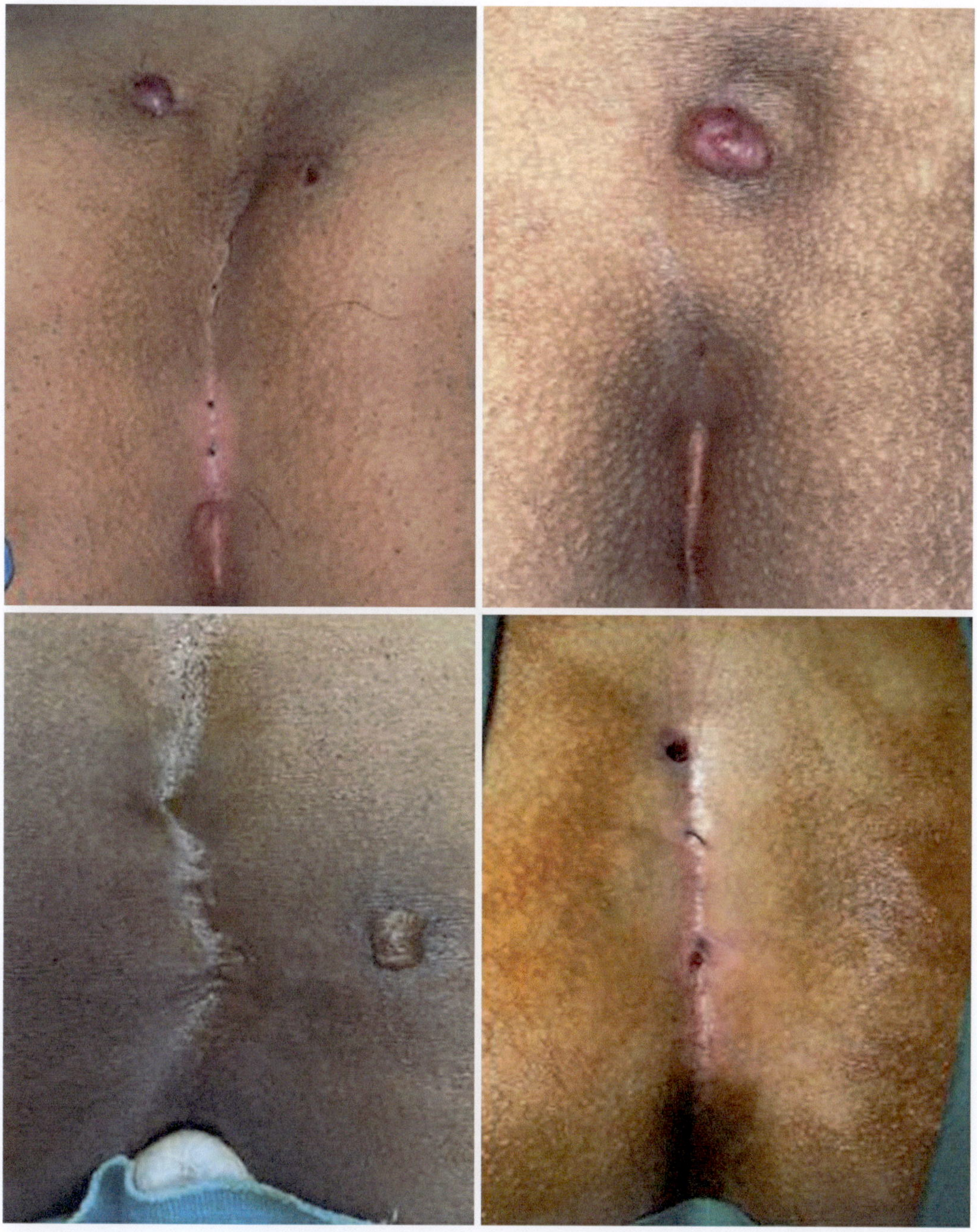

Fig. 24.1 Cases which were earlier managed by flaps can be easily managed with EPSiT/VAAPS with decreased morbidity and almost same short term recurrence

24.3 Contraindications

- Midline non-healing wounds larger than 1 cm (Fig. 24.3). Such patients need good skin cover.
- Midline wound failure after previous surgery (Fig. 24.4).
- Unusual cases as shown are better managed with flaps as of today (Figs. 24.5 and 24.6).

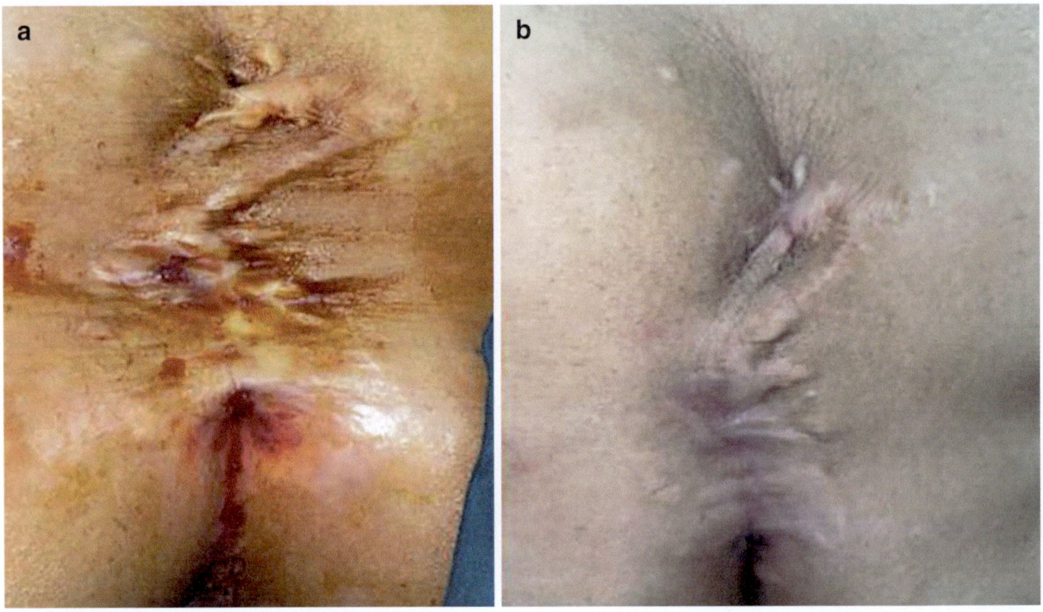

Fig. 24.2 (**a**) Case of recurrence after flap in a young lady. (**b**) Managed with LEPSiT

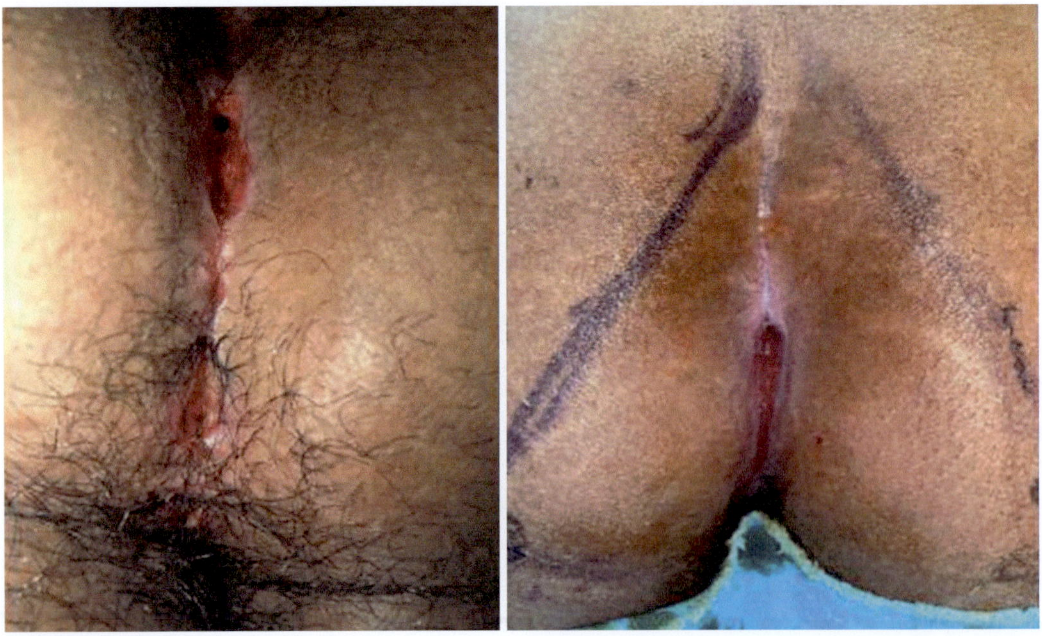

Fig. 24.3 Large midline non-healing wound (>1 cm) needs good skin cover by flap

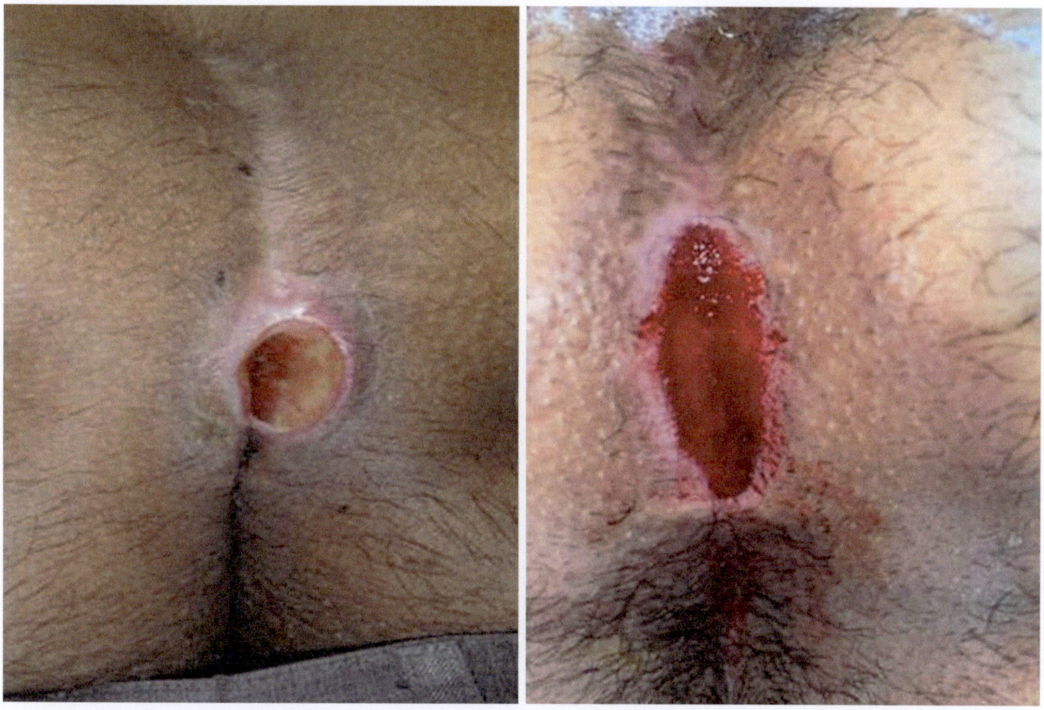

Fig. 24.4 Midline non-healing wounds after midline closure better managed with asymmetrical closure (Bascom cleft lift procedure)

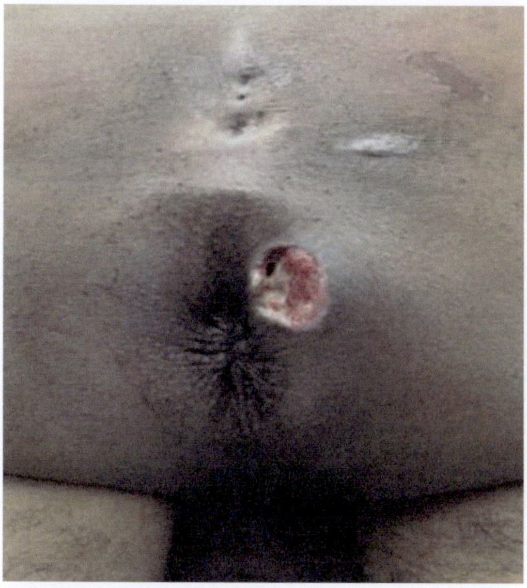

Fig. 24.5 PNS with large peri-anal ulcer managed by BASCOM 2. Fistula in ano ruled out

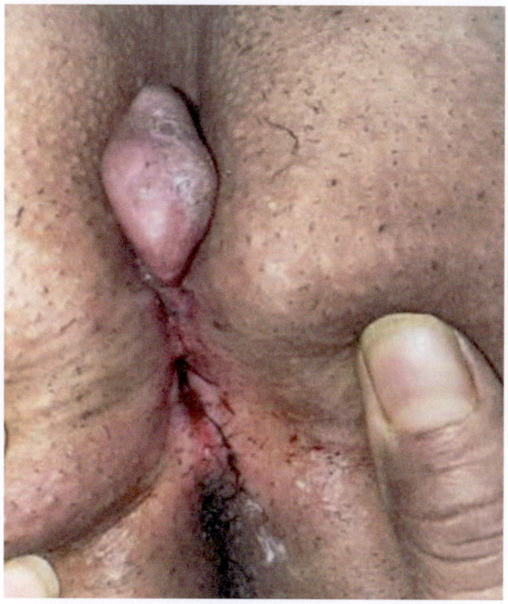

Fig. 24.6 PNS with large pedunculated inflammatory mass managed with BASCOM 2

24.4 Equipment

- Pads and sheets to make prone and prone-jack knife position.
- Sterile sheets.
- Skin biopsy punches.
- Meinero's scope (Figs. 24.7 and 24.8).
- Saline and glycine large packs/glycine and mannitol 1% solution.
- Endo forceps.
- Endo brush.
- Monopolar bug bee electrode.
- LASER machine and fibre optional.
- Volkman's scoupe.
- 4.0 nylon suture on cutting needle.
- Sterile dressing material.

See Video 24.1

Video showing Meinero's scope and instrumentation.

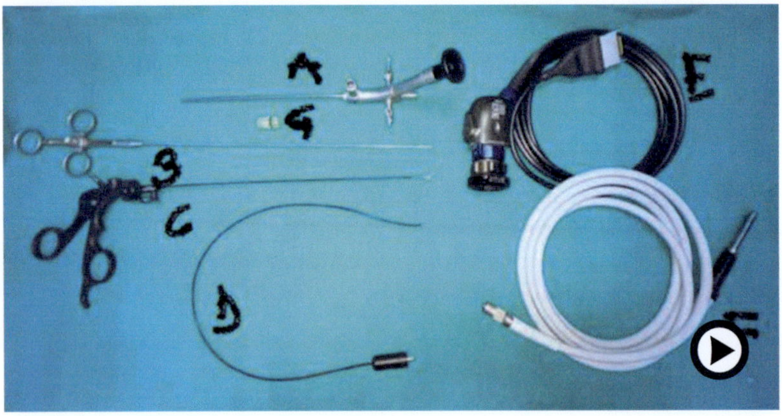

Fig. 24.7 Meinero's scope Storz (A) and associated accessories, brush (B), forceps (C), bug bee monopolar electrode (D), camera (E), fibroptic cable (F), water tight washer (G). Video 24.1 Meinero's scope and instrumentation (▶ https://doi.org/10.1007/000-hqg)

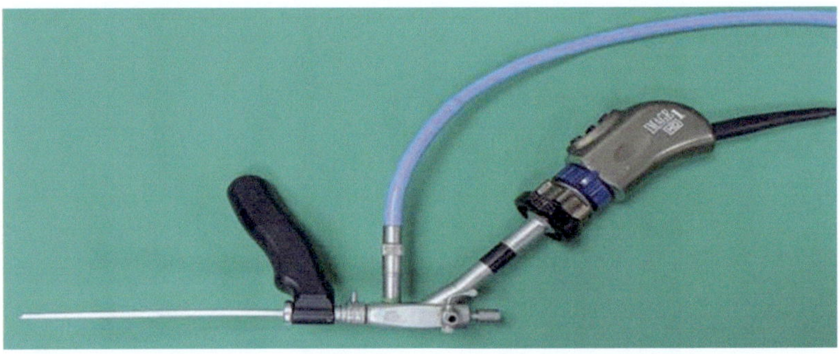

Fig. 24.8 New Meinero's scope has reversible handle which makes it easy to use in pilonidal sinus management

24.5 Procedure (Video 24.2 EPSiT Procedure) [1, 2]

- Pre-op epilation by epilatory cream.
- We always check for any hypersensitivity to cream by application of cream on inner side of forearm of non-dominant hand (patch test).
- Take a photograph of the area on mobile phone and then enlarge the picture to see all pits (Figs. 24.9 and 24.10).
- In endoscopic procedure, there is no need to mark navicular area.
- Patient lies prone with all bony prominences padded well.
- Prone-jack knife in case we want to assess anal opening for any suspicious connection with anal canal.
- General anaesthesia with endotracheal tube to protect the respiratory system.
- Though spinal anaesthesia can be given but it is uncomfortable for the patient if procedure gets prolonged.
- In case of very short tract, local anaesthesia can be instituted if patient's temperament allows.
- Prophylactic antibiotics ceftriaxone 1 g is given with induction of anaesthesia.
- Strap the area to wide open the natal cleft (Fig. 23.4).
- Sterile draping is done and is covered by water-proof sheet.
- Window is created in waterproof sheet to uncover operative area (Fig. 24.9).
- Suction is kept to prevent undue water spilling on sheets and in operation theatre.
- Attachment of camera and light source to endoscope is done.
- Attach tubing of fluid (either saline or glycine mannitol mixture) to inlet point of scope.
- White balancing is done.
- Set moon-crescent of obturator at 6 0' position.
- Planning on table is done as per position of pits and secondary openings.

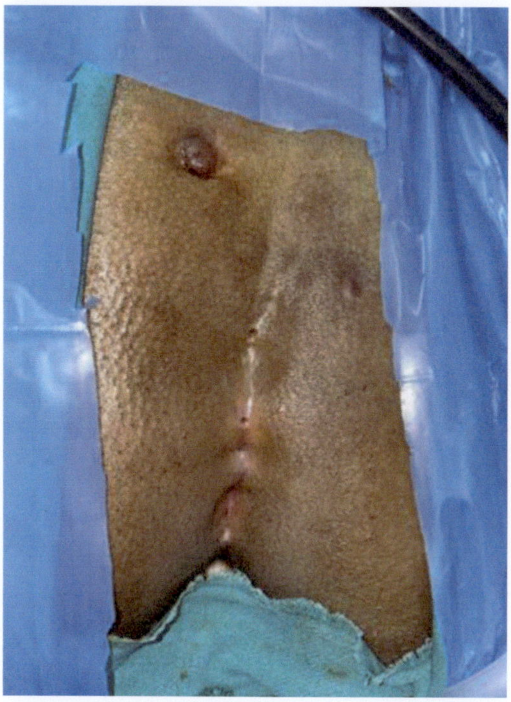

Fig. 24.9 Picture of the diseased area, patient prone with buttocks strapped. Note the window created in water proof sheet

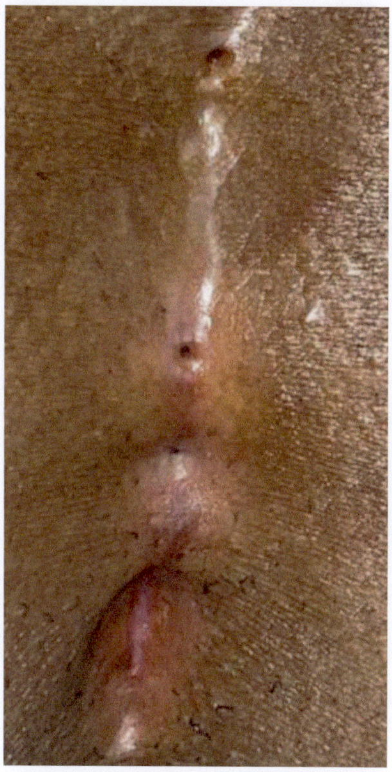

Fig. 24.10 Picture enlarged to see the pits clearly

24.5.1 Diagnostic Phase

- Opening of tract can be dilated with artery forceps, Haeger dilator or excised with cautery.
- Scope is inserted in the sinus tract with fluid running through the channel. One can use path-finder or pressure device in fluid bottle to maintain pressure in the tract to keep it open (see the instrumentation Video 24.1).
- Keep the scope at an acute angle with skin surface as disease is subcutaneous (Fig. 24.11).
- More obtuse angle at entry, can perforate the sinus wall and one may enter soft tissue around the tract (Fig. 24.12).
- Sinus cavity in visualised for hair, debris and inflammatory tissue lining.

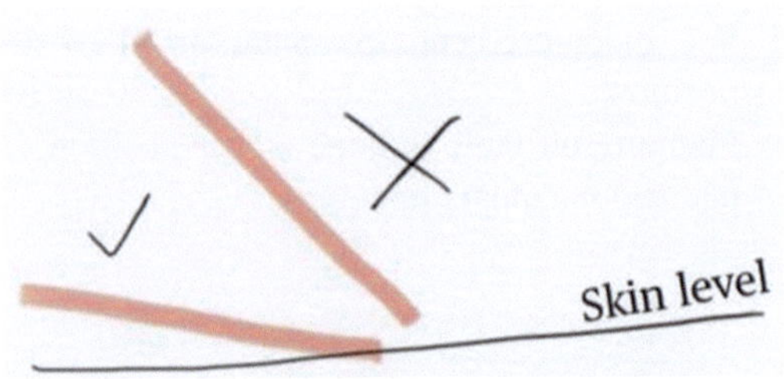

Fig. 24.11 Angle of the scope with skin should be acute as disease is subcutaneous

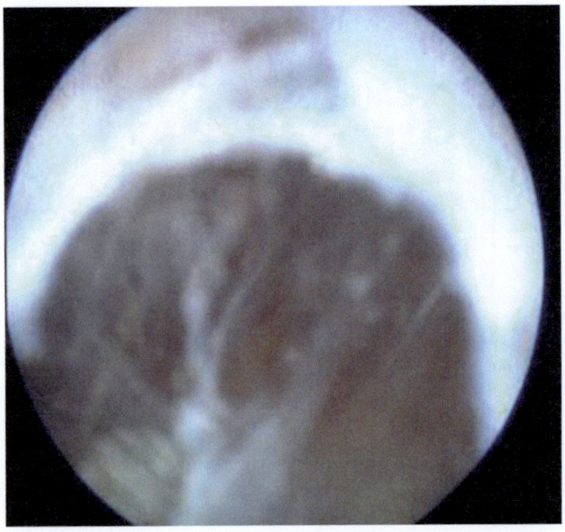

Fig. 24.12 Cobweb appearance on screen due to perforation of the tract

24.5.2 Therapeutic Phase

- Removal of hair and debris is done with endo forceps (Figs. 24.13 and 24.14).
- Embedded hair can be removed with endo brush.
- Fulgration of pseudo epithelium of the tract is done by bug bee monopolar electrode or LASER fibre (Fig. 24.15).
- Curettage is done with Volkman's scoupe.
- Tract is washed with saline and hydrogen peroxide mixture.
- Reinspection of the sinus tract is done to check any hair and debris.
- Re-fulguration, if required, is done.
- Excision of pits is done by skin punch (Fig. 24.16).

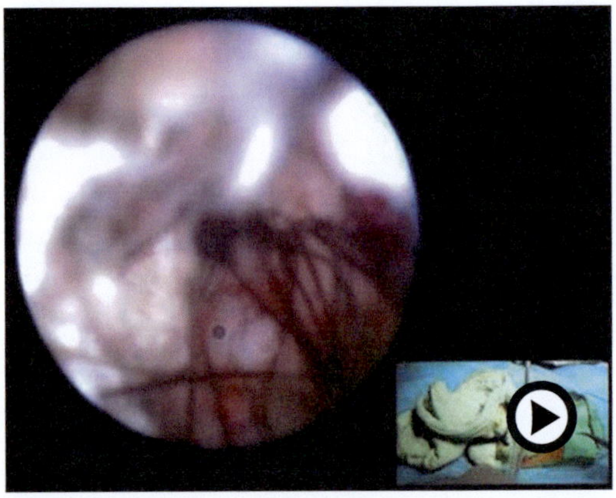

Fig. 24.13 Hair in PNS being removed with endo forceps. Video 24.2 EPSiT procedure (▶ https://doi.org/10.1007/000-hqf)

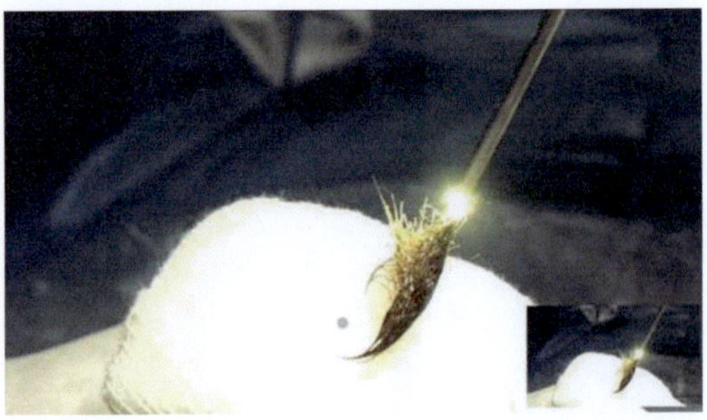

Fig. 24.14 Tuft of hair in endo forceps tip

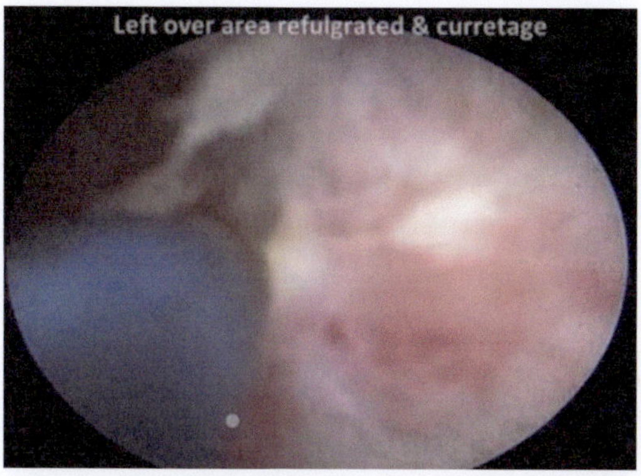

Fig. 24.15 Pseudo epithelium and granulation tissue fulgration by monopolar ball point tip/bug bee electrode

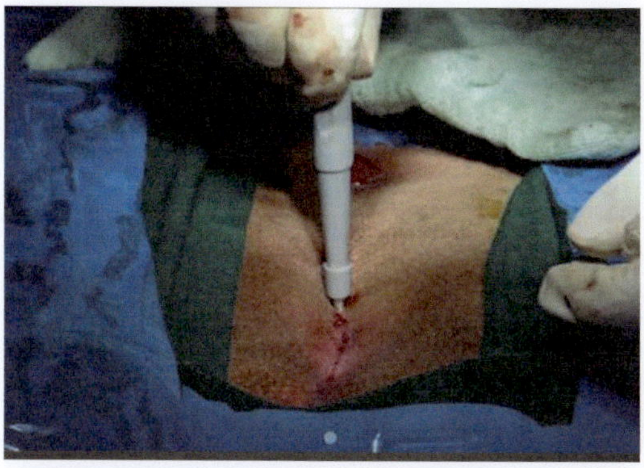

Fig. 24.16 Skin punch removes the pit by clear margins

- Insertion of scope is done from other side to have opposite side view of the tract.
- Check for any hair or debris and remove it.
- If there is history of drainage of abscess, check any residual tract on that side and one can punch out with large skin punch to fully explore the area with scope in bidirectional manner.
- Mid-line wounds created by excision of primary pits are closed with vertical mattress sutures of 3 or 4.0 nylon on cutting needle. Lateral wounds are kept open for drainage (Fig. 24.17).
- Pass sutures with straps on.

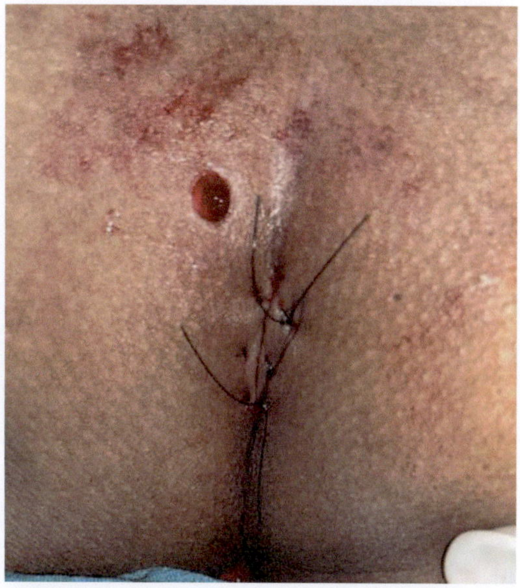

Fig. 24.17 Mid-line wounds closed with vertical mattress sutures of 3.0 nylon and lateral wound kept open

- Before tying the sutures, remove the straps to relax the skin margins.
- Dress the wound with application of ointment.
- Patient is advised to lie on back in contrast to flap surgery.
- *See* procedure Video 24.2

24.6 Post-operative Care of the Wound (Fig. 24.18)

- Avoid premature closure of lateral wound, use sterile earbuds to keep it open.
- Epilate the area till all wounds heal.
- Healing usually takes place within 14–20 days, though at times it may take longer time.
- To prevent long-term recurrence, LASER hair reduction in sacrococcygeal area with 10 cm diameter is suggested though evidence is not very strong.

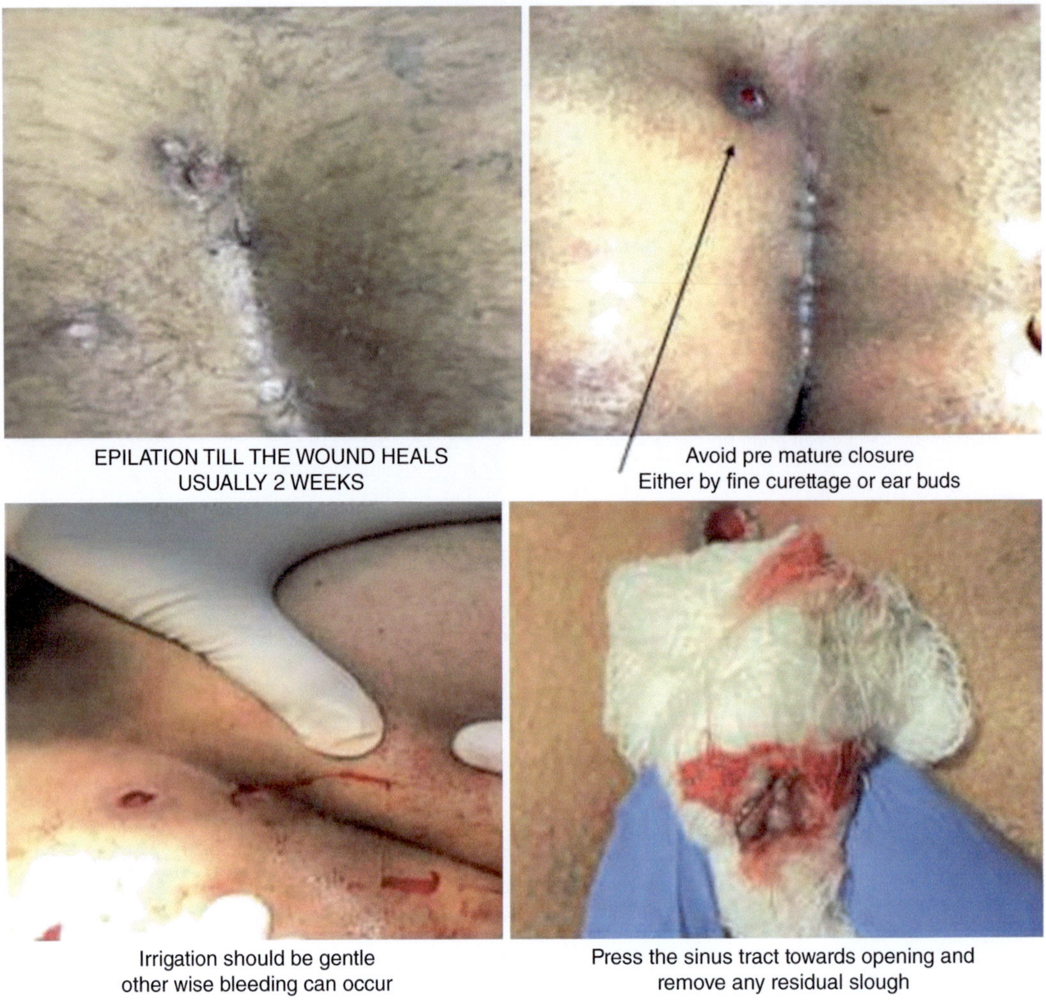

Fig. 24.18 Post-operative care of the wound after endoscopic management

24.7 Tips and Tricks

- Select your case well, non-healing mid-line wounds more than 1 cm in length are not good candidates for endoscopic management, better give good skin cover.
- Practice instrument attachment and navigation outside as for any new procedure.
- For use and care of scope and 2 mm instruments, one can refer to chapter on VAAFT.
- While inserting scope in the tract keep scope at an acute angle with the skin, as tract is subcutaneous. An obtuse angle may rupture the tract in the beginning with consequent fluid dispersing in buttocks.
- Debridement with endo-forceps helps in keeping area clean.
- If the tract is full of hair, there may not be any space inside for fluid to dilate the sinus cavity. Be gentle, slowly remove the hair and debris. Once space is created, irrigation fluid dilates the tract and visibility improves.
- If there is no exit to fluid, then also visibility may be an issue, punch out one pit. Or if there is no other pit or exit point, one can create one at other end over a probe.

- Keep monopolar electrode tip or LASER fibre tip 1 cm from lens of the scope to avoid thermal damage.
- Always wear LASER protective glasses even if you are working inside the tract, to prevent eye damage in case of inadvertent withdrawal of LASER fibre.
- Close mid-line wounds by vertical mattress sutures.
- Leave the lateral wound open and enlarged for drainage.
- Avoid premature closure of lateral wound, use sterile earbuds to keep it open.
- Epilate the area till all wounds heal.
- LASER hair reduction in the sacrococcygeal area is advised to decrease the reoccurrence.

24.8 Variations of the Technique

- In VAAPS Melieno used 4 mm hysteroscope.
- Instead of monopolar current one can use 1470 diode LASER energy in video endoscopic LASER ablation of pilonidal sinus (VELAP) aka LASER-assisted EPSiT (LEPSiT).
- With LASER, glycine is not required, instead one can use saline.
- Pass LASER fibre through the working channel, take fibre tip 1 cm out of the scope and start delivering energy 10 watts continuous wave while withdrawing scope and fibre assembly together @ 1 mm/second (Fig. 24.19; Video 24.3).
- It is good idea to decrease the saline flow to minimum so that walls of the sinus cavity fall upon the fibre.
- Another way is that after completion of diagnostic phase and removal of hair, remove the scope and put LASER fibre in the cavity without scope and fulgrate as in SiLaT. It speeds up the process (Fig. 24.20; Video 24.4).
- Then do check endoscopy and curette the tract.

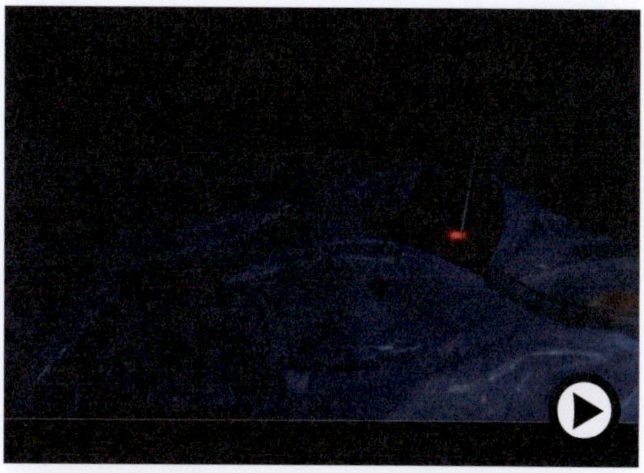

Fig. 24.19 LASER with scope. Video 24.3 LASER with scope (▶ https://doi.org/10.1007/000-hqe)

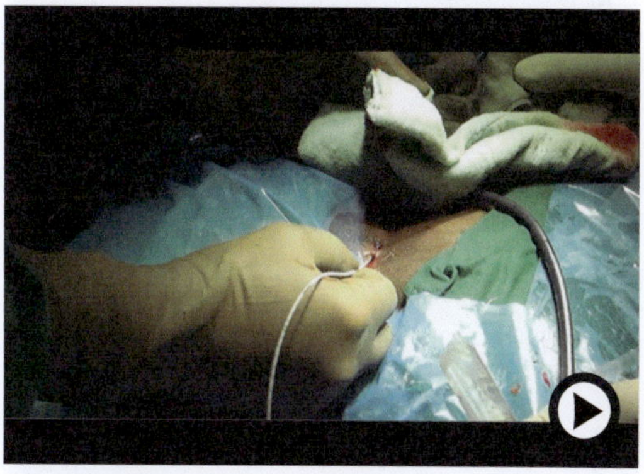

Fig. 24.20 Video Open LASER after scopy. Video 24.4 Open LASER after scopy (▶ https://doi.org/10.1007/000-hqh)

- Flush with saline thoroughly.
- Re-insert the LASER fibre to deliver LASER energy at 10 watts continuous wave, with drawing fibre @ 1 mm/second with an intent to contract the cavity and tracts.

24.9 Hybrid Approach

Combined endoscopic method with small-flap procedure in a case of PNS disease with sacrococcygeal pit led to successful management with minimum morbidity (Figs. 24.21, 24.22, and 24.23).

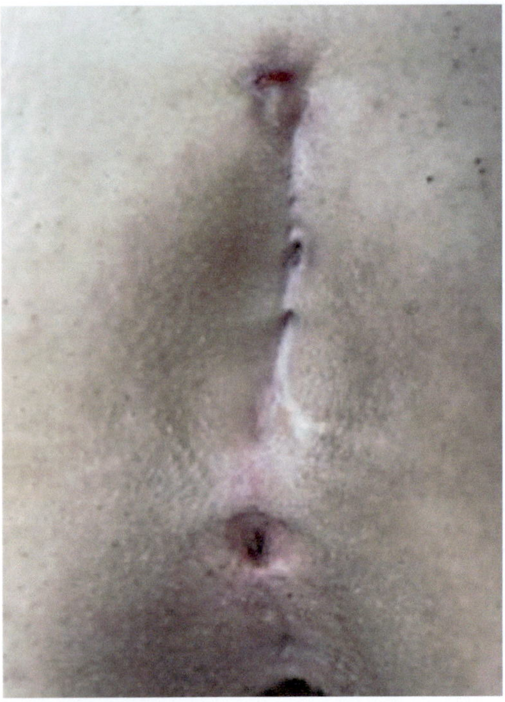

Fig. 24.21 PNS disease in a young lady with lower large pit which also contained hair but no communication with the main disease area

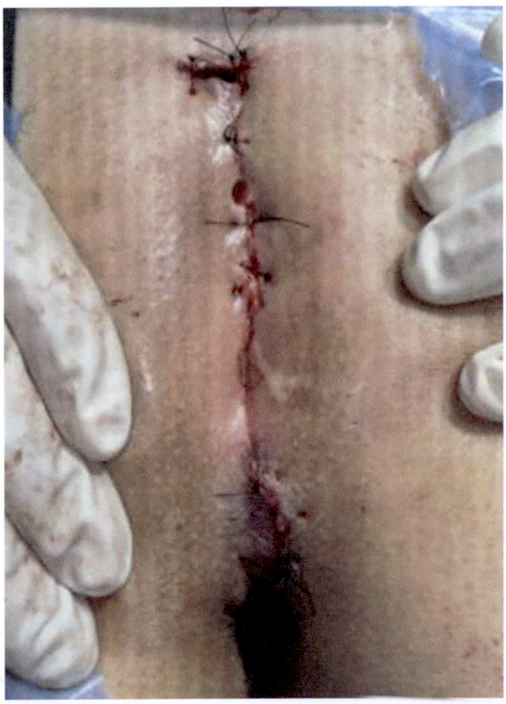

Fig. 24.22 PNS disease treated with endoscopic method and lower dimple pit filled by a small flap

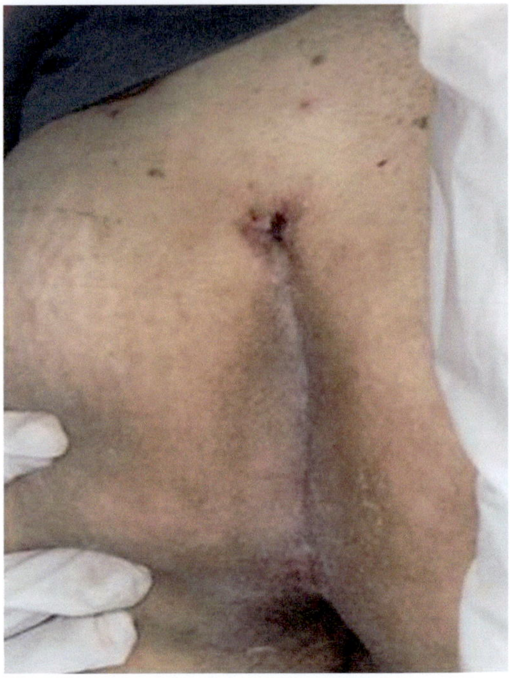

Fig. 24.23 Complete healing after 14 days

Table 24.1 Complications of endoscopic PNS treatment

Complications	Prevention	Management
Losing the tract appearance of cobweb on screen Fig. 24.12	Entry angle of scope should be acute with the skin Fig. 24.11	Stop infusing saline or glycine under pressure withdraw the scope and find the tract by visualising the granulation tissue
Thermal damage to skin while fulgration of ceiling of tract	If skin blanches stop energy transmission and pour cold saline on the skin	Lavage with cold saline free flow for 10 minutes
Premature closure of the opening of the side tract	To keep patency/open by earbud or gentle saline Wash	Reopen the mouth of the opening and do mild curettage

24.10 Complications (Table 24.1)

For complications of putting scope, small instruments and prevention of damage to instruments, one can refer to Table 15.1 in Chap. 15 on VAAFT.

Algorithm for Endoscopic Management of PNS

History and clinical examination
Define the role of MIS
Check Meneiro's scope and trolley for camera and monitor
Layout scope and accessories on separate trolley
Define the pits and secondary sinus
Dilate pit to accommodate tip of the scope
Rush glycine mannitol solution through the fluid channel
Do diagnostic phase of EPSiT
Define sinus cavity and tracts
Punch out the pits
Therapeutic phase
Remove hair and debris with endo forceps and endo brush
Put bug bee electrode through instrument channel
Keep tip of ball point/bug bee 1 cm out of the working channel
Fulgrate lining of sinus cavity with monopolar electrical current by withdrawing scope with electrode
Side to side movement of scope is also done
Check whole lining should be brown but not charred
Curette the cavity with Volkman's scoop and fine debridement with endo brush
Irrigate with H_2O_2 saline solution using syringe from water channel
Use suction tip to suck water flowing out from tract to avoid wetting of sheets and floor
Check for completeness of debridement under vision
Re-fulgrate left out areas of granulation and curette again if required
Wash thoroughly
Achieve haemostasis by bug bee
Enter scope from cranial as well caudal side or from side channel to ensure complete debridement under vision
Close mid line wounds with 3.0 nylon vertical mattress sutures
Apply water proof anti septic dressing

References

1. Meinero P, Stazi A, Carbone A, Fasolini F, Regusci L, La Torre M. Endoscopic pilonidal sinus treatment: a prospective multicentre trial. Color Dis. 2016;18(5):O164–70. https://doi.org/10.1111/codi.13322. PMID: 26946340.
2. Milone M, Fernandez LM, Musella M, Milone F. Safety and efficacy of minimally invasive video-assisted ablation of pilonidal sinus: a randomized clinical trial. JAMA Surg. 2016;151(6):547–53. https://doi.org/10.1001/jamasurg.2015.5233. PMID: 26819186.

Suggested Reading

Dönmez M, Uludag M. Evaluation of the early outcomes of laser-endoscopic pilonidal sinus treatment combination and comparison with the combination of cautery-phenol-endoscopic pilonidal sinus treatment. Cureus. 2022;14(7):e26948. https://doi.org/10.7759/cureus.26948. PMID: 35989794; PMCID: PMC9378937.

Giarratano G, Toscana C, Shalaby M, Buonomo O, Petrella G, Sileri P. Endoscopic pilonidal sinus treatment: long-term results of a prospective series. JSLS. 2017;21(3):e2017.00043. https://doi.org/10.4293/JSLS.2017.00043. PMID: 28904522; PMCID: PMC5592432.

Gulcu B, Ozturk E. Endoscopic pilonidal sinus treatment vs. laser-assisted endoscopic pilonidal sinus treatment: short-term results from a retrospective case-matched study. Tech Coloproctol. 2022;26(4):271–7. https://doi.org/10.1007/s10151-021-02568-8. Epub 2022 Jan 13. PMID: 35025023.

Gulcu B, Ozturk E. Minimally invasive pilonidal sinus treatment: EPSIT versus PEBAI method. Surg Laparosc Endosc Percutan Tech. 2024;34(1):48–53. https://doi.org/10.1097/SLE.0000000000001245. PMID: 37971236.

Huurman EA, Galema HA, de Raafi CAL, Wijnhoven BPL, Toorenvliet BR, Smeenk RM. Non-excisional techniques for the treatment of intergluteal pilonidal sinus disease: a systematic review. Tech Coloproctol. 2023;27(12):1191–200. https://doi.org/10.1007/s10151-023-02870-7. Epub 2023 Nov 6. PMID: 37930579; PMCID: PMC10638206.

Mahmood F, Hussain A, Akingboye A. Pilonidal sinus disease: review of current practice and prospects for endoscopic treatment. Ann Med Surg (Lond). 2020;57:212–7. https://doi.org/10.1016/j.amsu.2020.07.050. PMID: 32793341; PMCID: PMC7415633.

Milone M, Velotti N, Manigrasso M, Milone F, Sosa Fernandez LM, De Palma GD. Video-assisted ablation of pilonidal sinus (VAAPS) versus sinusectomy for treatment of chronic pilonidal sinus disease: a comparative study. Updat Surg. 2019;71(1):179–83. https://doi.org/10.1007/s13304-018-00611-2. Epub 2018 Dec 12. PMID: 30542957.

Milone M, Velotti N, Manigrasso M, Vertaldi S, Di Lauro K, De Simone G, Cirillo V, Maione F, Gennarelli N, Sosa Fernandez LM, De Palma GD. Long-term results of a randomized clinical trial comparing endoscopic versus conventional treatment of pilonidal sinus. Int J Surg. 2020;74:81–5. https://doi.org/10.1016/j.ijsu.2019.12.033. Epub 2020 Jan 9. PMID: 31926328.

Milone M, Gallo G, Grossi U, Pelizzo P, D'Amore A, Manigrasso M, Perinotti R, La Torre M, De Palma GD, Basso L. Endoscopic sinusectomy: 'a rose by any other name'. A systematic review of difierent endoscopic procedures to treat pilonidal disease. Color Dis. 2023;25(2):177–90. https://doi.org/10.1111/codi.16361. Epub 2022 Oct 29. PMID: 36217688.

Tam A, Steen CJ, Chua J, et al. Pilonidal sinus: an overview of historical and current management modalities. Updat Surg. 2024;76:803. https://doi.org/10.1007/s13304-024-01799-2.

25 Sacrococcygeal Pilonidal Sinus Disease (PSD): New Classification Proposed Including Endoscopic and LASER Treatment

Abstract

- Due to diverse presentations of the pilonidal sinus disease (PSD) treatment has to be tailored accordingly and no standard single treatment is available, for pilonidal sinus disease.
- Minimally invasive surgery (MIS) including endoscopy and LASER is getting popular in management of PSD.
- Based on the clinical presentation and management of 95 consecutive PSD cases under a set protocol, a novel classification of PSD is suggested.
- This is the first classification to include endoscopic and LASER in the treatment of PDS.
- Where, why and which minimal invasive surgical (MIS) method to do in PSD? Where the flap is required?
- Find answers from this classification.
- Sketches and clinical photographs showcase the different subsets of classification.
- Comparison with main existing classifications of PSD is presented in table form.
- The basis of classification and management revolves around either the presence or absence of large midline wound, in primary as well as in recurrent PSD.
- Very simple to understand and apply.
- Wide acceptance of this novel classification (Singla–Mital classification of PSD) may lead to universal standardisation in the treatment of pilonidal disease and will promote future targeted research.

25.1 Classification of Pilonidal Sinus Disease

Pilonidal sinus disease is an acquired disease of pilo-sebaceous gland origin, manifesting as subcutaneous infection in upper half of the gluteal cleft.

Pilonidal sinus disease (PSD) may present as acute abscess, lateral sinus disease or an indolent ulcer or midline non-healing wound after excision.

No standard single treatment is available for pilonidal sinus disease. Due to diverse presentations of the disease, treatment has to be tailored accordingly.

Recent data worldwide suggests role of minimally invasive procedures involving LASER and video endoscopic means in the effective treatment of pilonidal sinus disease [1–3].

The authors think that there is a need for proper classification of pilonidal sinus disease of natal cleft, a classification system which should be able to guide treatment, predict prognosis and provide opportunity for comparative analysis of such treatment for further research. It should also incorporate the new and widely getting popular treatments, in the form of endoscopic pilonidal surgery (EPSiT) [1–3] or pilonidal sinus LASER treatment (PiLaT or SiLaC) [4, 5] and when both are combined video endoscopic/video-assisted LASER ablation of pilonidal sinus or LASER-assisted EPSiT (VELAP/VALAP or LEPSiT). Ablation under vision will further improve the results.

S. K. Singla, K. Mital, *Operative Manual of Minimally Invasive and LASER Ano-proctology*,
https://doi.org/10.1007/978-981-96-6190-9_25

Table 25.1 Singla–Mital classification of pilonidal sinus disease (PSD)

Staging	Description	Treatment
P0	Pit is there but no inflammation ever	Observation and rule out sacrococcygeal dimple only
Pm	Minimal disease History of inflammation, at present no cellulitis or Induration, or stretched infected hair follicle only	Epilate and treat infected hair follicle if present
Pa	Acute abscess, primary or during recurrence	Incision 1 cm off the mid line, and drainage with curettage Try to locate midline pit, re-evaluate after 5 days when oedema subsides Punch out the pit
P1 Sub classified into P1a P1b	Chronic discharging, sinus or induration laterally, unilateral, bilateral, midline pits, *no skin loss in midline*	Minimal invasive procedures without flap
P1a	Straight tracts, no sinus cavities and *disease load not in midline*	Traditional minimal invasive techniques of sinusectomy, lay open, Gips, Bascom pit picking (Bascom 1) or SiLaT or EPSiT/LEPSiT Lay open and sinusectomy delay healing and need more dressings
P1b	Multiple tracts, sinus cavities or and *disease load in midline*	Gips, Bascom 1, SiLaT or EPSiT/LEPSiT Lay open and sinusectomy not advisable
P2	*Midline skin loss*, midline pits so large and extensive that their removal will make a *large wound in midline (>1 cm)* and unusual cases	Excision and off midline closure. In order of preference as per literature: modified Limberg's, Karydakis, BASCOM cleft lift or Z plasty We find Bascom's cleft lift (Bascom 2) more versatile flap
Pr1	Recurrence after previous surgery including flap surgery, *with out mid line skin loss*	EPSiT/LEPSiT
Pr2	Recurrence with *skin loss or non-healing midline wound*	Bascom's cleft lift (Bascom 2)

Note:
EPSiT and VAAPS are different names of similar technique
SiLaT, SiLaC and PiLaT are different names for same technique
LEPSiT and VELAP are names given to endoscopic method when LASER is used as energy source

We propose the following classification system (Singla–Mital classification of PSD) (Table 25.1).

25.2 Modifiable Predisposing Factors to be Noted in All Patients

Sitting hours per day.
Baths per week.
Body mass index [6].

- Our Novel Classification is based on different clinical presentations of PSD and their recent management.
- Clinical photographs and corresponding sketches explain the presentation (Figs. 25.1, 25.2, 25.3, 25.4, 25.5, 25.6, 25.7, 25.8, 25.9, 25.10, 25.11, 25.12, 25.13, 25.14, 25.15, and 25.16).
- Following pages unfold the novel classification.

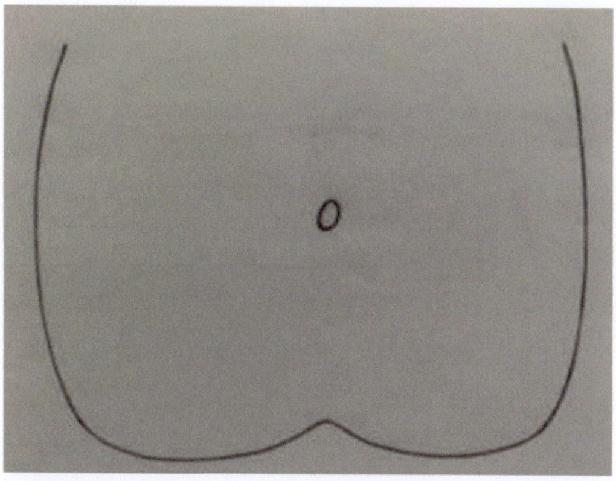

Fig. 25.1 (P0) No disease. Only pit, rule out sacrococcygeal dimple

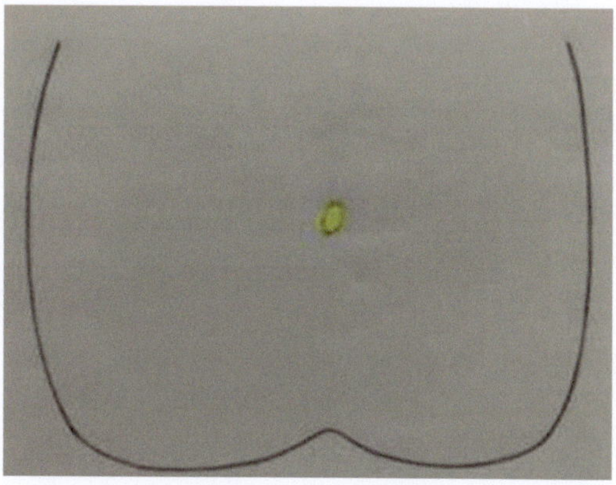

Fig. 25.2 (Pm) Minimal disease. History of inflammation, at present no cellulitis or induration, only stretched infected hair follicle

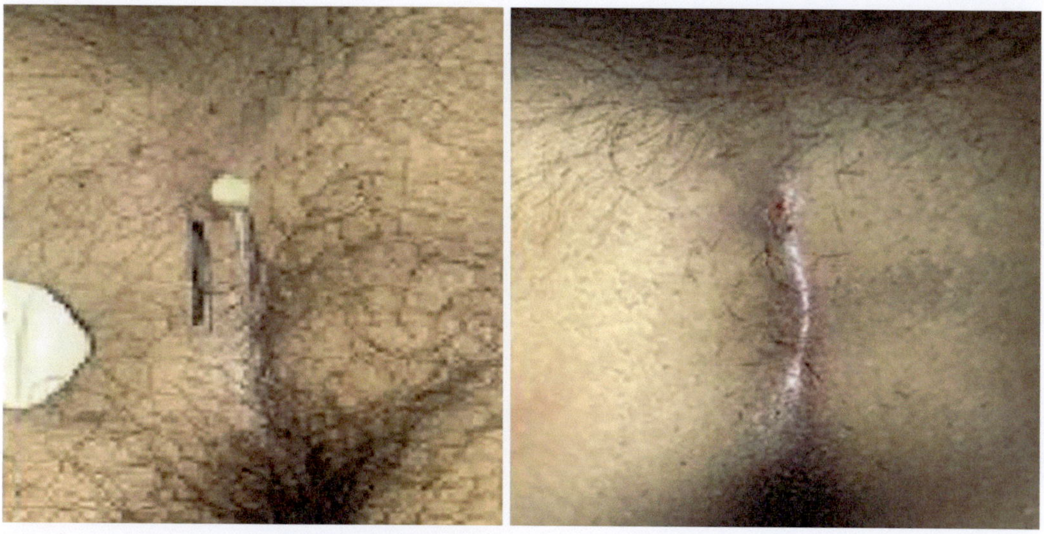

Fig. 25.3 (Pm) Minimal disease (on left), epilate and treat infected hair follicle

> (P0, PM) Only observation and epilation is advised. Treat infected follicle if present.

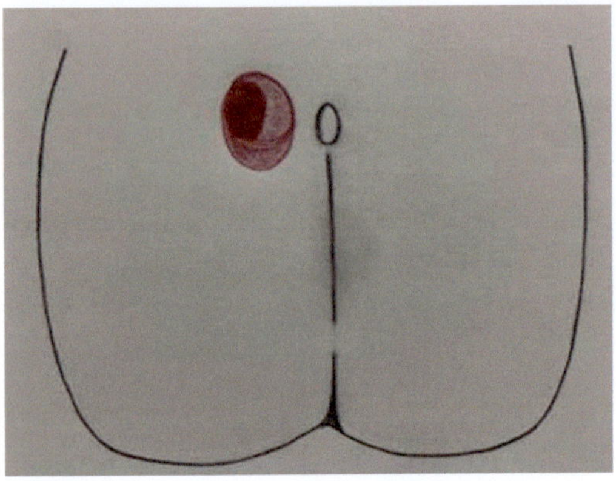

Fig. 25.4 (Pa) Abscess. Off the midline drainage

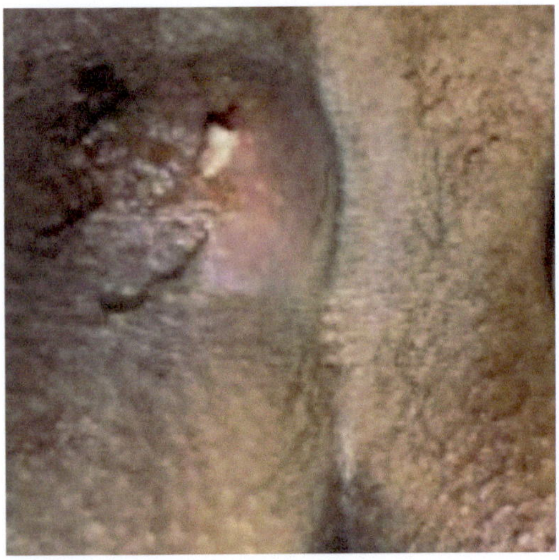

Fig. 25.5 Clinical picture of Pa

(PA) Abscess. Drain, off the midline and curette. Locate pits and punch them out to decrease recurrence.

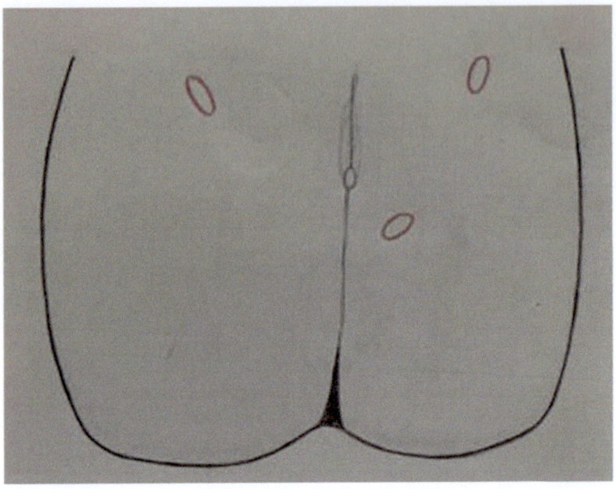

Fig. 25.6 (P1a) Pits with lateral sinus. Disease load not in midline

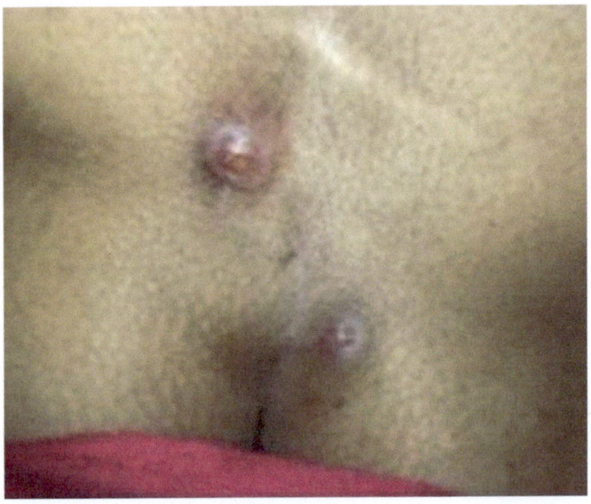

Fig. 25.7 Clinical picture of P1a

(P1A) Pits and straight tracts disease load not in midline. MIS advised. Lay open and sinusectomy can be done but prolong healing time we advise at least Gips method.

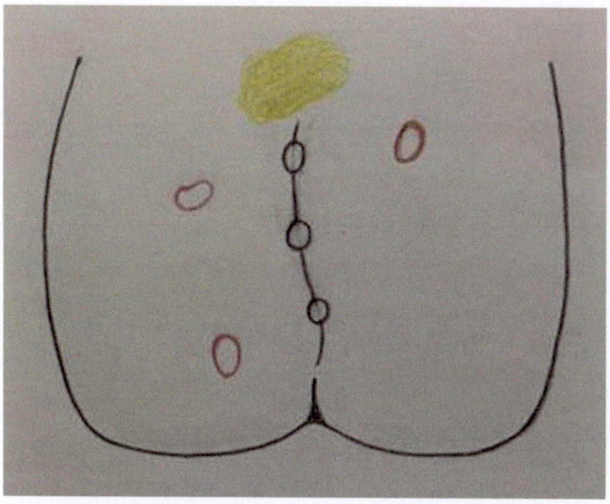

Fig. 25.8 (P1b) Pits with sinus. Disease load in midline and induration (yellow patch) of under lying abscess

Fig. 25.9 All these cases without large midline wound are grouped together as P1b

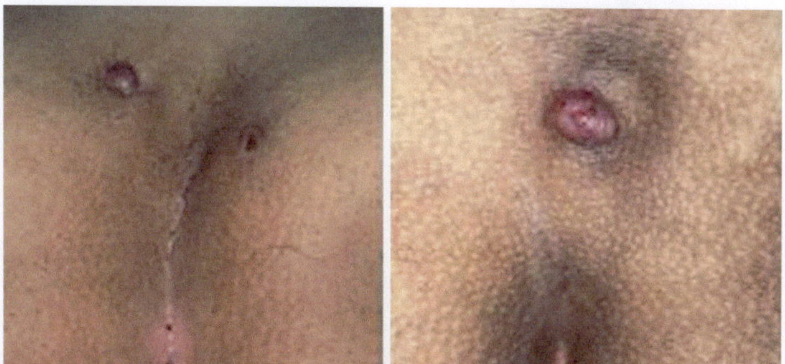

(P1) No midline large wound. MIS advised. (P1B) EPSIT/LEPSIT advised. Lay open and sinusectomy not advisable.

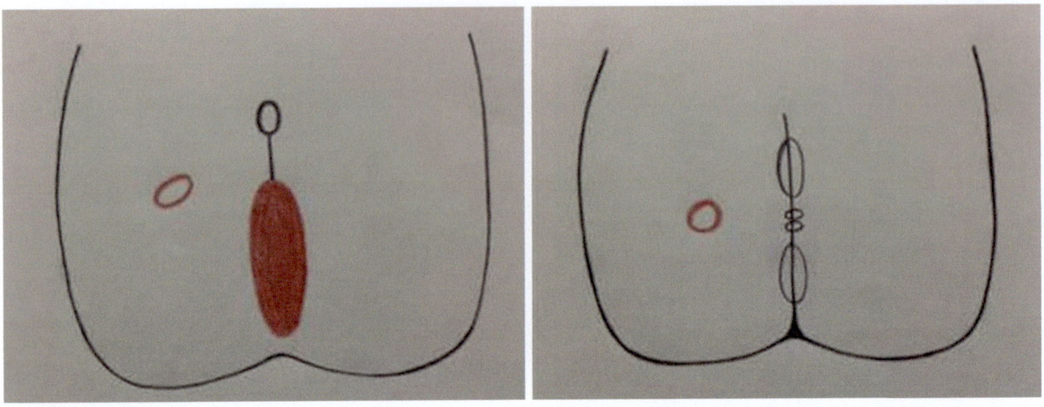

Fig. 25.10 (P2) Midline wound >1 cm or pits so large and close that excision will lead to large midline wound

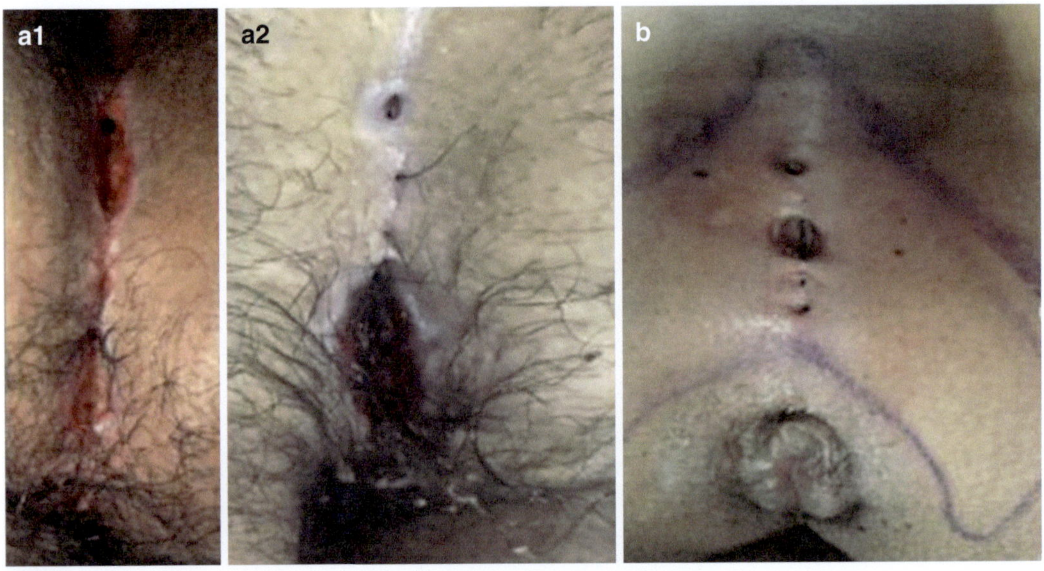

Fig. 25.11 Clinical photographs of P2 (**a**1, **a**2) large midline wound. (**b**) Pits large and close by, excision will lead to large midline wound

(P2) Large midline wound. Off the midline closure with a flap we find BASCOM 2, a versatile flap.

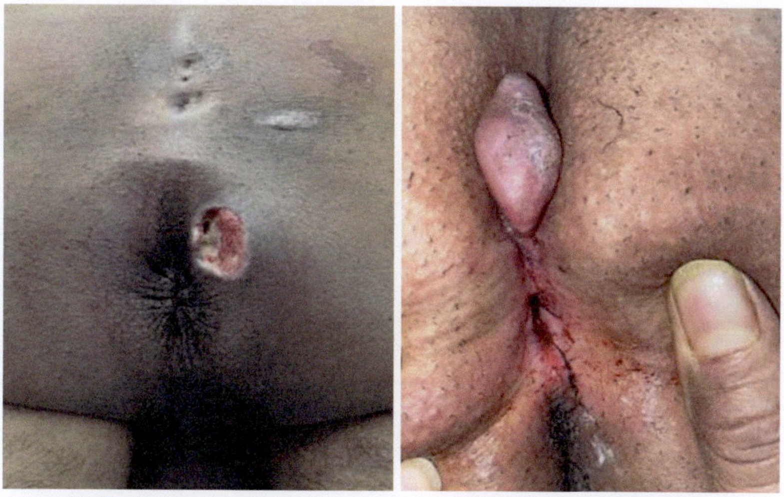

PNS with large peri anal ulcer managed by BASCOM 2. Fistula in ano ruled out.

PNS with large pedunculated inflammatory mass

Fig. 25.12 Unusual cases need flap surgery as of today categorised as P2, managed with Bascom 2

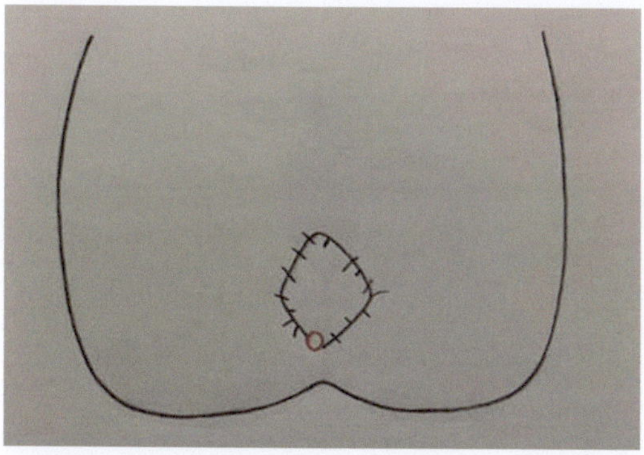

Fig. 25.13 (Pr1) Recurrence after flap or after MIS, without large midline wound

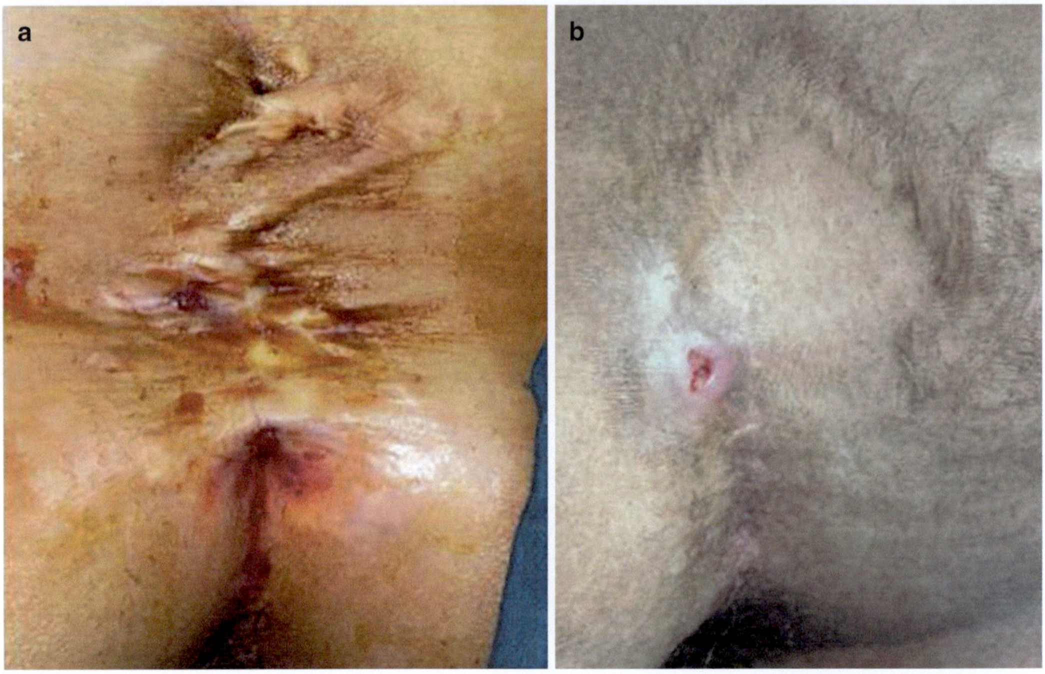

Fig. 25.14 (Pr1) Recurrence after flaps without skin loss in midline (**a**) after Z plasty (**b**) after Limberg flap

(PR1) No large midline wound EPSIT/ LEPSIT.

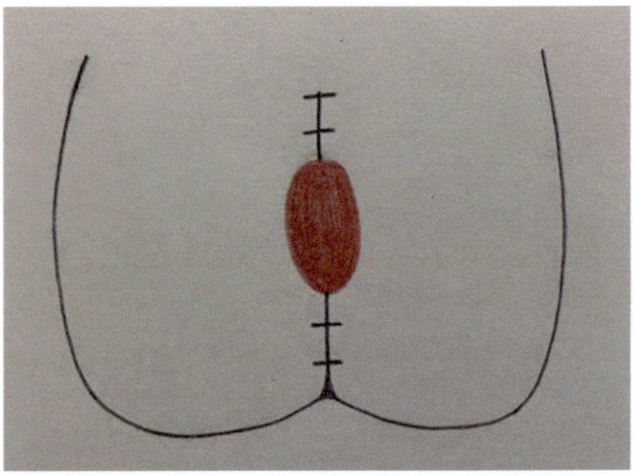

Fig. 25.15 (Pr2) Midline wound failure/recurrence with large midline wound after midline closure or flap

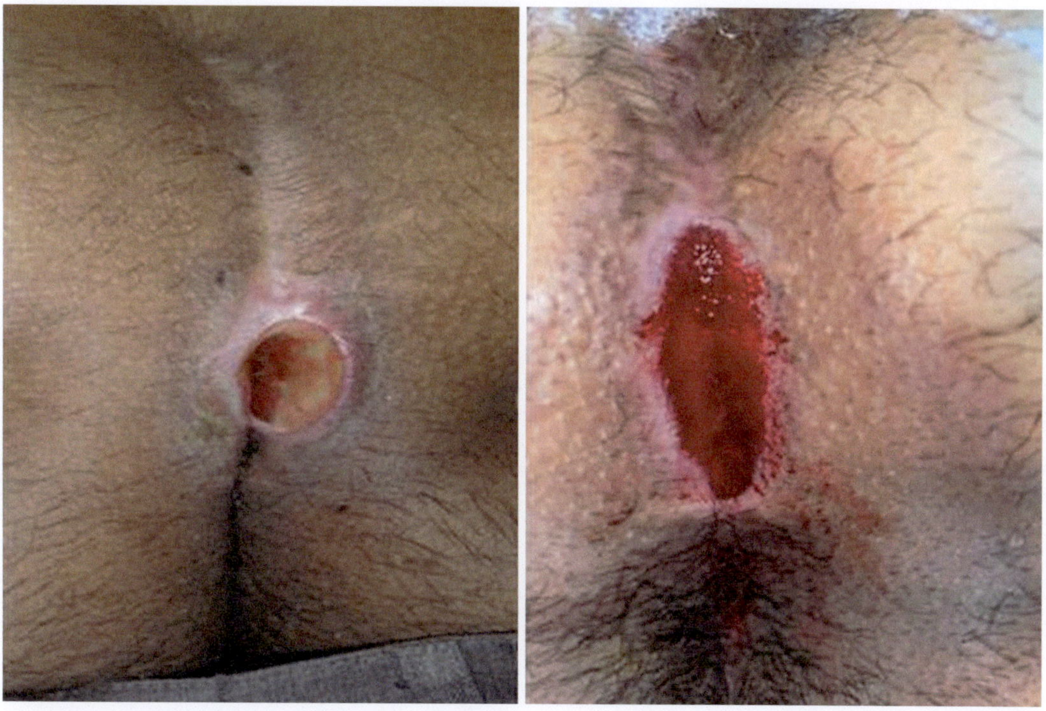

Fig. 25.16 Clinical photographs of Pr2

(PR2) Recurrence with large midline wound needs good skin cover with flap (BASCOM 2).

Points which make this classification unique:

- It is simple to apply.
- This classification incorporates newer modalities of treatment (endoscopic and LASER).
- Guides the treatment aspect.
- The classification can predict prognosis based on category and treatment.
- It gives opportunity for further research on comparative treatments within one category.
- There is no need to define navicular area or mark anal triangle. As endoscopic management is not affected by the lateral distance of sinus from midline or proximity of sinus to anal canal.
- It is based on the clinical management of consecutive 95 cases from 16 May 2019 to 14 August 2024. Operated at single centre of author SKS (Singla Hospital Bhiwani, Haryana, India).
- Nine patients required a flap and 2 patients were managed by hybrid technique of endoscopy and small flap. Rest of the 84 cases could be managed with endoscopic methods. Cases with minimal disease and abscess have been excluded from this calculation.
- Preliminary data of 82 cases along a procedural video (endoscopic management of PSD) was presented at AIIMS New Delhi on 27 April 2024.

25.3 Discussion

25.3.1 Predisposing Factors for Pilonidal Sinus Disease

- Familial tendency, hair stiffness, sitting hours per day, number of baths per week and body mass index have an influence on the disease [6].
- Last three can be modified with change in life style. Hair stiffness can be modified by hair conditioning and leave on hair serum on scalp and LASER treatment of hair around sacrococcygeal gluteal cleft. These methods need further studies and comparative analysis.
- Some recent case series report, decreased post-operative recurrence rates after pilonidal surgery when post-operative LASER depilation was used [7–9].
- Treatment for no active disease (P0), minimal disease (Pm) and acute abscess (Pa) are fairly established and need no further clarification [8, 10, 11].
- Other cases are broadly categorised into two types, i.e., without any skin loss in the cleft (P1) and cases with skin loss more than 1 cm in the midline have been labelled as (P2).
- All P1 cases (P1a and P1b) can be treated by endoscopic, LASER ablation or both. Similarly, some classical minimal procedures like Bascom 1, Pit picking [12–15] can also be used but without the clarity of under vision treatment. Simple laying open the tract [16] and sinusectomy [17] can be used if excessive disease load is not in the midline (P1a), but these methods delay the healing time if compared with Gips method and SiLaT.
- It means that for P1 cases, endoscopic and LASER are the best in terms of confidence in handling disease under vision, effectiveness, decreasing morbidity, time required off the work. Healing usually takes 2–3 weeks in endoscopic and LASER treatment, though few cases may take longer.
- All cases labelled as P2 need a flap procedure with off the midline closure.
- Midline closure should be abandoned in modern practice [18].
- In spite of success of Bascom cleft lift procedure in complicated cases [19, 20], commonly preferred flap procedures in medical literature are Limberg flap, Karydakis, Bascom's cleft lift and Z plasty in order of sequence [21, 22].
- Modified Limberg (lower angle towards the anus is not made in mid line but slightly off the midline) should be preferred over original Limberg flap.
- Unusual cases as shown in Fig. 25.12, pedunculated central mass and associated large ulcers in perianal area, which needs exploration for fistula in ano should be treated by excision and off the midline closure as of now. That's why unusual cases are categorised as P2.
- For recurrence also, our classification is simple, all cases with no skin loss, Pr1 can be managed by endoscopic [23] and LASER treatment and non-healing mid line wounds, central skin loss, i.e., Pr2 should be managed by flap procedures with off the midline closure, as of now [20–22].
- One should always rule out fistula in ano, if tract from lower pit is going caudal [10].
- Following tables compare our classification with some known classification systems (Tables 25.2 and 25.3).
- Some recent studies used fibrin glue mostly in conjunction with some type of minimal excision of midline—pits with healing rates around 96% after two fibrin treatments [25].
- Phenol has also been used as sole treatment or in combination with endoscopic management in some studies [26, 27] though in German

Table 25.2 Comparison of classification system of pilonidal sinus disease PSD

Disease category	Tezel classification	Berlin 17 classification	Our proposed classification
Asymptomatic	I	–	Po
Abscess	II	–	Pa
Solitary midline sinus	–	1a	P1a
Midline sinuses only	–	2a/2b	P1b
Long midline ulcerated wound	–	1b	P2
2° sinus in navicular area–unilateral	III	3a	P1b
2° sinus in navicular area–bilateral	III	3b	P1b
Abscess drainage scar	–	3c	–
2° sinus(es) outside navicular area	IV	3d	P1b
Caudal secondary sinus	IV	4a/4b	P1b
Recurrent disease	V	5a–d	Pr1
Unhealed surgical wound	–	5a–d	Pr2
Hirsute	–	–	–
Male	–	–	–
Overweight	–	–	Yes
Duration >6 months	–	–	–
Size >0.5 cm	–	–	Yes
Length from distal to proximal sinus	–	–	–
Infection	–	–	–
Stiffness of hair	–	–	Yes
Sitting hour	–	–	Yes
Bath per day	–	–	Yes

Modified from Tezel et al. [24]

guidelines, phenol is not recommended for the fear of its toxicity.

- We use 40% liquid phenol on a very thin swab on a probe to touch in the tract in case there is a delay in healing for more than 3 weeks after MIS.
- In conclusion, a clear trend towards minimally invasive techniques and off-midline procedures is recognisable in all international guidelines—Italian, American and German [28].
- Our novel classification further guides where to perform minimally invasive methods and where to perform off the midline closures with flaps. It is simple to apply and there is no need to define navicular area or mark anal triangle, as endoscopic management is not effected by the lateral distance of sinus from midline or proximity of sinus to anal canal. Wide acceptance of this novel classification may lead to universal standardisation in the treatment of pilonidal disease and will promote future targeted research.

Table 25.3 Comparison of treatment in different classifications

Tezel type	Berlin type 2017	Disease type description	Treatment option	Sub type description of Berlin 2017	Our proposed classifications	Our description type	Our treatment options
Type 1	–	Asymptomatic	Observe	–	Po and Pm	Pit is there but no inflammation ever and no abscess at present but pits with history of inflammation there	Observation and rule out sacrococcygeal dimple only & epilation only, preferably by LASER
Type 2	–	Abscess	Lateral incision + drainage	–	Pa	Acute abscess, primary or during recurrence	Incision off the mid line at least 1 cm and drainage with curettage
Type 3	Type 1	Single midline pit/ sinus/wound only (above tip of coccyx; no previous surgery)	Pit excision or sinusectomy ± phenol	Single midline pit/sinus	P1a	Straight tracts, no sinus cavities and disease load not in midline	Traditional minimal invasive techniques of sinusectomy, lay open, Gips, Bascom pit picking or SiLaT or EPSiT\ LEPSiT
				Single midline long wound	P2	Midline skin loss, midline pits so large and extensive that their removal will make a large wound in midline (1 cm)	Excision and off midline closure modified Limberg9s, Karydakis, BASCOM cleft liftor Z plasty
	Type 2	Multiple midline pit/ sinus/wound only (above tip of coccyx; no previous surgery)	Tailored/modified Limberg flap	Midline sinuses 2 or 3	P1a	Straight tracts, no sinus cavities and disease load not in midline	Traditional minimal invasive techniques of sinusectomy, lay open, Gips, Bascom pit picking or SiLaT or EPSiT\ LEPSiT
				Midline sinuses 4 or more	P1b	Multiple tracts, sinus cavities or and disease load in midline	Gips, Bascom 1, SiLaT or EPSiT/LEPSiT
	Type 3	Midline plus lateral openings (above tip of coccyx; no previous definitive surgery)	Cleft lift (Bascoms original description) Cleft lift with Pit excision or sinusectomy ± phenol (for pits in anal triangle) Karydakis flap	Bilateral lateral extension within navicular area	P1b	Multiple tracts, sinus cavities or and disease load in midline	Gips, Bascom 1, SiLaT or EPSiT/LEPSiT
				Abscess scar within navicular area	P1b	Multiple tracts, sinus cavities or and disease load in midline	Gips, Bascom 1, SiLaT or EPSiT/LEPSiT

				Superior/ lateral extension beyond navicular area	P1b	Multiple tracts, sinus cavities or and disease load in midline	Gips, Bascom 1, SiLaT or EPSiT/LEPSiT
	Type 4	Primary disease extending below tip of coccyx (no previous definitive surgery)	Tailored/modified Limberg flap Cleft lift (Bascoms original description) Cleft lift with Pit excision or sinusectomy ± phenol (for pits in anal triangle) Karydakis flap ± subcutaneo us fistulectomy	Midline pit(s)/ sinus(es)/ wound Lateral extension	P1b if large wound then P2	Multiple tracts, sinus cavities or and disease load in midline if large wound than Midline skin loss, midline pits so large and extensive that their removal will make a large wound in midline (1 cm)	Endoscopic and/or LASER ablation if large wound then Excision and off midline closure. modified Limberg's, Karydakis, BASCOM cleft lift or Z plasty
Type 4	Type 5	Defect after definitive surgery present for more than 3 months	Tailored/ modified Limberg flap Cleft lift (Bascoms original description) Cleft lift with Pit excision or sinusectomy ± phenol (for pits in anal triangle) Karydakis flap ± subcutaneo us fistulectomy	Unhealed wound above tip of coccyx	P2	Midline skin loss, midline pit so large and extensive that their removal will make a large wound in midline (1 cm)	Excision and off midline closure modified Limberg's, Karydakis, BASCOM cleft lift or Z plasty
				Recurrence above tip of coccyx	Pr1/Pr2	Recurrence with small sinus/ Recurrence with skin loss or non-healing midline wound	EpsiT or VELAP/Modified Limberg's, Ka rydakis, BASC OM cleft lift or Z plasty
				Unhealed wound below tip of coccyx	Pr2	Recurrence with skin loss or non-healing midline wound.	Modified Limberg's, Ka rydakis, BASC OM cleft liftor Z plasty
				Recurrence below tip of coccyx	Pr1	Recurrence with small sinus	EpsiT or VELAP
Type 5		–	Phenol only Pit excision only cleft lift Tailored/modified Limberg flap	–	–	–	–

Modified from Tezel et al. [24]

Algorithm to Treat PSD as per Our Classification

Po = Observation

Pm = Epilation observe treat infected Hair follicle

Pa= Incision off the mid line and curettage

P1 = MIS traditional or EPSiT/LEPSiT

P2 = Flap

Pr1 = EPSiT/LEPSiT

Pr2 = Bascom cleft lift (Bascom 2)

References

1. Meinero P, Stazi A, Carbone A, Fasolini F, Regusci L, la Torre M. Endoscopic pilonidal sinus treatment: a prospective multicentre trial. Color Dis. 2016;18:O16430170.
2. Gabriela G, Claudio T, Mostafa S, et al. Endoscopic pilonidal sinus treatment: long-term results of a prospective series. JSLS. 2017;21(3):e2017.00043. https://doi.org/10.4293/JSLS.2017.00043.
3. Emile SH, Elfeki H, Shalaby M, Sakr A, Giaccaglia V, Sileri P, Wexner SD. Endoscopic pilonidal sinus treatment: a systematic review and meta-analysis. Surg Endosc. 2018;32(9):375433762.
4. Georgiou GK. Outpatient laser treatment of primary pilonidal disease: the PiLaT technique. Tech Coloproctol. 2018;22:7733778.
5. Pappas AF, Christodoulou DK. A new minimally invasive treatment of pilonidal sinus disease with the use of a diode laser: a prospective large series of patients. Color Dis. 2018;20:O2073O214.
6. Harlak A, et al. Sacrococcygeal pilonidal disease: analysis of previously proposed risk factors. Clinics (Sao Paulo). 2010;65(2):125–31.
7. Conroy FJ, Kandamany N, Mahafiey PJ. Laser depilation and hygiene: preventing recurrent pilonidal sinus disease. J Plast Reconstr Aesthet Surg. 2008;61:106931072.
8. Ganjoo A. Laser hair reduction for pilonidal sinus my experience. J Cutan Aesthet Surg. 2011;4:196.
9. Oram Y, Kahraman F, Karincaoglu Y, et al. Evaluation of 60 patients with pilonidal sinus treated with laser epilation after surgery. Dermatologic Surg. 2010;36:88391.
10. Johnson EK, Vogel JD, Cowan ML, Fein Gold DL, Steele SR. The American Society of Colon and Rectal Surgeons' clinical practice guidelines for the management of pilonidal disease. Dis Colon Rectum. 2019;62:146–57. https://doi.org/10.1097/DCR.0000000000001237. © The ASCRS 2019.
11. Doll D, Friederichs J, Boulesteix AL, Dflsel W, Fend F, Petersen S. Surgery for asymptomatic pilonidal sinus disease. Int J Color Dis. 2008;23:8393844.
12. Bascom J. Pilonidal disease: origin from follicles of hairs and results of follicle removal as treatment. Surgery. 1980;87:5673572.
13. Nordon IM, Senapati A, Cripps NP. A prospective randomized controlled trial of simple Bascom's technique versus Bascom's cleft closure for the treatment of chronic pilonidal disease. Am J Surg. 2009;197:1893192.
14. Iesalnieks I, Deimel S, Kienle K, Schlitt HJ, Zfllke C. Pit-picking surgery for pilonidal disease. Chirurg. 2011;82:9273931.
15. Gips M, Melki Y, Salem L, Weil R, Sulkes J. Minimal surgery for pilonidal disease using trephines: description of a new technique and long-term outcomes in 1,358 patients. Dis Colon Rectum. 2008;51:165631662.
16. Garg P, Menon GR, Gupta V. Laying open (deroofing) and curettage of sinus as treatment of pilonidal disease: a systematic review and meta-analysis. ANZ J Surg. 2016;86:27333.
17. Soll C, Dindo D, Steinemann D, Haufic T, Clavien PA, Hahnloser D. Sinusectomy for primary pilonidal sinus: less is more. Surgery. 2012;150:99631001.
18. Al-Khamis A, McCallum I, King PM, Bruce J. Healing by primary versus secondary intention after surgical treatment for pilonidal sinus. Cochrane Database Syst Rev. 2011:CD006213.
19. Bascom JU. Repeat pilonidal operations. Am J Surg. 1987;154:1183122.
20. Bascom J, Bascom T. Failed pilonidal surgery: new paradigm and new operation leading to cures. Arch Surg. 2002;137:114631150; discussion 1151.
21. Enriquez-Navascues JM, Emparanza JI, Alkorta M, Placer C. Meta-analysis of randomized controlled trials comparing different techniques with primary closure for chronic pilonidal sinus. Tech Coloproctol. 2014;18:8633872.
22. Boshnaq M, Phan YC, Martini I, Harilingam M, Akhtar M, Tsavellas G. Limberg flap in management of pilonidal sinus disease: systematic review and a local experience. Acta Chir Belg. 2018;118:78384.
23. Meinero P, La Torre M, Lisi G, et al. Endoscopic pilonidal sinus treatment (EPSiT) in recurrent pilonidal disease: a prospective international multicenter study. Int J Color Dis. 2019;34:7413746.
24. Tezel E, Leventoglu S, Wysockı AP. Trends toward a tailored approach for pilonidal sinus disease. Coloproctology. 2019;41:1213126. https://doi.org/10.1007/s00053-018-0314-0.
25. Sian TS, Herrod PJJ, Blackwell JEM, et al. Fibrin glue is a quick and effective treatment for primary and recurrent pilonidal sinus disease. Tech Coloproctol. 2018;22:7793784. https://doi.org/10.1007/s10151-018-1864-4.

26. Gan X-X, Liu P, Chen S-H, Li J, Zhao X, Chen W, Zhang J, Yang C-P, Wang M-X, Wang L-W, Zhang D, Xin X, Dai G-Y. A meta-analysis comparing phenol treatment with surgical excision for pilonidal sinus. Asian J Surg. 2024;47(1):8–15. ISSN 1015-9584, https://doi.org/10.1016/j.asjsur.2023.06.111. https://www.sciencedirect.com/science/article/pii/S1015958423009673.
27. Gecim IE, Goktug UU, Celasin H. Endoscopic pilonidal sinus treatment combined with crystalized phenol application may prevent recurrence. Dis Colon Rectum. 2017;60(4):405–7. https://doi.org/10.1097/DCR.0000000000000778.
28. Iesalnieks A, Herold OA, Doll D. Systematic reviews and meta-analyses German National Guideline on the management of pilonidal disease: update 2020. Langenbeck's Arch Surg. 2021. Published: 05 May2021. https://doi.org/10.1007/s00423-020-02060-1. https://link.springer.com/article/.

26 Transanal Minimal Invasive Surgery (TAMIS)

Abstract

- Proctectomy with total mesorectal excision (TME) provides effective local tumour control and is considered as standard of care in rectal cancer. Though it is associated with a significant risk of perioperative morbidity, and a small risk of mortality.
- Ability to detect early rectal neoplasms due to screening programmes, coupled with efficacy of modern neoadjuvant therapies, there is significant increase in the proportion of rectal cancers potentially amenable to local excision.
- Predominantly there are two transanal rectum-sparing approaches: transanal endoscopic microsurgery (TEM) and transanal minimally invasive surgery (TAMIS).
- TAMIS has gained more popularity because of short learning curve, versatility and ability to use conventional laparoscopic instruments.
- Present and possible indications of the procedure are enumerated.
- Steps of the procedure using GelPOINT Path platform (Applied Medical, Rancho Santa Margarita, CA) are explained in detail by clinical photographs and video.
- Complications, their prevention and management are compiled in a table form, for ready reference.
- Algorithm for TAMIS has been developed for ready reference on way to operation theater (OT).
- "References" and "Suggested Reading" sections are available for a more inquisitive reader.

Supplementary Information The online version contains supplementary material available at https://doi.org/10.1007/978-981-96-6190-9_26. The videos can be accessed individually by clicking the DOI link in the accompanying figure caption or by scanning this link with the SN More Media App.

26.1 What One Should Know Before the Procedure

- Transanal minimally invasive surgery (TAMIS) is a type of surgery where pathological conditions of the rectum are managed transanally by using principles and equipment of minimally invasive surgery.
- TAMIS term was first coined by Sam Atallah in 2010 [1]. He performed six cases of trans-anal excision using a single incision laparoscopic surgery (SILS) port. He titled his paper as "Trans anal minimally invasive surgery: a giant leap forward".
- Trans-anal excision (TAE) in modern sense was first described by Park and Stuart in 1970 in a series of 30 patients having villous adenomas of the rectum. These were open procedures [2].
- Gerhard Buess from Germany in 1984 used the TEM (trans-anal endoscopic microsurgery) platform to perform transanal surgeries in a minimally invasive manner. He used specialised rectoscope and curved instruments to perform TEM [3]. However, due to the costly equipment, fixed platform, need for specialised instruments and steep learning curve, its

S. K. Singla, K. Mital, *Operative Manual of Minimally Invasive and LASER Ano-proctology*,
https://doi.org/10.1007/978-981-96-6190-9_26

use did not spread wide. Though many surgeons continued to be trained and inspired by him but its worldwide popularity remained limited [4].

- TAMIS, however, gained rapid popularity because of the simplicity of its platform and instruments. Its invention coincided with the introduction of SILS port for laparoscopy. One could use conventional laparoscopic instruments with which most of the surgeons doing laparoscopy were familiar with [5].
- Specialised platforms are now available in the market which have been specially designed for transanal surgery. Special curved instrumentation is also available, however, in the authors experience conventional laparoscopic instruments and energy sources are sufficient [5].
- With TAMIS technique one can have access to the proximal and mid-rectum:
  - For resection of benign and early-stage malignant rectal lesions.
  - For non-curative intent surgery of more advanced lesions in patients, unfit for radical surgery.
  - TAMIS matches TEMS in view of conversion rate, re-operation rate, and complication. It scores over TEMS-in technique learning time and operation set up time.
  - TAMIS results in less short-term anal sphincter dysfunction than TEM, as has been shown using the rigid 40-mm TEM scope [6].
- So TAMIS is an easily accessible, technically feasible, cost-effective and more versatile alternative to TEM.
- Adequate resection margin of the lesion without fragmentation of the specimen, is the goal.
- The same TAMIS platform has been used for transanal NOTES surgery, a technique originally performed with TEM. The proctectomy is completed in a "reverse" approach. This overcomes the difficulty of the narrow pelvis especially in male patients and tackles the trouble of the distal margin. Because the dissection is started from below, the distal margin is never in question. It may also provide better dissection of the circumferential margin of the distal mesorectum [7].
- No surprise TAMIS is being utilised in various other conditions like pelvic abscess drainage, rectal stenosis, recto urethral fistula, treatment of anastomotic dehiscence and control of post-operative anorectal bleeding.
- Appropriate training, applications of right technique and continuous assessment of results must be ensured for growth of this technique.

26.2 Indications for TAMIS

Indications for benign and malignant anorectal lesions.

26.2.1 Benign Lesions

- Adenomas of rectum.
- Hemartamatous polyps.
- Bleeding.
- Retrieval of foreign body.
- Stricturoplasty.
- Mucosal advancement flaps for anal fistula.
- For any new surgical procedure indications stretch as safety profile is established. Some more recent indications are as below:
- Recto urethral fistula.
- Drainage of pelvic abscess pouting in rectum, under vision.
- Still other investigators have used TAMIS to control post-operative anastomotic bleeding and to provide access for suture closure of an anastomotic leak [8].
- Suturing hole in iliococcygeus after coring in case of suprasphincteric fistula may be an indication for use of TAMIS platform.

26.2.2 Malignant Lesions [9–11]

- National comprehensive cancer network (NCCN) describes the following indications for trans anal excision in rectal cancers: lesion should occupy <30% of rectal circumference. It should be < 3 cm in size, mobile, not fixed. Within 8 cm from anal verge or higher for TEM and TAMIS [10, 11].

- T1 lesions confined to submucosa only—favourable histological features like no lymphovascular invasion, or perineural invasion. Moderate to well-differentiated adenocarcinoma, no lymphadenopathy on imagining.
- TAMIS is also indicated when patients with advanced cancers have a near complete response (nCR) after neoadjuvant therapy but refuse to undergo standard TME [10, 12, 13].
- For patients with questionable T1 versus T2 lesions with no evidence of nodal metastasis, a TAMIS resection can serve as an "excisional biopsy," guiding further treatment with the final pathology report.
  - T1 tumours with poor pathological features or T2 tumours need more radical surgery in the form of an low-anterior reaction (LAR) [14, 15].
- Patients with more advanced lesions (T3) can be considered for TAMIS resection when they are medically unfit to have a more radical surgery.
- The indications for TAMIS can also be broadened to include local excision of clinical TO (cTO) lesions in patients with locally advanced rectal cancer after neoadjuvant therapy for the purpose of confirming mural pathological complete response. cPR (ypT0) [16–18].

  This can be considered a valid option, as the risk of occult node positivity for ypT0 lesions is predictably low, at 3–6% [19–21].

26.3 Pre-operative Requisition: Staging and Counselling

26.3.1 Clinical Examination and Proctoscopy

- For an anorectal lesion, perform DRE and rigid proctoscopy to assess the tumour for location, size, mobility, circumferential involvement and vertical distance from the anal verge.
- Do colonoscopy to exclude any synchronous lesions and take biopsy.
- If histopathology reports malignancy, further workup for local invasion is done with either endorectal ultrasound (ERUS) or magnetic resonance imaging (MRI) of the rectum. Endorectal ultrasound (ERUS) is a good modality for differentiating T1 from T2 cancers and for superficial lesions.
- Computed tomography (CT) scan of the chest, abdomen, and pelvis should be performed to exclude distant metastasis.
- A good chat with local radiologist where both surgeon and radiologist are watching the scan on the computer is highly recommended as it makes anatomy clear to the surgeon and is a good way to give feed back to the radiologist.

26.3.2 Counselling

- Patients should be made to understand by adequate counselling that all these efforts are being done to get rid of the malignancy and at the same time to preserve the anorectal function and continence post-operatively.
- Patients should understand that they have curative intent surgery by TAMIS for their early lesion if histo-pathology report returns as a T1 lesion with favourable characteristics but that they may still need a formal oncologic resection in the form of low-anterior resection (LAR) if the pathology returns as a T2 lesion or poor histopathology features (lymphatic/vascular/perineural invasion, poor differentiation, tumour budding), positive margins or deeper invasion (submucosal levels: Sm3) as defined by the Kikuchi classification which may mean potential metastasis to lymph nodes [15, 21].
- Patients with spread to nodes and other viscera should be evaluated by institutional cancer board and treated accordingly.
- All these patients need close follow-up.

26.4 Pre-operative Preparation

- Informed consent is taken after explaining the alternatives to the procedure.
- Bowel preparation is started and patient put on clear liquid diet a day before. A split prep with 4 L of polyethylene glycol is preferred by the author.
- We follow standard surgical care improvement project (SCIP) protocols for colon surgery, including perioperative antibiotics, β blockers and deep venous thrombosis prophylaxis.
  - A prophylactic antibiotic dose is administered. 1 g Ertapenem single dose is a good choice and covers both aerobic and anaerobic bacteria and need not to be repeated till 24 h.
  - A Foleys catheter is inserted to decompress the urinary bladder and monitor urine output.
  - Sequential compression device (SCD) sleeves are placed to prevent deep vein thrombosis (DVT).

26.4.1 Equipment

- Skin preparation agent—povidine iodine solution.
- Sterile drapes and sheets.
- Trolley of general instruments—as required for haemorrhoidectomy.
- Device for transanal access:
  - There are two FDA-approved devices for transanal access with the TAMIS procedure:
    1. SILS Port (Covidien, Mansfield, MA).
    2. GelPOINT Path (Applied Medical, Rancho Santa Margarita, CA).

    Both easily sit transanally and allow insufflation for pneumorectum through a designated channel. With the advent of transanal specific platforms like GelPOINT Path it is possible to access all the quadrants of rectum easily though lesions located posteriorly are more easily dealt with. One can change the position of the patient depending upon the location of the lesion; however, it is rarely necessary. With TEM platform, the position has to be decided before fixing the platform as it cannot be altered later.
- We use GelPOINT Path (Figs. 26.1 and 26.2).
- Laparoscopic tower with camera processor, insufflator with CO_2 for insufflation and video monitor.
- Trolley for laparoscopy instruments usually required for lap. Cholecystectomy.
- Laparoscopic needle holder.
- Monopolar L hook with suction is preferable.
- Stirrups for lithotomy—Candy cane or Allen Stirrup.
- Allen stirrup is preferable in case abdominal access is required.

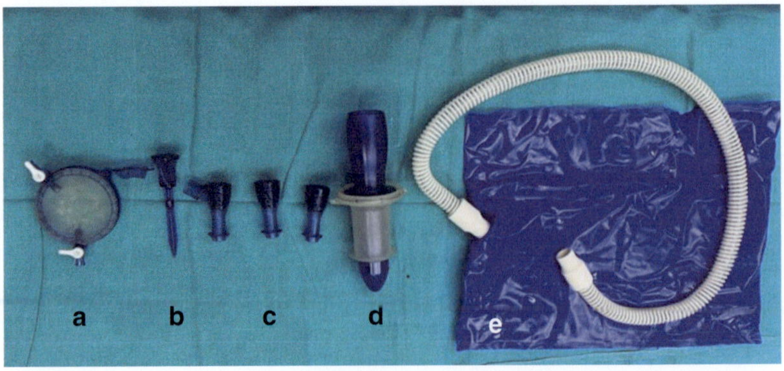

Fig. 26.1 Equipment for TAMIS (GelPOINT Path). (A) GelPoint Cap, (B) Obturator, (C) Trocars, (D) Silicon Channel with Obturator, (E) Reservoir bag

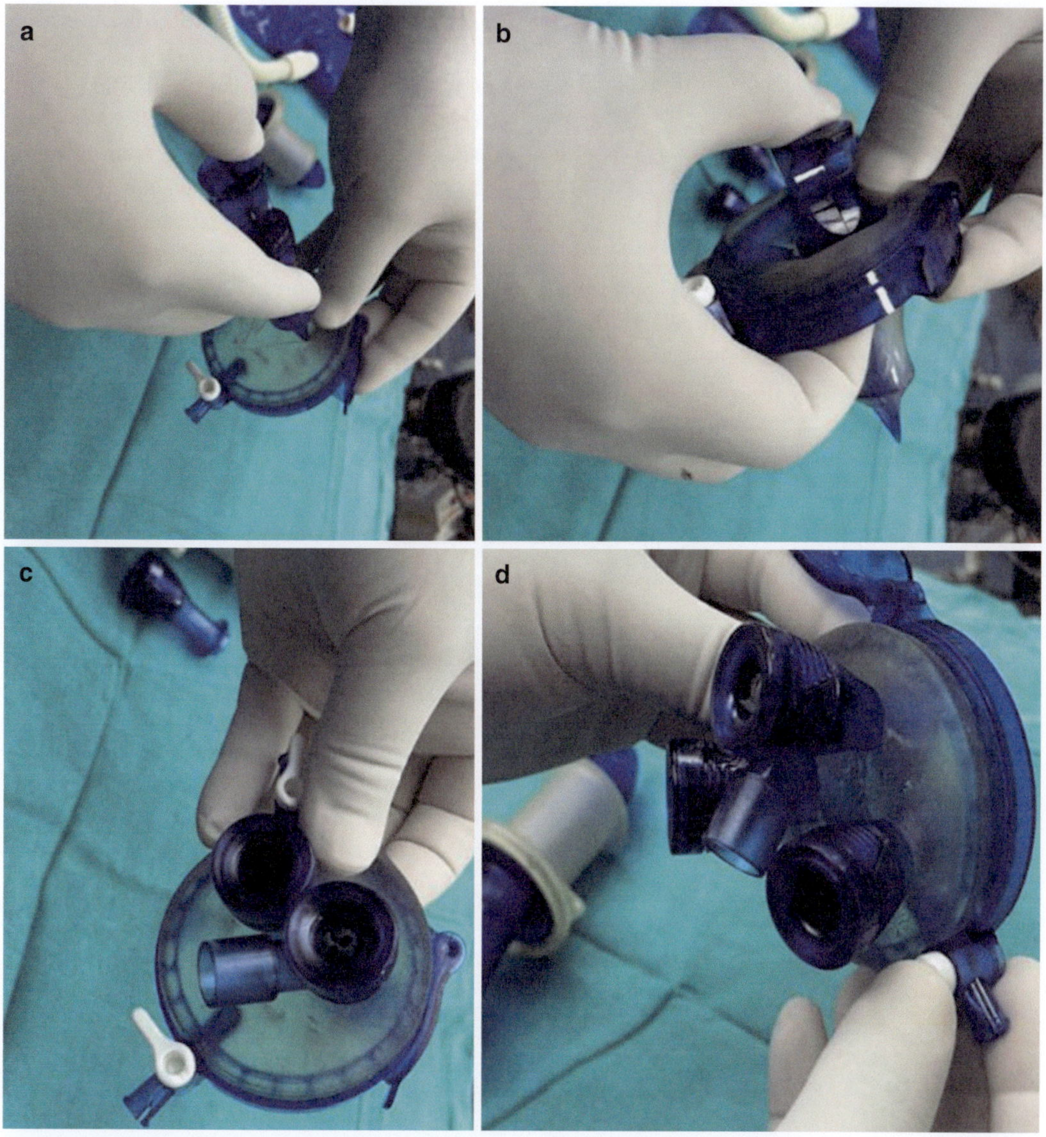

Fig. 26.2 Steps to fix ports in the cap in a triangular manner: (**a**) port with obturator kept at one point, (**b**) sharp tip of obturator is thrust in the cap, (**c**) two ports fixed on the cap, (**d**) all three ports—in a triangle configuration fixed on the cap

26.4.2 Anaesthesia

We prefer and recommend general endotracheal anaesthesia (GETA) with muscle paralysis to avoid collapse of the rectal wall which often occurs with diaphragmatic excursion. Also in case of creation of pneumoperitoneum one has better control and safety.

26.4.3 Position

- Lithotomy with slight Trendelenburg position with patient low on table and legs high enough to give surgeon and team, the working space.
- A video monitor just between the patient's legs over the abdomen in front of the surgical team is best suited for hand and eye coordination.

- It is authors' preference to paint-drape the abdomen from start, in case a pneumoperitoneum gets created especially in high-anteriorly located lesions.

26.5 Procedure (Video 26.1)

- A digital rectal examination is performed. This is followed by insertion of anal dilator which comes with GelPoint path (Applied Medical).
- After this, Lone star hooks are placed to retract anal margins (Fig. 26.3). This is a very important step as it makes insertion of the silicon channel easy (Fig. 26.4).

26.5.1 Fixation of the GelPOINT Path

- Once GelPOINT Path platform's silicon channel is inserted, it is secured with N0 1 silk suture to the perianal skin. Ports are inserted in the cap in a triangular manner, before fixing it to the flange of the silicon channel (Figs. 26.5 and 26.6).
- In case a SILS port is used, ports are inserted after fixing the channel as it has no cap.
- Pneumo-rectum is createdby connecting the CO_2 gas to the reservoir bag or else an Airseal system is used depending on availability.
- Pressure is kept at 15 mm Hg.

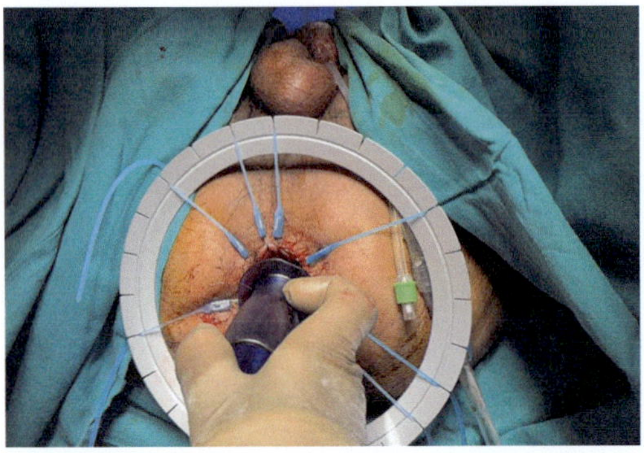

Fig. 26.3 Anal dilator insertion and application of Lone Star retractor

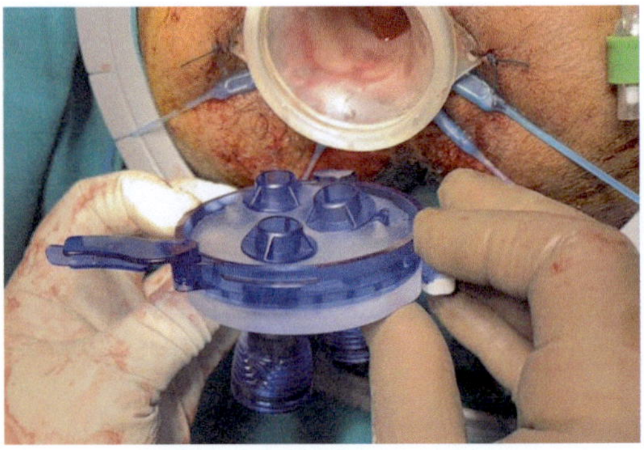

Fig. 26.5 Cap with ports inserted in triangular manner ready to be fixed to flange of silicone channel, which is already secured to perianal skin by sutures

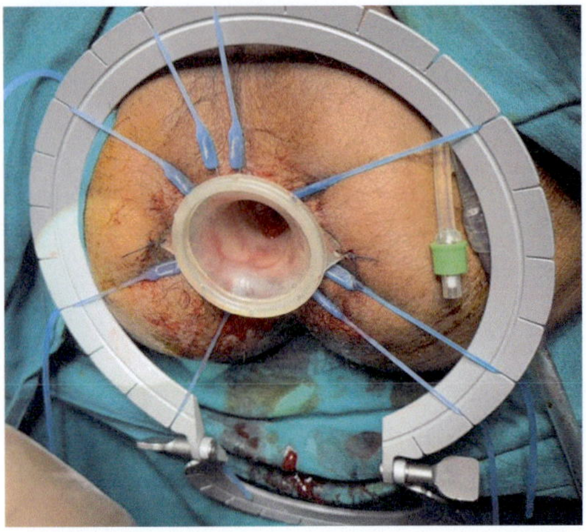

Fig. 26.4 After application of Lone Star retractor, lubricated silicon channel is inserted in the anal canal and fixed by silk sutures

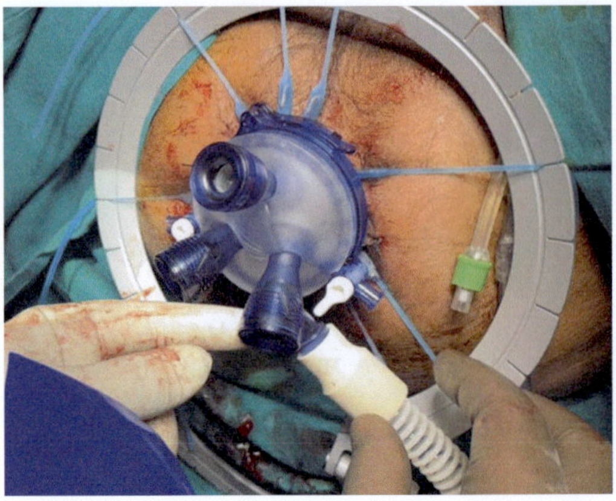

Fig. 26.6 GelPOINT Path platform inserted in anal canal and fixed to perianal skin. Note: one port has side channel for CO_2 gas from reservoir bag

26.5.2 Diagnostic Rectoscopy (Fig. 26.7)

Rectoscopy is done using 30° 5 mm laparoscope through one port.

26.5.3 Scoring the Lesion (Fig. 26.8)

Lesion is scored 1 cm around the margins with L laparoscopic hook. This will ensure maintaining a negative and adequate margin during the dissection.

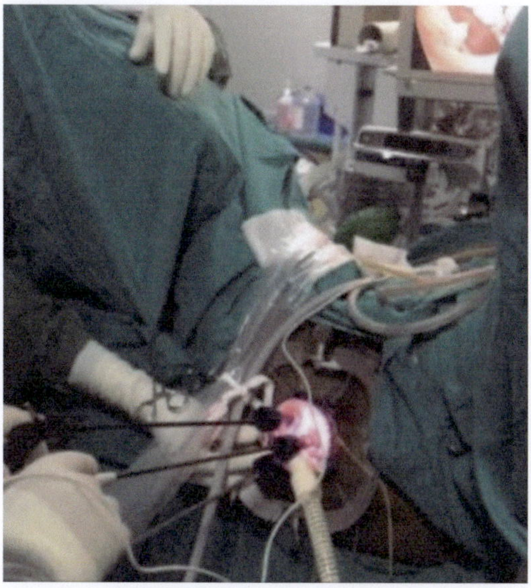

Fig. 26.7 Assistant holds the scope and surgeon operates with both hands. L hook in the right hand and grasper in the left hand

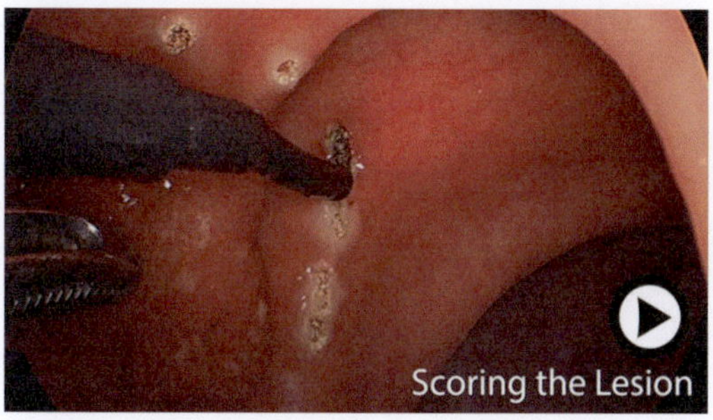

Fig. 26.8 Lesion is scored 1 cm around the margin with L hook. Video 26.1 TAMIS procedure (▶ https://doi.org/10.1007/000-hqj)

An atraumatic bowel grasper is used to retract the lesion and deepen the dissection.

Grasping the lesion with graspers is avoided to prevent inadvertent crushing, fragmentation and spillage of the tumour cells. Back of grasper is used to retract the lesion.

26.5.4 Full Thickness Dissection (Fig. 26.9)

- Dissection is deepened with the L hook till perirectal fat is seen (Fig. 26.9). Care must be taken to remain perpendicular to the tumour so as not to compromise the deep margin.
- At this point, the edge of the dissected lesion can be grasped with the grasper and retraction given (Fig. 26.10).
- Dissection is done in this manner circumferentially.
- CO_2 insufflation provides a natural "pneumo-dissection" and helps in controlling minor blood ooze thereby maintaining the clarity of the planes during dissection.

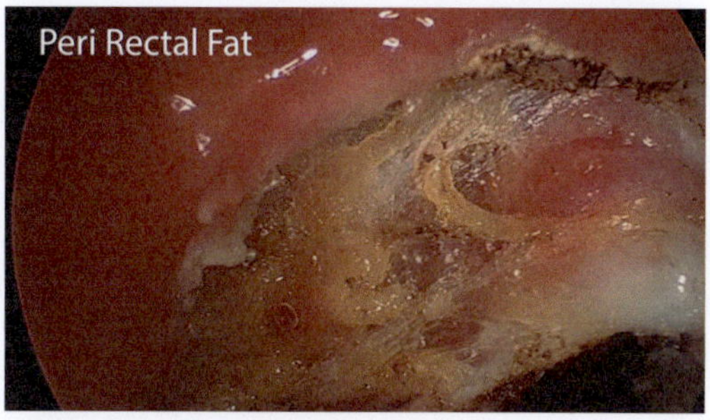

Fig. 26.9 Perirectal fat seen after full thickness excision

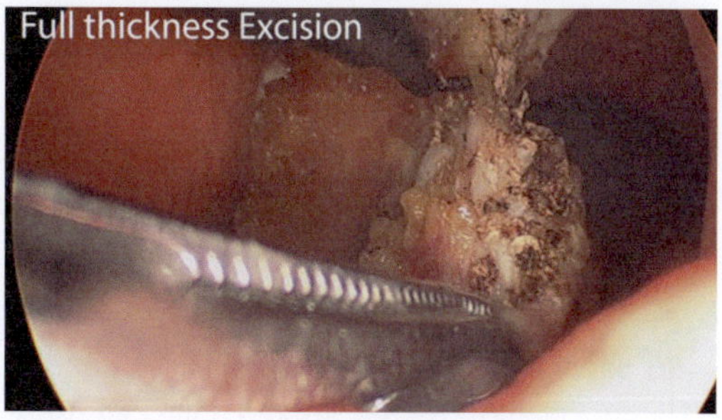

Fig. 26.10 Edge of the lesion is grasped for deep dissection

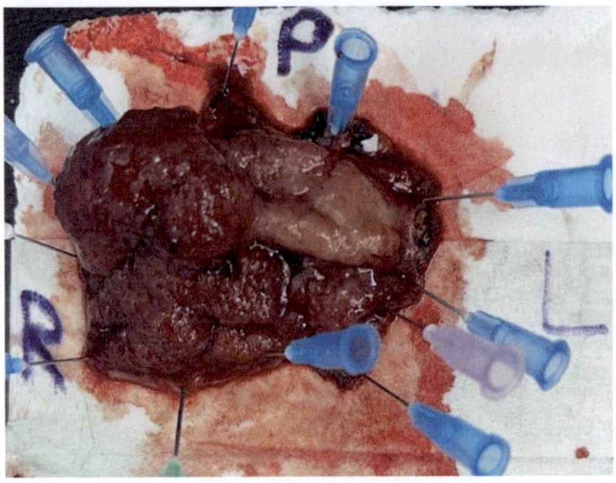

Fig. 26.11 Specimen is fixed on board with free margins pinned and oriented (P) proximal, (R) right, (L) left

- If pneumo-peritoneum is created during dissection, a Veress needle can be inserted to decompress the peritoneal cavity, as is done in case of total extra peritoneal (TEP) repair in hernia. The hole in peritoneum is sutured transanally.
- The specimen is delivered per anus holding the inferior edge of the specimen.
- *Fixation of specimen on a flat board for orientation.*
- Specimen then placed on a card board or thermocol and oriented and marked. Its free margins are pinned with 22G needles (Fig. 26.11).
- It is sent to a pathologist, or pathologist is requested to take it from OT.
- Pathologist is suggested to vertically section the specimen so that depth of invasion can be assessed in case of suspected cancers. Specimen orientation should be done before dealing with the defect in the rectum as the surgeon may forget the orientation, latter.

A new pair of sterile gloves are donned after dealing with the specimen.

26.5.5 Handling the Rectal Defect After Resection of the Lesion

- Now attention is paid to the rectal defect. Due to pneumorectum the defect usually appears large. Haemostasis is checked. One can use L hook or energy source of one's choice to achieve haemostasis.

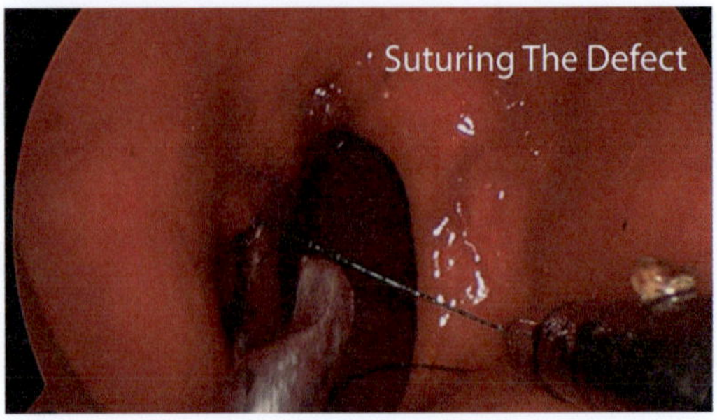

Fig. 26.12 Suturing the defect with barbed suture

- There are two ways to deal with the rectal defect. Surgeon can either leave it open or close it.

26.5.6 Suturing the Rectal Defect (Fig. 26.12)

- The author prefers to close it because keeping defect open is associated with higher rates of rectal bleeding. In one of our patients we had to take the patient back to OT twice. Pneumo-rectum pressure should be kept at 10 mm Hg to facilitate the closure.
- A barbed 3.0 suture is used to close the defect in running manner. If the defect is large then two threads are run from each corner.
- Always aim to close the defect perpendicular to the lumen. After closing the defect suture line is examined.
- Cap of the port is removed and the stay sutures are cut. Channel is removed.
- It is good habit to inject local anaesthetic in the perianal region to give post-operative pain relief.
- A pyramidal sterile guaze dressing is done. No anal packing is done.
- Patient is then kept in supine position, extubated and shifted to post-operative ward in a stable condition.

26.6 Post-operative Management

- TAMIS is a well tolerated operation. Patients usually complain of some anal pain due to stretching and placement of Lone Star hooks. Pain is mild and managed with analgesics for first day. Rarely analgesia is required on subsequent days.

- However, if the lesion was close to dentate line and dissection involved crossing it distally then patients have more pain and its good idea to inject solution of methylene blue 1% and bupivicane 0.25% in 1:5 ratio to prolong the analgesia.
- Clear liquid diet is started on the day of surgery. Diet is advanced when patient passes flatus, usually on the second post-operative day.
- If the case is done in the morning and patient is comfortable, has passed urine and there is no abdominal distention, then one can be discharged by evening. Patients done in the afternoon or evenings are usually kept overnight.
- No antibiotics are necessary and we do not advise routine complete blood count (CBC) unless indicated.
- No sitz bath is recommended. However, stool softeners are advised.

26.7 Complications of the Procedure

- TAMIS is a well-tolerated operation with good short- and long-term outcomes [22, 23]. It has few complications (Table 26.1).
- Mortality rates are low, with a mean value of 0.29% [22].

Table 26.1 Complications of TAMIS

Complications	Prevention	Management
Acute urinary retention (4.9%) [24]	Do not over load. However, our policy is to catheterise all patients before the procedure and catheter is taken out next day after the patient passes flatus. Rarely, it becomes necessary to discharge the patient on catheter	Catheterisation of bladder
Rectal bleeding (2.2%) [24]	Suture the rectal defect	If bleeding does occur post-operatively then a repeat visit to OT is usually required. The defect can be sutured if not done before. Packing is usually not helpful in these situations
Suture line disruption	Do not close the rectal defect under tension. Avoid superficial bites take adequate depth along all layers while suturing the defect	If associated bleeding is there, suture the defect. If patient has no bleeding then he can be just given stool softeners. Give antibiotics if there is high white cell count or fever
Abscesses are unusual <1%	Avoid dead space and do not crush the tissue while suturing the rectal defect	MRI [24] Transanal drainage
Peritoneal perforations (5%) Evident by loss of pneumo-rectum	Observe haemostasis during dissection to enable identification of planes. Happens while dissecting anteriorly placed lesions	Suture with 3.0 braided suture Diagnostic laparoscopy is seldom necessary but should not be hesitated if thought of [24]
Rectovaginal fistula <1% [15]	Rectovaginal breech if detected during surgery, immediate repair should be done	Manage like any other rectovaginal fistula. Status of the tumour will also affect the management

Algorithm for TAMIS Using Gel Point Path Platform

Indication/contraindications
History, clinical examination and DRE proctoscopy and colonoscopy as per requirement
GETA and lithotomy position
Lithotomy in Allen stirrups
Clean drape peri anal site and abdomen
Fix gel point trocars with ports on cap in a triangular fashion
Anal dilatation by obturator
Application of Lone star retractor
Insertion and fixation of silicon channel mount cap with prefixed ports on flange of silicone channel
Start flow of CO_2 and maintain pressure of 15 mm of Hg
Put 5 mm 30 degree scope in central port
Do diagnostic rectoscopy
Put 5 mm tissue retractor through left hand port and L hook dissector through right port
Lesion is scored and dissected with 1 cm margin on surface as well in depth
Dissect completely and check haemostasis
Retrieve specimen
Remove cap along, to avoid any crushing
Rectal defect created after dissection is closed with help of laparoscopic needle holder in right hand and Mary land in left hand
Use 3.0 barbed suture
Check for haemostasis
Remove gelpoint path assembly
Patient position is changed from lithotomy to supine
Anaesthesia reversal, shift to post op care area

Acknowledgment We acknowledge with great humility the contribution of Dr. Sheikh Mohammad Taha Mustafa MBBS, MS, MRCS (Glasg) Head of Colon and Rectal Surgery Sir Ganga Ram Hospital, New Delhi, in preparing and revising this chapter.

References

1. Atallah S, Albert M, Larach S. Transanal minimally invasive surgery: a giant leap forward. Surg Endosc. 2010;24:2200–5.
2. Parks AG, Stuart AE. The management of villous tumours of the large bowel. Br J Surg. 1973;60:688–95.
3. Buess G, Hutterer F, Theiss J, Böbel M, Isselhard W, Pichlmaier H. A system for a transanal endoscopic rectum operation. Chirurg. 1984;55:677–80.
4. Saclarides TJ. Transanal endoscopic microsurgery. Clin Colon Rectal Surg. 2015;28:165–75.
5. Sheikh MTM. How I do it?-Transanal minimally invasive surgery. Indian J Colo-Rectal Surg. 2019;2:3–5.
6. Martin-Perez B, Andrade-Ribeiro GD, Hunter L, Atallah S. A systematic review of transanal minimally invasive surgery (TAMIS) from 2010 to 2013. Tech Coloproctol. 2014;18:775–88.
7. Atallah SB, Larach S, deBeche-Adams TC, Albert MR. Transanal minimally invasive surgery (TAMIS): a technique that can be used for retrograde proctectomy. Dis Colon Rectum. 2013;56:931.
8. deBeche-Adams T, Nassif G. Transanal minimally invasive surgery. Clin Colon Rectal Surg. 2015;28(3):176–80. https://doi.org/10.1055/s--0035-1555008. PMID: 26491410; PMCID: PMC4593921.
9. Morson BC, Bussey HJ, Samoorian S. Policy of local excision for early cancer of the colorectum. Gut. 1977;18:1045–50.
10. NCCN July 1st, 2024 Guidelines for local excision of T1 rectal cancer.
11. Albert MR, Atallah SB, deBeche-Adams TC, Izfar S, Larach SW. Transanal minimally invasive surgery (TAMIS) for local excision of benign neoplasms and early-stage rectal cancer: efficacy and outcomes in the first 50 patients. Dis Colon Rectum. 2013;56(3):301–7.
12. Optimisation of response for organ preservation in rectal cancer: neoadjuvant chemotherapy and radiochemotherapy vs. radiochemotherapy. [cited Aug 3, 2015]. Available from https://ClinicalTrials.gov/show/NCT02514278.
13. Smith FM, Waldron D, Winter DC. Rectum-conserving surgery in the era of chemoradiotherapy. Br J Surg. 2010;97(12):1752–64.
14. Qi Y, Stoddard D, Monson JR. Indications and techniques of transanal endoscopic microsurgery (TEMS). J Gastrointest Surg. 2011;15:1306–8. [PubMed] [DOI].
15. deBeche-Adams T, Hassan I, Haggerty S, Stefanidis D. Transanal Minimally Invasive Surgery (TAMIS): a clinical spotlight review. Surg Endosc. 2017;31:3791–800. [PubMed] [DOI].
16. Garcia-Aguilar J, Shi Q, Thomas CR Jr, Chan E, Cataldo P, Marcet J, Medich D, Pigazzi A, Oommen

S, Posner MC. A phase II trial of neoadjuvant chemoradiation and local excision for T2N0 rectal cancer: preliminary results of the ACOSOG Z6041 trial. Ann Surg Oncol. 2012;19:384–91. [PubMed] [DOI].
17. Kundel Y, Brenner R, Purim O, Peled N, Idelevich E, Fenig E, Sulkes A, Brenner B. Is local excision after complete pathological response to neoadjuvant chemoradiation for rectal cancer an acceptable treatment option? Dis Colon Rectum. 2010;53:1624–31. [PubMed] [DOI].
18. Kim CJ, Yeatman TJ, Coppola D, Trotti A, Williams B, Barthel JS, Dinwoodie W, Karl RC, Marcet J. Local excision of T2 and T3 rectal cancers after downstaging chemoradiation. Ann Surg. 2001;234:352–8; discussion 358. [PubMed] [DOI].
19. Bedrosian I, Rodriguez-Bigas MA, Feig B, Hunt KK, Ellis L, Curley SA, Vauthey JN, Delclos M, Crane C, Janjan N, Skibber JM. Predicting the node-negative mesorectum after preoperative chemoradiation for locally advanced rectal carcinoma. J Gastrointest Surg. 2004;8:56–62; discussion 62. [PubMed] [DOI].
20. Bujko K, Nowacki MP, Nasierowska-Guttmejer A, Kepka L, Winkler-Spytkowska B, Suwiński R, Oledzki J, Stryczyńska G, Wieczorek A, Serkies K, Rogowska D, Tokar P, Polish Colorectal Study Group. Prediction of mesorectal nodal metastases after chemoradiation for rectal cancer: results of a randomised trial: implication for subsequent local excision. Radiother Oncol. 2005;76:234–40. [PubMed] [DOI].
21. Yeo SG, Kim DY, Kim TH, Chang HJ, Oh JH, Park W, Choi DH, Nam H, Kim JS, Cho MJ, Kim JH, Park JH, Kang MK, Koom WS, Nam TK, Chie EK, Lee KJ. Pathologic complete response of primary tumor following preoperative chemoradiotherapy for locally advanced rectal cancer: long-term outcomes and prognostic significance of pathologic nodal status (KROG 09-01). Ann Surg. 2010;252:998–1004. [PubMed] [DOI].
22. Sheikh MTM. Transanal minimally invasive surgery (TAMIS): short and mid term outcomes. Original article accepted for publication in Indian J Colo Rectal Surg. 2020;3:35–7.
23. Bambrule P, Sheikh MTM, Mittal T, Dey A, Kumar A, Kanuri H, Malik VK. Transanal minimally invasive surgery – initial experience. Curr Med Res Pract. 2019;9:196–200.
24. Aracil XS, et al. Management of intra- and postoperative complications during TEM/TAMIS procedures: a systematic review. Minevera Surg. 2021;76(4):343–9. https://doi.org/10.23736/S2724-5691.20.08405-9. Epub 2021 Jan 12.

Suggested Reading

Duggan WP, Heagney N, Gray S, et al. Transanal minimally invasive surgery (TAMIS) for local excision of benign and malignant rectal neoplasia: a 7-year experience. Langenbeck's Arch Surg. 2024;409:32. https://doi.org/10.1007/s00423-023-03217-4.

Kim MJ, Lee TG. Transanal minimally invasive surgery using laparoscopic instruments of the rectum: a review. World J Gastrointest Surg. 2021;13(10):1149–65. https://doi.org/10.4240/wjgs.v13.i10.1149. PMID: 34754384.

Lee SG, Russ AJ, Casillas MA Jr. Laparoscopic transanal minimally invasive surgery (L-TAMIS) vs robotic TAMIS (R-TAMIS): short-term outcomes and costs of a comparative study. Surg Endosc. 2019;33:1981–7. [DOI].

Rimonda R, Arezzo A, Arolfo S, Salvai A, Morino M. TransAnal Minimally Invasive Surgery (TAMIS) with SILS™ port versus Transanal Endoscopic Microsurgery (TEM): a comparative experimental study. Surg Endosc. 2013;27(10):3762–8. [PubMed] [Google Scholar].

Correction to: Operative Manual of Minimally Invasive and LASER Ano-proctology

Correction to:
S. K. Singla, K. Mital, *Operative Manual of Minimally Invasive and LASER Ano-proctology*, https://doi.org/10.1007/978-981-96-6190-9

The original version of this book was published with an incorrect table, figure, and few minor errors. This has now been corrected and "About the Author" section has been included in the foreword.

The updated version of this book can be found at
https://doi.org/10.1007/978-981-96-6190-9

S. K. Singla, K. Mital, *Operative Manual of Minimally Invasive and LASER Ano-proctology*,
https://doi.org/10.1007/978-981-96-6190-9_27

Appendix

S. K. Singla, K. Mital, *Operative Manual of Minimally Invasive and LASER Ano-proctology*, https://doi.org/10.1007/978-981-96-6190-9

LASERS in Surgery and Specifically in Ano-proctology

Introduction

LASER is an acronym for Light Amplification by Stimulated Emission of Radiation. A LASER machine emits intense light with a single wavelength in a very thin, parallel beam that may be concentrated onto a very small area. Einstein initially put forth the theoretical underpinnings of this process in 1917. It was first used with microwaves, was named as "MASERS", which stands for Microwave Amplification by Stimulated Emission of Radiation (1952–53). In 1958, Schaum and Townes demonstrated that the concept could be applied to the visible spectrum. That led to the invention of LASER by Maiman in 1960. He created the first functional LASER by employing a ruby as the lasing medium. Townes, Basov and Prokhorov were awarded the Nobel Prize in Physics for their contributions on LASERS in 1964.

Soon after, LASER beams were created with varying wavelengths using materials other than rubies and several groundbreaking applications quickly emerged. Three years after Theodore Maiman's accomplishment, a study on the surgical applications of LASER was published, raising hopes that the technology will revolutionise medicine as it has done in other sectors. However, development has been slower than many anticipated.

Still, there are now numerous distinct applications of LASERS in surgery. The following pages provide a broad overview of the main areas of interest, especially in ano-proctology.

Technical Facts

How LASER Beam Is Produced with Its Unique Properties

In LASER physics, amplification or gain is a process where the medium transfers part of its energy to the emitted electromagnetic radiation, resulting in an increase in optical power.

Electrons in a lasing medium leap to higher energy levels when light or an electric current is applied (Stimulated absorption) (Fig. 1). Electron

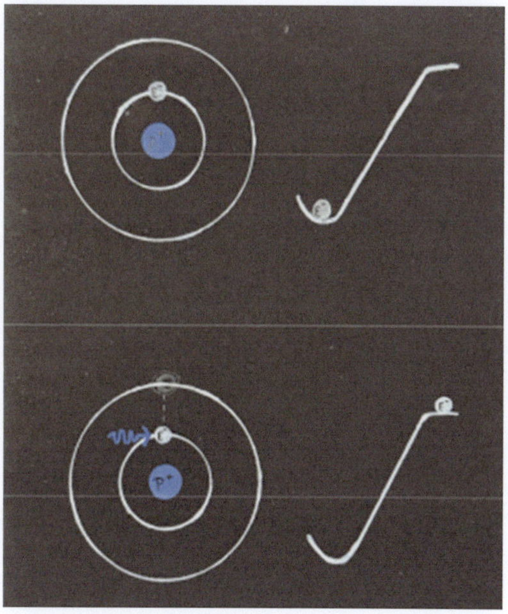

Fig. 1 Stimulated absorption

S. K. Singla, K. Mital, *Operative Manual of Minimally Invasive and LASER Ano-proctology*, https://doi.org/10.1007/978-981-96-6190-9

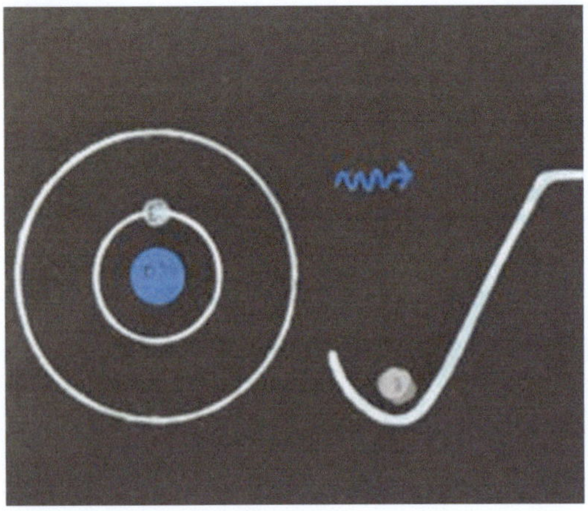

Fig. 2 Spontaneous emission

in a high-energy state tend to decay to a stable state, releasing photon of energy referred to as spontaneous emission (Fig. 2). When an electron in a high-energy state is struck by a photon (the quality of which depends on lasing media), it decays to a lower energy level and releases another photon. The wavelengths of the first and second photons are identical, and the two waves are in phase with one another, called coherent (Stimulated emission) (Fig. 3).

The unique feature of lasing media, which can be crystal, gas, liquid dyes or a semiconductor, is that more atoms can be obtained in an excited, high-energy state than in the baseline stable state—a phenomenon referred to as "population inversion" (Fig. 4).

More and more photons are released when the emitted light is reflected back and forth through the medium by mirrors at either end. A beam of light that is collimated (parallel), coherent (waves all in phase) and monochromatic (single wavelength) (Fig. 5) will emerge if there is a light outlet, such as a central hole in one of the mirrors or one mirror that is only semi-reflective.

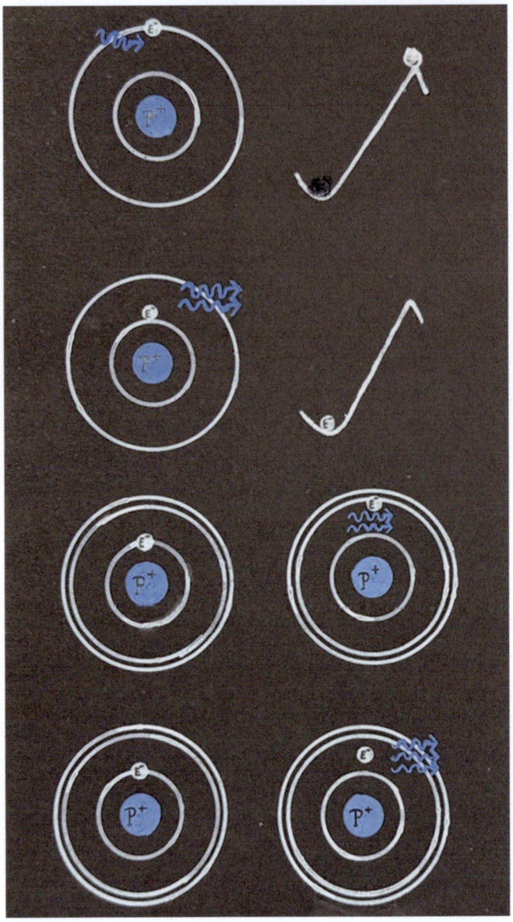

Fig. 3 Stimulated emission

The beam's ability to produce coherent light allows for the achievement of extremely high energy concentrations.

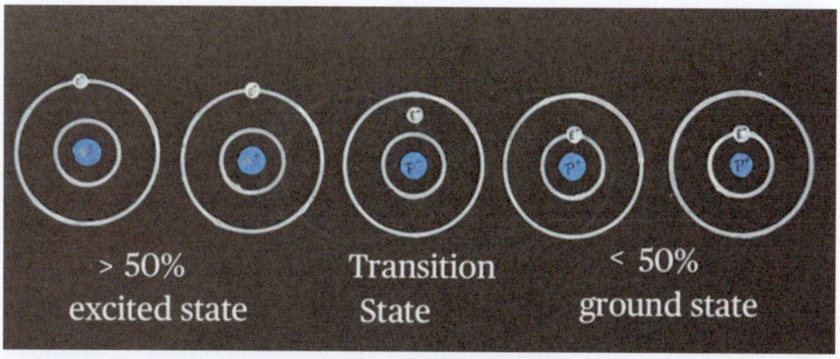

Fig. 4 Population inversion

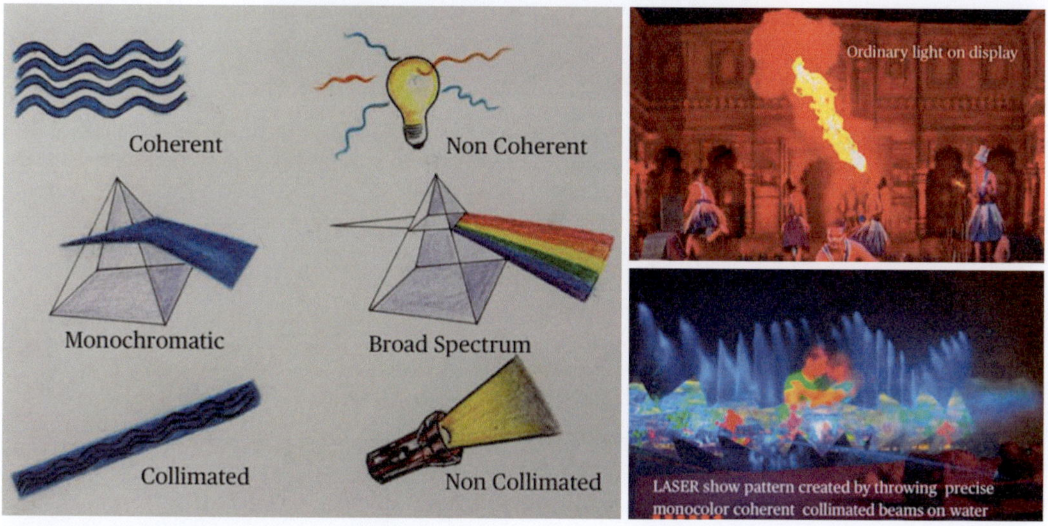

Fig. 5 Physical characteristics of LASER beam in comparison to white light

LASERS Used in Surgery

LASERS get their name from the lasing material they contain because it determines their specific properties, like power and wavelength. Multiple LASERS are used now a days in different surgical branches, which are enumerated in a table (Table 2) at the end of the chapter.

Let's have A look at LASER, in which we as ano-proctologists are interested.

Diode LASER

Similar to a light-emitting diode, a LASER diode (LD) or injection LASER diode (ILD), aka semiconductor LASER, is a semiconductor device that can produce lasing conditions at its junction when a diode is directly pumped with electrical current (Fig. 6).

The doped (*doping is the process of adding some impurity atoms in a pure or (intrinsic) semiconductor so as to increase the conductivity of a semiconductor*) p-n transition uses voltage to recombine electrons with holes. As electrons decay from higher to lower energy levels, they emit radiation in the form of photons. This is a spontaneous emission. Continuing the procedure can result in stimulated emission, which produces light with the same phase, coherence and wavelength. The wavelength of the output beam in LASER diodes is determined by the semiconductor material used, which can range from infrared (IR) to ultraviolet (UV).

Diode LASERS can be used for a variety of applications, which include surgery also.

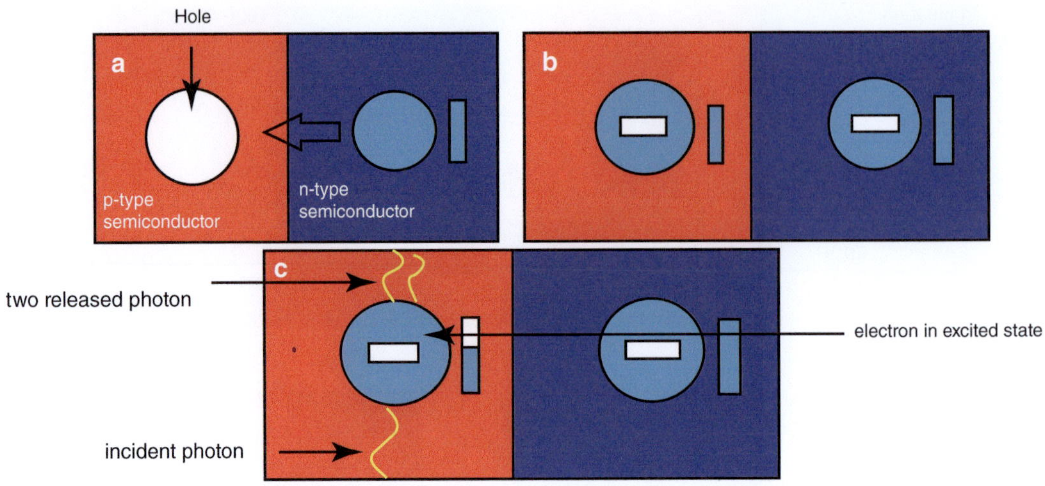

Fig. 6 (**a**) Movement of electron from n-type to p-type semiconductor after passing current. (**b**) Hole (vacancy in valance band of an atom where electron is missing) filled with electron after passing current. (**c**) Excited electron hit by a photon, it decays and liberates two photons with same frequency and polarisation that are identical to the incident one

LASER Beam Tissue Interaction (Fig. 7)

LASER is a light wave, so it obeys all rules of optics when exposed to a surface of another medium:

- Reflection (Beware this property of LASER can cause unexpected harm also.).
- Refraction and scattering.
- Absorption (depends on chromophores).
- Transmission.

Of course, interaction depends on the characteristics of the medium on which LASER energy falls (Tissue in our case).

Whatever energy is absorbed by the tissue leads to certain effects that are utilised in surgery.

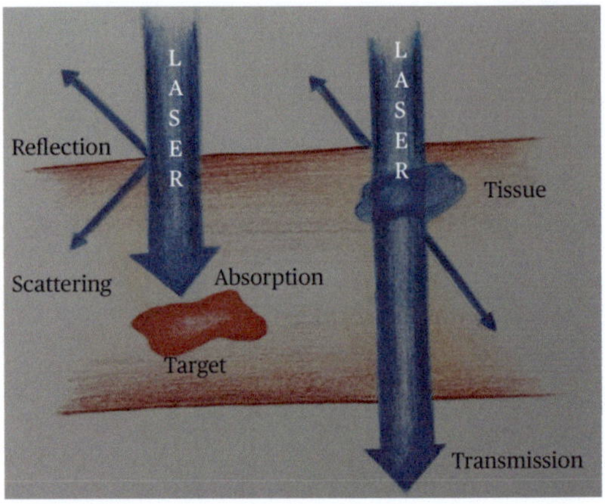

Fig. 7 LASER beam-tissue interaction follows principles of light wave

Effect on Tissues

The Effects of LASER Light Are Determined By

- Wavelength of the LASER beam.
- Spot size created.
- Total energy applied *(the product of power and exposure time-energy in Joules = power in watts multiplied by time in seconds; e.g. when we deliver 6 watts of energy for 3 second pulse at a spot in case of LASER haemorrhoidoplasty, it means we are delivering 18 joules of energy at one spot).*
- Optical characteristics of the target tissue, such as its vascularity or pigmentation.
- Water content is another determinant for the LASER effect on human organs.

Here Comes the Concept of Chromophores (Fig. 8)

A chromophore is a material that is either endogenous to the tissues or exogenous, meaning it is brought from outside. It absorbs specific wavelengths of light, depending on its absorption coefficient.

Examples of endogenous chromophores are melanin, haemoglobin, (oxy-haemoglobin, deoxy-haemoglobin and meth-haemoglobin), water, protein, peptide bonds, aromatic amino acids, nucleic acid, urocanic acid and bilirubin. A 1470-nm diode LASER is used in ano-proctolgy as its well absorbed by water as well as blood, i.e. haemoglobin (*water and haemoglobin are chromophores here*), which makes it more versatile as compared to the 980 nm wavelength, which is not absorbed by water so well.

Exogenous compounds like different colours of tattoo-ink also act as chromophores (Fig. 8).

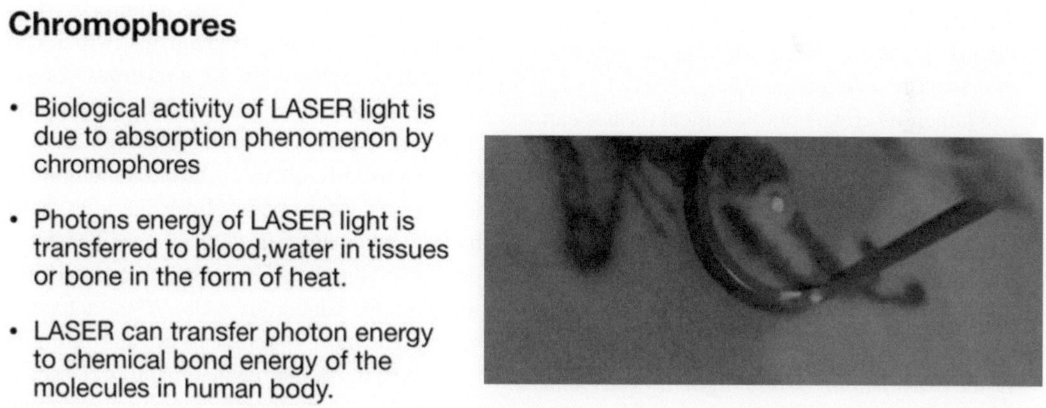

Fig. 8 Mechanism of LASER application on chromophores in a tissue. Diode LASER in use to remove tattoo, black-ink pigment serves as chromophore

Effect of LASERS
LASER VS Tissue

- Hyperthermia
- Thermal effects depend energy density
- Photo coagulation
- Photo vaporisation
- Photo ablation

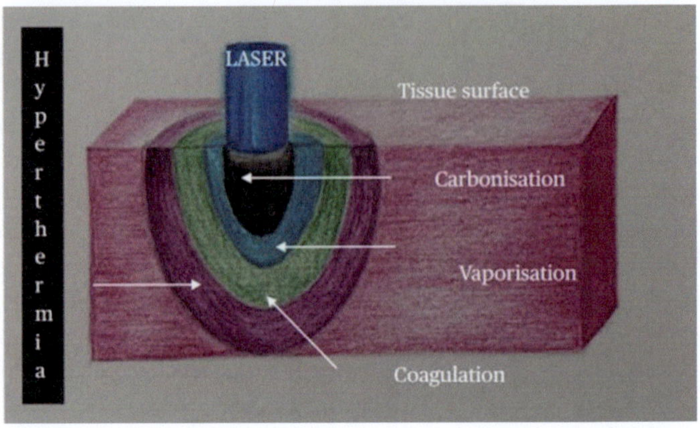

Fig. 9 Primary effect of LASERS on tissue

Primary Effect on the Tissues (Fig. 9)

- Thermal tissue damage is the primary result. Hyperthermia, protein denaturation, tissue contraction from changes in fibrous tissue proteins, and finally cell water-boiling occur as the target tissue is heated by the beam. Additionally, there are local intracellular heat effects, pressure effects and elastic rebound effects of the energy.

  Numerous effects on biological tissues can be achieved by utilising these modifications.

In order to create haemostasis, local swelling, protein denaturation and fibrous tissue contraction might block small capillaries. The heat may also thrombose the blood inside vessels, intensifying the impact.

If the wavelength of the light is such that blood pigment selectively absorbs it, it can sclerose veins with minimal change to the surrounding tissues- for instance, the blue-green light from an argon laser; nowadays, we prefer 1470 nm or 1980 nm for endo venous laser ablation (EVLA), as it is absorbed by both water and haemoglobin, producing better results.

Cells can be vaporised to steam with no charring or harm to other cells if the wavelength is one that water absorbs well (such as the infrared output of a carbon dioxide laser). This is because the energy is absorbed by the latent heat of water vaporisation. This technique allows for the removal of small tissue areas, and as the surface cells are vaporised, the beam progressively penetrates deeper, enabling precise control over the depth of the effect while being visible, unlike diathermy or cryotherapy. By moving the beam across the tissue, a linear incision can be created.

- Additionally, LASERS can eliminate cells through non-thermal mechanisms, which can be applied selectively to cancerous tissue. Malignant cells have a preference for porphyrins, and exposure to ultraviolet light causes porphyrins to fluoresce, offering a method for identifying such cells. Investigations have been conducted on a derivative of haematoporphyrin, known as HpD, which is especially selective for cancerous cells. When activated by LASER light, it generates cytotoxic singlet oxygen within the cells, enabling targeted destruction of malignant tumours, provided that the surrounding healthy tissue has a low affinity for HpD.

Concept of Pulse Wave and Continuous Wave (Fig. 10)

LASER energy, when delivered in pulse mode e.g. a 3-second pulse means energy is delivered for 3 seconds, and then the machine automatically stops delivering energy. Again, on pressing the foot plate, machine delivers a burst of energy for 3 seconds.

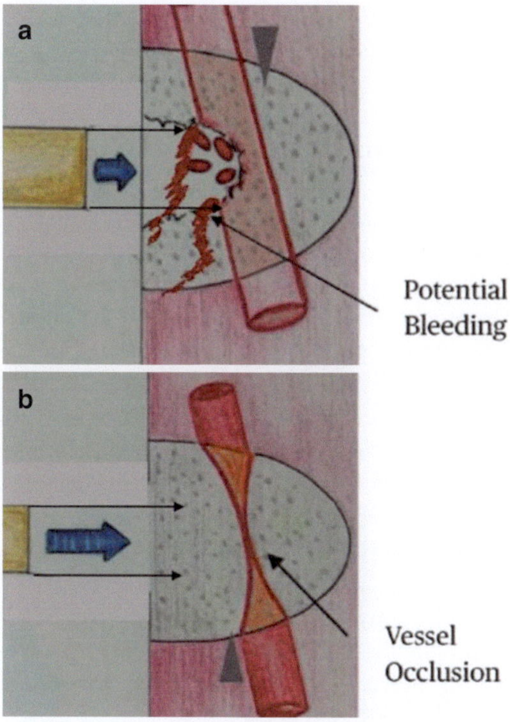

Fig. 10 (**a**) Continuous mode LASER potential bleeding. (**b**) Pulse mode vessel thermo occlusion, arrow heads show coagulated tissue

No energy is delivered in between the two bursts of energy for a specified period, this causes effective shrinkage of underlying tissue as tissue gets time (Thermal Relaxation time) to cool in between.

Thermal Relaxation Period

The duration required for a target to emit approximately 63% of its thermal energy is referred to as the thermal relaxation period. It ranges from a few nanoseconds (tattoo particles) to hundreds of milliseconds (leg venules), contingent on the size of the target chromophore. The greater the chromophore, the longer the thermal relaxation period, because vast regions take a long time to cool. Pulse mode prevents evaporation and charring due to burning. This effect is utilised in LASER haemorrhoidoplasty.

Continuous waves do not allow tissue to cool; instead, they heat the tissue beyond its thermal relaxation time, which causes a cell's temperature to rise abruptly to the point where intracellular water boils and vaporises, causing the cell to burst and produce cleavage, ablation and cutting. This effect is utilised in case of bare fibre delivering energy in a forward direction to incise the tissue. Excess heat may spread to nearby tissues to cause collateral damage.

A continuous wave is also delivered to avoid skip areas while withdrawing radial fibre at a slow, predetermined speed in case of a tract such as a vein or sinus. By withdrawing the fibre, we control the time of energy exposure at one site, thereby controlling total energy at a particular site. Tissue near to the fibre leads to ablation, and deeper tissue gets less heat and causes coagulation and contraction.

Advantages of Utilising LASERS

Accuracy and Precision

Incision with traditional knives can bring disruptive and drag effects due to mechanical energy, while a LASER beam delivery system, when operated manually, can precisely aim the narrow beam at small targets and move it across tissues to create an incision. The level of accuracy is further enhanced with the use of an operating microscope and a micromanipulator.

Less Lateral Damage

Lateral damage is less than what occurs with heat, generated by diathermy. Additionally, diathermy currents can travel along blood vessels, potentially leading to thrombosis and further damage to surrounding tissues due to ischemia.

Accessibility

The beam can be transmitted through flexible optical fibres, and when combined with flexible endoscopes, it allows entry to areas like the gastrointestinal tract or the bronchi. The beam itself does not obstruct visibility, so when it is passed through a rigid tube, such as a bronchoscope or laryngoscope, it does not hinder the visual access to the target. The laser also enables access to regions like the inside of the eye through the clear cornea.

Flexible optical fibres can be fixed in handles to work like a knife in hand and can be put in sinus or fistula tracts with bends. For safety purposes, flexible fibres can be passed through hollow tubes in tracts, like passing diode LASER fibre through infant feeding tube, already placed in a sinus or fistula tracts.

No Touch Technique

As the instrument does not make contact with the target tissue, the risk of bacterial contamination is minimised. Other haemostasis techniques, like diathermy, often dislodge a blood clot when the instrument is removed, which does not occur with the LASER.

Targeted for Specific Cells

The output from the argon LASER is preferentially absorbed by blood, leaving nearby non-pigmented cells relatively unharmed. The demonstration or elimination of malignant cells containing haematoporphyrin derivatives stands out as an exciting illustration of how LASERS can specifically act on particular cells.

Wound Healing and Pain

Several additional benefits of using LASERS for various surgical procedures have been asserted, namely, LASER cuts are less painful than traditional cuts and that they heal more swiftly. Healing does seem to be faster, compared to incisions made by diathermy, but likely not quicker than those made with a conventional knife, and differences in pain levels have yet to be substantiated.

LASER Surgery for Malignant Tumours

LASERS have been suggested to possess unique anti-cancer properties by obstructing lymphatics and encapsulating cancer cells during tumour removal; however, there is no supporting evidence for this claim, and it seems that LASERS do not increase the chances of spreading cancer cells.

Precautions While Using LASERS

LASER radiation poses a potential threat to patients, operators and bystanders, necessitating adherence to strict safety regulations. The Department of Health and experts on LASER use have issued guidelines regarding these safety measures.

The eyes are particularly vulnerable to LASER radiation. Incorporating filters in the eyepiece of optical devices and providing protective goggles for both the operator and observers significantly enhance safety.

Utilising non-reflective instruments helps minimise stray radiation.

Employing signs and locks on doors is essential to prevent unauthorised entry into areas where LASERS are in operation.

Additionally, the eyes of patients must be diligently safeguarded.

Fire represents another serious risk, which can be mitigated through the use of non-volatile anaesthetics, wet swabs, non-reflective tools, and ensuring that all materials that the LASER beam could potentially contact are non-flammable.

Applications in Ano-proctology

Diode LASER energy can be transmitted through Fibre optic cable.

Bare fibre mounted on a handle can be used to deliver LASER energy in a forward direction. Energy is best utilised when it falls perpendicular on the target tissue (Fig. 11).

When used in a continuous mode, bare fibre is used to give incision and excise small areas of target tissue, like in case of sentinel tags, fissure-margins, and incising the internal sphincter in a fissure.

Different tips can be mounted over a bare fibre to change the directions of the flow of energy and ease the negotiation of the fibre in the tissue.

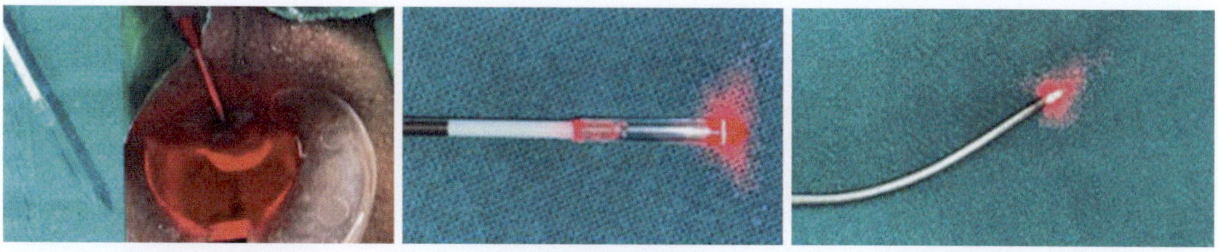

Fig. 11 Type of LASER fibres with different tips suitable for varied uses

In conical fibre, a conical tip is mounted over optical fibre to help negotiate the sub-mucosal cushion and deliver energy in a fan shape to effectively coagulate the tissue and prevent counter perforation of mucosa (Fig. 11).

In radial fibre, a special round tip is mounted on optical fibre, which has a blunt end but a circumferential side window to release LASER energy all around as 'corona' in case of a vein, sinus and fistula. Round blunt end makes entry into a tract comfortable and safe (Fig. 11).

Selection of Wave Length of Diode LASER Energy

Earlier in the haemorrhoid LASER procedure operation, a Doppler probe was inserted into the anal canal through a dedicated disposable proctoscope to identify the terminal branches of superior haemorrhoidal arteries, approximately 3 cm above the dentate line.

A 980-nm diode LASER-pulsed shot was used for tissue shrinkage. The depth of shrinkage was regulated by the power and duration of the LASER beam. Through a 1000-micron conical LASER fibre, five pulsed laser shots were delivered to each identified artery trans-anally through the mucosa with a proctoscope to close the terminal branches.

A 980-nm diode LASER is absorbed by blood more as compared to water, so when applied through mucosa, it spares the mucosa and affects the blood vessels.

In the procedure termed as LASER haemorrhoidoplasty, LASER energy is delivered in sub-mucosal cushions.

A 1470-nm diode LASER is absorbed both by water and blood efficiently, so it is not delivered from the mucosal surface, but instead put in the sub-mucosal cushion to have the desired effects of coagulating blood vessel as well as coagulating matrix tissue around sinusoids.

A 1980-nm diode LASER, though, is absorbed better by water than 1470 nm and is used for endovenous LASER ablation of varicose veins. It produces less bruising and less cord effect in the initial 5 days, but the overall effect is the same.

A machine delivering 1980 nm is almost double the cost of a 1470-nm diode machine, so for general surgery and ano-proctolgy use, the 1470-nm diode LASER is sufficient and more versatile as of today.

Dosage of 1470-nm diode LASER for various procedures in ano-proctology are shown in Table 1.

How to Clean the LASER Fibre Tip Whenever LASER energy is delivered in continuous mode, due to a rise in temperature, carbonisation occurs at the tip of LASER fibre. It increases resistance to further transmission of energy. This carbon deposition should be wiped off by a swab soaked in diluted H_2O_2 while moving the swab from tip to body of the fibre. Wiping in the reverse direction, i.e. from body to tip, may loosen the tip, which may get dislodged from the body of the fibre.

Table 1 LASER fibre and dosage for ano-rectal procedures

Purpose	Type of LASER and fibre	Energy in watts	Mode of transmission
Haemorrhoids (A) To puncture anoderm for entry in to sub-mucosal cushion	1470 Diode LASER *Conical fibre*	6	Pulse mode (A) 1 s pulse
(B) Delivery of energy in the cushions		6	(B) 3 s pulse[a]
Fissure	1470 Diode LASER *Bare fibre*	7	Continuous mode
Fistula	1470 Diode LASER *Radial fibre*	10	Continuous mode. Fibre withdrawal @ 1 mm/s
Pilonidal sinus	1470 Diode LASER *Radial fibre*	10	Continuous mode. Fibre withdrawal @ 1 mm/s

[a]Total amount of LASER energy to be delivered in LASER haemorrhoidoplasty
Total of $6 \times 3 = 18$ joules at one point
One cushion 9 points in fan shape manner at three stations = $18 \times 9 = 162$ joules
Three cushions or total in anal canal delivered energy does not exceed 500 joules

Table 2 LASERS used in surgery

Branch of surgery	LASER used	Application	Wavelength in nm	Reference
Orthopaedics	Holmium LASER	Meniscal tear, chondral disease, arthroscopic surgery, coagulate and vaporise tissue	2100	[1]
	Nd:YAG LASER	Bone formation, osteoblast proliferation and eliminating bacteria	1060	
	Argon LASER	Bleeding control and bone ablation	448 (Blue), 514 (Green)	
Urology	Nd:YAG LASER	Bladder carcinoma, urethral bleeding, urolithiasis, superficial penile carcinoma, bladder haemangioma and urethral stricture disease	10	[2]
	Ho:YAG LASER	Stone fragmentation, tumour resection, urethral and ureteral strictures, prostate surgery and circumcision	2140	
	CO_2 LASER			
	KTP	Bladder neck incision	532	
	LBO	Large prostate glands	532	
	Diode LASER		980	
	Thu:YAG LASER	Prostate surgery, kidney stone management and BOO and bladder tumours	2000	
Gynecology	HeNe	Finder beam	633	[3]
	CO_2 LASER	Cutting and vaporising	10,600	
	Nd:YAG LASER	Coagulation of gastrointestinal tract bleeding & hysteria optic surgery	1064	
	Argon LASER	Mild, moderate and severe endometriosis	532 & 514	

(continued)

Table 2 (continued)

Branch of surgery	LASER used	Application	Wavelength in nm	Reference
Opthalmology	Infrared diode LASER	Retinopathy of prematurity (ROP), retinal photocoagulation, LASER tissue welding, bladeless LASIK	806–810	[4]
	Ultraviolet excimer LASER	Photorefractive keratectomy, situ keratomileusis	193	
	Femtosecond LASER	Cataract surgery, corneal refractive surgery & corneal transplantation	1028–1053	
	KrCI excimer LASER	Tissue removal & reshaping the cornea	222	
	Nd:YAG LASER	Posterior capsulotomy, vitreolysis, pupillary sphincter, IOL surface, IOL position & retinal conditions	1064	
	Argon LASER	Diabetic retinopathy, retinal detachment, glaucoma, angle-closure glaucoma, macular degeneration & pterygium	514	
	Diode LASER	Retinopathy of prematurity (ROP), glaucoma & pain control	780–850	
	Double frequency Nd:YAG LASER	Corneal vascularisation, retinal conditions, corneal stromal reinforcement & subhyaloid haemorrhage	832	
	Krypton red LASER	Branch retinal vein occlusion (BRVO), macular oedema, retinal neovascularisation, chorodial neovascularisation (CNV), retinal tears, diabetic retinopathy & wet macular degeneration	647	
General surgery	CO_2 LASER	Tissue cutting, excising vascular lesions, treating scars, treating premalignant lesions and treating airway and digestive tracts	10,600	[5]
	Nd:YAG LASER	Coagulation, endoscopy and intraoral soft tissue surgery	1060	
	GaAlAs LASER	Removing tumours, sealing blood vessels, sealing lymph vessels, treating skin conditions, precise incision and laryngeal surgeries	750–900	
	HF LASER	Reduce blood loss, decrease discomfort, reduce risk of infection, better wound healing & minimise surgery	2600–3000	
	Diode LASER	Oral surgery, nasal cavity and skull base tumour surgery, hysteroscopy & pyogenic granuloma removal	810–1064	
	Excimer LASER	–	193	
ENT surgery	CO_2 LASER	Removing lesions and tumours, treating cancer, treating paediatric airway lesions, treating ear ailments, improving hearing, improving the airway, treating epistaxis & breaking up salivary stones, benign/malignant tonsils	980–10,600	[6]
	KTP LASER	Cholesteatoma, vocal fold lesion treatment, endoscopic sinus surgery & cochlear implant surgery, obstructive sleep apnoea	532	
	Aqua Lase-E	Targeted tissue interaction, reduce thermal injury, minimized blood loss & less invasive procedure,	1470	

(continued)

Table 2 (continued)

Branch of surgery	LASER used	Application	Wavelength in nm	Reference
Oncology surgery	Nd:YAG	Treating internal organs, treating lungs cancer & treating bladder carcinoma	1064	[7]
	KTP-YAG	Treating cutaneous vascular lesions, treating subglottic haemangiomas, vaporising prostatic adenomatous tissue, enucleating bladder tumours & treating chronic radiation proctopathy	532	
	CO_2 LASER	Skin cancer, head and neck cancer & localised scar tissue	10,600	
	Thulium LASER	Bladder cancer, upper urinary tract carcinoma & airway stenosis	2016	
	Ho:YAG LASER	Endoscopic fragmentation, ablation and resection, urethral and ureteral strictures, benign prostatic hyperplasia & upper-tract urothelial carcinoma(UTU C)	2100	
	Diode LASER	Brain tumour surgery, laryngeal cancer, non-muscle-invasive bladder cancer and partial nephrectomy	800–980	
	Visible LASER	LASER ablation, photodynamic therapy (PDT), LASER interstitial thermal therapy (LITT) & sealing nerve endings	430–680	
	Mid-IR LASER	Destroying tumours, shrinking tumours, treating cancer symptoms, treating cancer side effects & sealing nerve endings	1900–3000 or 9300–10,600	
	IR LASER	Thermotherapy, photoimmunotherapy, laser interstitial thermal therapy (LITT) & near infrared fluorescence imaging	1300–1600	
Vascular surgery	Pulsed dye LASER	Vascular malformations, port-wine stains & basal cell carcinoma	577, 585, 590 & 595	[8]
	Nd:YAG LASER	Broken capillaries and spider veins, port-wine stains & haemangiomas	1064	
	KTP LASER	Vascular malformations & port-wine stains	532	
	Argon LASER	Cutaneous lesions, intraoral lesions, congenital vascular lesions & colon lesions	488 & 514	
	Copper LASER	Mucosal venous malformation, cherry and spider angiomas, angiokeratomas & pygenic granulomas	578	
	Krypton LASER	Vascular lesions & macular vascular lesions	568	
	CO_2 LASER	Haemostasis, reduce bleeding, rapid healing & sterile treatment	10,600	
	Diode LASER	Remove vascular lesions, treating venous malformations, treating haemangiomas & EVLA	800 1470–1980	
	Alexandrite LASER	Vascular lesions	755	

(continued)

Table 2 (continued)

Branch of surgery	LASER used	Application	Wavelength in nm	Reference
Dermatology	KTP LASER	Vascular lesions, pigmented lesions, tattoo removal & rejuvenation	532	[9]
	Pulsed Dye LASER	Vascular lesions, warts & non-vascular skin lesions	585–595	
	Nd:YAG LASER	Skin rejuvenation, pigmentation removal, vascular lesions removal, hair removal & skin tumour removal	1060	
	LP ruby LASER	Tattoos, pigmented lesions, nevus of Ota & nevus of Ito	694	
	LP alexandrite LASER	Hair removal, vascular lesions, pigmented lesions, venous lakes of lip, recalcitrant viral warts & basal cell nevus syndrome	755 & 800	
	CO_2 LASER	Skin tags, sunspot, warts, acne scars, premalignant lesions and skin cancer, hamartomas, wrinkles, photodamage, birthmarks & rhinophyma	10,600	
	Erbium: YAG LASER	Skin lesions, skin resurfacing, skin rejuvenation & skin texture	2940	
Ano-proctology	Diode LASER	Haemorrhoids, fistula in ano, pilonidal sinus disease and fissure	980, 1470	

Use of Putting Ice-Coat After LASER Surgery in Case of LASER Haemorrhoidoplasty (LHP)

Applying a glove finger-coat filled with ice in the anal canal for 10 minutes is good to relieve oedema and associated inflammation after giving LASER energy in closed space.

Operating LASER Machine

Before operating the LASER machine, the operator should know the process and ensure that he is properly trained and knows about the medical effects and risks associated with the use of LASER.

The operator ensures that the LASER machine is properly working, and if there is any damage, the device should not be used.

Before using the LASER machine, the operator should check all the connections, power supply and accessories.

In the operating room, enough protective goggles should be available for the operator, assistants and observers.

While working, the foot pedal of the LASER machine should be operated only by the surgeon. The pedal should be in a locked position while not in use, to prevent any thermal injuries.

The LASER machine is switched to ready mode before use and switched back to standby mode after use.

Position of LASERS in Mind of Patients

Expectations of people from LASERS are quite high, and a common person does not differentiate between procedures done by LASER and endoscopes, especially laparoscope. For them, everything is the same, but different from open surgery with a large incision.

The LASER procedure is positioned in mind of prospects as a procedure that offers the following benefits:

- It is completely painless.
- It does not require recovery time.
- It carries zero risk of complications.

- It provides instant cure for haemorrhoids with no recurrences.
- It involves no cut, bleeding or anaesthesia.
- It does not require hospitalisation.
- Just short of self-medication and taking a pill.

Industry wants to propagate it in a similar way for obvious reasons.

The time has come to reposition the LASER in minds of prospects and medical professionals.

- LASER is no magic wand.
- LASER is another energy source, to be used judiciously.
- LASER has a precise role in combination with other elements of minimally invasive surgery with significant advantages.
- We need to standardise the procedures.
- The medicos should learn all the known procedures to handle anorectal problems in minimally invasive ways.

Acknowledgement We acknowledge the contribution of Dr. Nitish Jawar for this thought of position of LASER in mind of patients and Dr. Sakshi for contributing Fig. 8 on removal of tattoo.

References

1. Li CL, Fisher CJ, Burke R, Andersson-Engels S. Orthopedics-related applications of ultrafast laser and its recent advances. Appl Sci. 2022;12:3957. https://doi.org/10.3390/app12083957.
2. Zarrabi A, Gross AJ. The evolution of lasers in urology. Ther Adv Urol. 2011;3(2):81–9. https://doi.org/10.1177/1756287211400494. PMID: 21869908; PMCID: PMC3150070.
3. DeLeon F, Baggish M. Glob Libr Women's Med (ISSN: 1756-2228). 2008. https://doi.org/10.3843/GLOWM.10023.
4. https://web.stanford.edu/~palanker/publications/Ophthalmic_Laser_Therapy.pdf.
5. Azadgoli B, Baker RY. Laser applications in surgery. Ann Transl Med. 2016;4(23):452. https://doi.org/10.21037/atm.2016.11.51. PMID: 28090508; PMCID: PMC5220034.
6. Orgain C, Rothholtz V, Wong BJF. Laser/light applications in otolaryngology. In: Nouri K, editor. Lasers in dermatology and medicine. Cham: Springer; 2018. https://escholarship.org/content/qt26g7k4d0/qt26g7k4d0_noSplash_cc36dc10498795b8cbe7f-ce6c43ec 547.pdf?t=rq8dlx.
7. Schena E, Saccomandi P, Fong Y. Laser ablation for cancer: past, present and future. J Funct Biomater. 2017;8(2):19. https://doi.org/10.3390/jfb8020019. PMID: 28613248; PMCID: PMC5492000.
8. Srinivas CR, Kumaresan M. Lasers for vascular lesions: standard guidelines of care. Indian J Dermatol Venereol Leprol. 2011;77:349–68.
9. Gianfaldoni S, Tchernev G, Wollina U, Fioranelli M, Roccia MG, Gianfaldoni R, Lotti T. An overview of laser in dermatology: the past, the present and ... the future(?). Open Access Maced J Med Sci. 2017;5(4):526–30. https://doi.org/10.3889/oamjms.2017.130. PMID: 28785350; PMCID: PMC5535675.

Suggested Reading

Ambe PC. Laser interventions in coloproctology. A plea for standardized treatment protocols. Tech Coloproctol. 2023;27(10):953–5. https://doi.org/10.1007/s10151-023-02859-2. Epub 2023 Aug 28. PMID: 37639034; PMCID: PMC10485080.

Choi B, Welch AJ. Analysis of thermal relaxation during laser irradiation of tissue. Lasers Surg Med. 2001;29(4):351–9.

Cochrane JPS. Chapter 2: Lasers in surgical practice. In: Russell RCG, editor. Recent advances in surgery 12. Churchill Livingstone; 1986.

Cochrane JPS, Beacon JP, Creasey GH, Russell RCG. Wound healing after laser surgery: an experimental study. Br J Surg. 1980;67:740–3.

Coldren LA, Corzine SW, Mashanovitch ML. Diode lasers and photonic integrated circuits. Wiley; 2012. ISBN 978-1-118-14817-4. https://books.google.com/books?id=D6Ub126rtPoC.

Dover JS, Arndt KA, Geronemus RG, et al. Illustrated cutaneous laser surgery: a practitioner's guide. Norwalk: Appleton & Lange; 1990.

Mulgaonkar AP, Hubschman JP, Bourges JL, Jordan BL, Cham C, Wilson JT, Tsao TC, Culjat MO. A prototype surgical manipulator for robotic intraocular micro surgery. Stud Health Technol Inform. 2009;142:215–7.

Patil UA, Dhami LD. Overview of lasers. Indian J Plast Surg. 2008;41(Suppl):S101–13. PMID: 20174534; PMCID: PMC2825126.

Index

S. K. Singla, K. Mital, *Operative Manual of Minimally Invasive and LASER Ano-proctology*,
https://doi.org/10.1007/978-981-96-6190-9

R

S

T

MIX
Papier aus verantwortungsvollen Quellen
Paper from responsible sources
FSC® C105338

If you have any concerns about our products,
you can contact us on
ProductSafety@springernature.com

In case Publisher is established outside the EU,
the EU authorized representative is:
Springer Nature Customer Service Center GmbH
Europaplatz 3, 69115 Heidelberg, Germany

Printed by Libri Plureos GmbH
in Hamburg, Germany